*What the experts are saying:*

"Dr. Winnifred Cutler uses her profound knowledge of women's sexual and reproductive systems to impart knowledge and insights you will not find anywhere else. Her information is extremely thorough, well-supported in the scientific literature, and also very wise. If you are thinking about a hysterectomy, recovering from one, or wanting to find unique new insights on the wisdom of your body, be sure to read this book."
—Sadja Greenwood, M.D., author of *Menopause, Naturally* and *Medical Self-Care Book of Women's Health*

"Essential information for every woman who is faced with a decision about hysterectomy; and when hysterectomy is necessary, the information she needs to help cope with surgery and heal optimally in spirit and body."
—Felicia H. Stewart, M.D., coauthor of *Understanding Your Body*

"Dr. Cutler's book is invaluable for all peri- and post-menopausal women who wish to maximize their cardiovascular, gynecological, and general health."
—Elizabeth Genovese, M.D., Clinical Associate Professor of Internal Medicine, Graduate Hospital, Philadelphia

"Extremely well-written and researched, providing a thorough overview useful to both physicians and their patients. . . . Gynecologists would be well served by reading this very thorough review of hysterectomy side-effects and their treatment modalities."
—*Fertility News*, a newsletter of the American Fertility Society

"This book contains the best chapters on exercise and nutrition for women that I have seen."
—Lawrence K. Spitz, M.D., Assistant Professor of Diagnostic Medicine, University of Pennsylvania Medical School

"A great source of information for mature women."
—Celso Ramon Garcia, M.D., Professor of Obstetrics and Gynecology, School of Medicine, University of Pennsylvania

"Very important! By clearly outlining options to patients, Dr. Cutler's book aids in individuation of patient care. That is what both a patient and her physician strive for."
—Millicent Zacher, D.O., Reproductive Surgeon, Albert Einstein Medical Center, Philadelphia, Pennsylvania

"Very objectively looks into alternatives and side effects of one of the most commonly performed procedures on women in this country."
— Phil Alberts, M.D., Fellow American College of Obstetrics and Gynecology, Portland, Oregon

## What readers are saying:

"It is with profound gratitude that I write to you. . . . Reading your book gave me a sense of validation, and with that, some self-esteem. I'm not crazy. . . . all those things I've felt intuitively are true after all. That feels really good."
— 36-year-old woman from Washington

"My wife had a hysterectomy with removal of ovaries 3½ years ago. . . . We read *Hysterectomy: Before and After* and feel it is the very best on the subject. You've done us and many others a great service."
— a supportive husband from New York

"If I had listened to the first doctor I would have a complete hysterectomy. . . . From your book I was able to find a [new] doctor and eliminate the need for hysterectomy through alternative treatment. . . . [My] prognosis is just fine . . . Thank you again for helping me."
— a woman from Florida

"You're so right about vitamins helping postoperatively. Before my operation, I upped my vitamin C intake to 1 gram a day . . . the whole [hospital] staff couldn't believe how fast and well my recovery was. How can I thank you for the health- and life-saving knowledge you gave me? I hope more women and doctors read your book."
— 33-year-old woman from Pennsylvania

"After reading *Hysterectomy: Before and After,* I now realize that many, many other women are going through the same thing because of surgery. You have helped to eliminate my guilt feelings, [and] helped me to realize that what I have suffered is very real, and that I did nothing to bring it upon myself."
— 51-year-old woman from Pennsylvania

# Winnifred B. Cutler, Ph.D.

# Hysterectomy: Before & After

*A Comprehensive Guide to Preventing, Preparing For, and Maximizing Health After Hysterectomy*

HarperPerennial

*A Division of HarperCollinsPublishers*

The author welcomes queries and comments. Please address all correspondence to:

Dr. Winnifred B. Cutler
Athena Institute for Women's Wellness Research
30 Coopertown Road
Haverford, PA   19041

Grateful acknowledgment is made for permission to reprint: Material on pages 345–359 is from *Fertility and Sterility*. Reproduced by permission of the publisher, the American Fertility Society. Excerpt on page 317 is from *Dietary Fibre, Fibre-Depleted Foods and Disease*, edited by Trowell, Burkett, and Heaton. Reprinted by permission of Academic Press, Orlando, Florida, and the author, Dr. Philip James. Excerpts on pages 340–341 are from "Pat Croce's Advice on Selecting Athletic Shoes," in the *Philadelphia Inquirer* on May 24, 1987. Reprinted by permission. Excerpt on pages 277–278 is from the *Journal of the International College of Surgeons,* 1956. Reprinted by permission of The International College of Surgeons. Table 8 on page 188 is from "Calcium Supplements Are Not All Equal," by Dr. Ralph Shangraw, copyright © 1988 by The New York Times Company. Reprinted by permission. Table 14 on pages 298–299 is by Elizabeth J. Johnson and Dr. Judith Marlett, copyright © *American Journal of Clinical Nutrition,* American Society for Clinical Nutrition. Table 3 on page 81 is from *Understanding Your Body* by Felicia H. Stewart, M.D., copyright © 1987. Reprinted by permission of Bantam Books, all rights reserved. Table 2 on page 78 by W. Budd Wentz, M.D., is from *Gynecologic Oncology,* 1974, vol. 2. Reproduced by permission of the author. Table 5 on pages 148–151 is from *Estrogen Replacement Therapy* by R. Don Gambrell, Jr., M.D. Reprinted by permission of the author.

First PERENNIAL LIBRARY edition published 1990.

*Artist: Pamela Sinkler Todd*

*The Library of Congress has catalogued the hardcover edition as follows:*

Cutler, Winnifred Berg.
    Hysterectomy: before and after.

    Bibliography: p.
    Includes index.
    1. Hysterectomy—Popular works. I. Title.
RG391.C87   1988        618.1′453        87-46132
ISBN 0-06-015916-2

ISBN 0-06-091629-X (pbk.)

02 03 04 05  RRD            26 27 28 29 30

*This book is dedicated
to improving the quality of health care to women
and
to Thomas E. Quay, Esq.,
for his significant efforts toward that end.*

# Contents

# List of Tables

## A note to the reader

A simple reference system is used throughout the book to direct medical professionals and interested lay readers to the published studies that form the basis for the information provided. The bibliography, beginning on page 367, lists approximately 1,000 published articles, each preceded by a number. Those numbers are inserted in the text as references to the studies.

# Hysterectomy: Before & After

*Hysterectomy: Before and After* has been written as a general guide for women who are considering having a hysterectomy or have already had one. It is intended to be informational and by no means should be considered a substitute for sound advice from a medical practitioner. Rather it is intended to provide women with information so that they will know what questions to ask and what alternatives to seek. Readers are also urged to consult with their physicians regarding drug therapy discussed herein.

# Women's Wellness:
## Securing Your Healthrights

*A woman in her late twenties is told that her uterine lining has a tendency to be overgrown with excess tissue and that, since this can lead to cancer, she will ultimately need a hysterectomy. She is advised that if she wants to have children, she should have them now, before it's too late.*

*Intense abdominal pain sends a 35-year-old woman to her doctor, who diagnoses endometriosis, a condition in which tissue from the lining of the uterus becomes attached to the ovaries and other parts of the abdomen. The prescription: hysterectomy.*

*A 45-year-old woman with a history of depression complains to her psychiatrist of abnormal bleeding. When the therapist sends her to a surgeon, her bleeding is not measured, yet she is told she should have a hysterectomy.*

*A 39-year-old woman begins to experience the symptoms of menopause. It dawns on her that the hysterectomy she had three years ago may be responsible for this early change of life.*

*A woman in her mid-fifties came through hysterectomy surgery in good physical health, but two years later she feels "blue" most of the time and doesn't have the energy for her daily tasks or even for the friendships she once had. Psychotherapy doesn't help.*

*A woman of 58 fractures her hip and fears that her hysterectomy has made her bones brittle and vulnerable. Hoping to resume an active life after recuperating, she wants to know what to do to prevent further bone deterioration.*

These vignettes represent but a handful of the stories of the millions of women in the United States who have had direct involvement with surgery to remove their uterus (hysterectomy), with or without removal of their fallopian tubes (salpingectomy) and ovaries (ovariectomy or oophorectomy).

Approximately 550,000 hysterectomies are performed every year in the United States, a country in which a woman has about a 50 percent chance of having a hysterectomy before she dies.* The situation in Canada appears to closely parallel that in the United States. In contrast, in Sweden a woman has about a 10 percent chance of having her uterus removed.[53, 341, 342] In the United States, the average age for premenopausal hysterectomy is 35;[214] in Scandinavia, the average age is 46.[457] Women in the United States have a five times higher rate of hysterectomy by the age of 44 (21 percent) than women in six European countries, where the rate is 4 percent.[265, 909](The population rates of hysterectomy are startlingly different in different regions of the United States. Women in the southern and central parts of the country have hysterectomies two to three times more often than women in the Northeast and on the West Coast.[174]) Ovariectomy is also an extremely common procedure in the United States, occurring in about half the women over age 40 who undergo hysterectomy.[215]

Why is the rate of pelvic surgery so huge in this country? The answer is difficult to search out because the reasons for surgery are rarely reported. One study evaluated data collected in the United States between 1978 and 1981 in an attempt to catalog the conditions leading to hysterectomy in women from 15 years to 44 years old. Although cancer is the only diagnosis for which

---

*Many of the studies are listed in the References, beginning on page 367. They include numbers 114, 115, 533, 729, 839, 887.

hysterectomy is automatically mandated, the study found that surgery was performed in response to cancer or a precancerous condition in only 10.6 percent of the cases.[214] But the propriety of such a high hysterectomy rate has long been questioned.

In a landmark paper published in 1957 in *The Proceedings of the Royal Society of Medicine,* Dr. Katerina Dalton reported that as time passed after hysterectomy, women became increasingly dissatisfied with having had the surgery. She found that during the time when a physician will usually follow up a postsurgery patient, women were satisfied; for example, within one year after the operation, 83 percent were satisfied. However, when women were questioned one to five years following surgery, only 41 percent were still satisfied with the operation. And at six to ten years, only 33 percent were satisfied.[182]

What accounts for the continued high incidence of hysterectomy? Despite Dalton's findings more than thirty years ago, many women and their doctors today erroneously believe that the uterus has no importance beyond enabling the bearing of children. Further, there remains within some areas of the medical community a lack of perception and awareness of the often serious physical and emotional problems experienced by women who undergo hysterectomy and ovariectomy.

## THE RISKS OF HYSTERECTOMY

Hysterectomy is a serious surgical procedure. Hysterectomy with the removal of the fallopian tubes and ovaries (bilateral salpingo-ovariectomy) is even more serious. In recent years, hundreds of scientifically valid research studies have been published that document the profound risks of hysterectomy.

When it will improve a woman's health, surgery is an appropriate and beneficial alternative. When surgery will cause more problems than it solves, it should be avoided.

The effects induced by hysterectomy include:

• *An alteration in the hormonal environment.* Hysterectomy alters a woman's circulating levels of estrogen, progesterone, testosterone, androstenedione, luteinizing hormone, follicle-stimulating hormone, and the beta endorphins.

- *Earlier aging.* On average, premenopausal women who lose their uterus enter menopause (the time when the ovaries shut down their "egg factory" and the estrogen and progesterone supplies are severely diminished) five years earlier than those who do not; ovariectomy produces menopause immediately. Postmenopausal women are similarly affected by the surgeries: they age more rapidly.
- *A high likelihood of serious postoperative depression.* Hysterectomy significantly increases the risk for depression, which often emerges as much as two years after surgery.
- *A deterioration of bone health.* Unless women take specific action to prevent this risk, hysterectomy will accelerate the loss of bone mass and increase the likelihood of developing osteoporosis.

In one study, within two years after ovariectomy, women who did not take replacement sex hormones had already lost 20 percent of their spinal bone mass.[299] Likewise, the first study to look at the effects of hysterectomy on bone loss, published in 1988, also provided data to suggest that hysterectomized women lose spine bone earlier than intact women.[163]

- *Decreased cardiovascular health.* In the early 1980s, approximately 485,000 women died each year from cardiovascular disease, compared with 60,000 women who died from cancer of the breast, uterus, cervix, or ovary, and with 21,000 women who died from diabetes.

Cardiovascular disease claims the lion's portion of deaths for women in the United States, yet premenopausal intact (nonhysterectomized) women rarely suffer from heart disease. The Framingham Study, which evaluated a large population of healthy people as they matured, found in investigating approximately 8,500 premenopausal person-years' experience that no premenopausal women developed a heart attack or died of coronary heart disease. Such events were common among postmenopausal women.[316]

Moreover, hysterectomy increases the risk of atherosclerosis and coronary heart disease three- to sevenfold over that of age-matched women who have not had the surgery.

There is a well-documented increased incidence of heart attack in women with early menopause. In one study, 33 percent of mature women who had entered menopause early (that is, from surgery) versus 12 percent of women who entered menopause naturally had heart attacks.[52]

- *Reductions in sexual functioning.* Hysterectomy very often reduces several dimensions of sexuality, including libido, arousal, vaginal lubrication, and orgasmic capacity.
- *Increased incidence of urinary incontinence.* After hysterectomy many women suffer from an inability to contain their urine.

While the overall outlook for health (without special treatments) after hysterectomy is not good, not every woman suffers every effect, and the degree of difficulty from particular effects differs from woman to woman.

What needs to be most strongly emphasized is that not all of the aftereffects of hysterectomy are obvious. Cardiovascular problems and osteoporosis progress silently, often making themselves known only when serious conditions have developed. In fact, the silent conditions caused by hysterectomy can be developing even when the more apparent ones are not present. A woman who is not depressed or who does not suffer from hot flashes may still be experiencing a progressive loss of bone mass and the beginnings of coronary heart disease *without any obvious symptoms.*

The effects of hysterectomy usually do not become apparent immediately. Approximately half the women who have had their uterus removed but who have retained their ovaries eventually suffer from a premature lack of ovarian production of hormones, but this effect often does not occur until two years after the surgery. At that point, when a woman complains of depression, for example, her physician may not connect the problem to her earlier hysterectomy and thus may fail to treat the hormonal imbalances that are the result of the surgery.

For women who face the possibility of hysterectomy, the good news is that the surgery can often be avoided. For women who have had a hysterectomy, the good news is that its effects are treatable and that it is never too late to reap the benefits of the wide range of treatment approaches now available.

## UP-TO-DATE INFORMATION IS ESSENTIAL

Many of the problems for which hysterectomy and ovariectomy are prescribed are still not well understood. While the state of the art of knowledge about women's reproductive physiology systems is advancing rapidly, much remains unknown.

Much of the information presented in this book has come to light since 1983, and much of it has not yet emerged in many medical schools, medical practices, and health centers. When a woman has a problem and seeks help from a physician, she may be unaware that even the well-informed doctor may have a limited ability to provide an effective answer.

A doctor generally bases his or her conclusions on knowledge gleaned from medical courses, the study of textbooks, and, ideally, from newly published research studies. Every month, hundreds of journals around the world produce an enormous proliferation of articles and studies that focus on aspects of uterine physiology, sexual physiology, hormonal effects, cardiovascular health, bone physiology, biochemical aspects of depression, hormonal involvement in the sense of well-being, nutritional influences on health and disease, and other subjects relevant to hysterectomy. Each study sets out to test one or two questions by gathering a particular sample of women, asking questions, and evaluating the results of the data. Each can produce only a tentative answer to a limited area of inquiry. The knowledge is built piece by piece, as investigators publish hundreds of research studies and other scholars synthesize that knowledge.

After a mosaic of thousands of studies has been published,

consensus is sometimes reached about the most effective ways to deal with a particular health issue, although this knowledge is still almost always tentative, limited, and subject to change. Most responsible physicians can barely keep up with a narrow slice of these studies, which are critically important for the health decisions surrounding hysterectomy.

Limitations to the systematic development of scientific knowledge are humbling to biomedical investigators who are working to improve the quality of health care for women, and scientists and physicians face serious problems and frustrations. Yet, as researchers publish results and knowledge expands, the accumulating evidence indicates a much greater role for the uterus and ovaries in a woman's total health than had been previously suspected.

Despite the fact that medical knowledge is imperfect and incomplete, women cannot wait for definitive answers when they have problems that must be addressed. Fortunately, there exists a large body of research results that can be synthesized to improve the quality of health care for women.

The statements made in this book are based upon a systematic review of some 3,000 scientific studies. Approximately 1,000 are specifically cited (and referenced within the text), providing a composite of the studies most relevant to issues surrounding hysterectomy as well as an extensive review of our best and newest information about hormonal replacement therapy (HRT), nutrition, exercise physiology, and other areas relevant to women's health as we age.

In many cases, this synthesis may introduce new ideas that have the potential of altering, for the better, biomedical approaches to the health care of women. That is, in fact, the mission of the book: to improve the quality of health care for women.

Women who face the prospect of surgery and those who have already endured it can gain from this book an awareness of what hysterectomy implies in order to successfully cope with its effects. It is never too late to improve your health, and it is never too early. The sooner you start, the more you will be able to participate in the decisions that are made about your body and your well-being.

## TEN PRINCIPLES OF WOMEN'S WELLNESS

The perspectives that inform *Hysterectomy: Before and After* can be expressed as ten simple principles.

1. *The functioning of a woman's body is elegantly symphonic in nature.* The exquisite intricacy of the body's internal orchestration is dependent upon the uterus and the ovaries. Because good health relies upon the complex, interrelated contributions of the various parts of a woman's body, it is naive to believe it possible to remove any of them with impunity. Likewise, the emotional well-being of a woman has a basis in her physical health.

2. *The uterus is valuable.* In addition to its capacity for gestating babies, the uterus plays a powerful role in keeping the ovaries working. It produces substances that affect brain function and that reduce the risk of cardiovascular disease, and it is a sexually responsive organ.

3. *The ovaries are valuable.* At every age and stage of life, ovaries are vital organs. In addition to their life-giving function of holding the eggs for the next generation, ovaries contain a "factory" for the production of hormones, as well as a great many other substances.

4. *Even when a hysterectomy should be considered, there is rarely a need to rush into surgery.* A significant body of research supports the wisdom of a conservative approach. Even in cases of disease that may mandate hysterectomy, several months' delay will rarely increase the risk of further problems. Women have time—and should take the time—to obtain an accurate diagnosis.

   *Note:* Emergencies are different. Some women have an emergency need—such as profuse bleeding or a ruptured uterus—that doesn't allow time for the slow, reasoned approach suggested for most women before they agree to a hysterectomy. Fortunately these emergency procedures are rare, probably accounting for less than 5 percent of the hysterectomies that are performed.

5. *Even if a problem may ultimately lead to hysterectomy, it is wisest not to start with surgery.* To overcome pathology while maximizing overall health now and for the future, women should begin with the mildest approach before agreeing to a more radical procedure, such as hysterectomy. Very often a nonsurgical treatment solves the problem.

6. *If surgery is necessary, it is best to take the least invasive option.* Most diseases of the lining of the uterus can be reversed with hormone treatments. Benign tumors can usually be removed, sparing the uterus. The ovaries and cervix can almost always be preserved unless they are diseased.

7. *The two categories of problems that women experience after hysterectomy are real and have a significant impact on their wellness.* Hysterectomized women suffer from important *apparent* problems, such as hot flashes, depression, urinary incontinence, and sexual distress, and from *silent* life-threatening diseases, such as osteoporosis and the degeneration of cardiovascular health.

8. *Hormonal replacement therapy is a magnificent option for most posthysterectomized women.* Dosage levels and balances have been refined to eliminate the risks for cancer that were found to be present in the earliest days of HRT. Today properly managed prescriptions for HRT do not increase the risk for cancer and in fact can decrease the risk.

Hormone therapies can now be given safely to improve the general health of most hysterectomized women. For example, when women start taking the proper doses of estrogen and progesterone, in most cases their bones stop deteriorating, their blood pressure drops, and their joy in life increases.

9. *Proper attention to nutrition and exercise can maximize a woman's health.* In combination with HRT, a balanced diet of healthful foods—with attention to fats, fiber, vitamins, and minerals—can help alleviate the effects of hysterectomy. Likewise, exercise has a beneficial effect on many body systems.

10. *With the proper information, women can take charge of their health.* By studying the results of research and working in open dialogue with compassionate physicians, women can enter a new age of participation in the decisions regarding their health care.

## *A WOMAN'S HEALTHRIGHT*

A woman should use the medical community as a resource that exists to serve her. She should approach professionals with a sense of personal dignity—not in a state of awe, but as a competent person who understands her body, who has a sense of what is going on in the research fields relevant to her health, and who wants to take advantage of the excellent options that have recently become available. This is every woman's healthright. It is never too early and never too late to begin improving your health.

In participating in your health care, you may need to overcome:

- An inbred lack of confidence in your own perceptions. Freeing yourself from feelings of intimidation and insecurity requires an active process of learning to believe in yourself, in your perceptions and your knowledge.
- A medical community that has often been trained to discount what women say. This situation can usually be overcome by firm courtesy coupled with a possession of knowledge and facts.
- A medical community that often cannot keep up with current research. Compassionate physicians often find that their energies are consumed by the demands of their patients, leaving

them without time to study new discoveries. Your knowledge of the facts can be critical in securing excellent health care.

I believe that health care for women has the potential to surge forward into a period of greatly improved quality. In this new era, physicians and patients must develop a mutually respectful exchange in which together they explore the problem or condition at hand, evaluate the various options for treatment, and then await the patient's decision. We are approaching an age of informed consent, in which women and the medical community will cooperate in improving the quality of health care for women. Patients must learn to understand their options and relieve their physicians of the potential harassment inherent in unreasonable medical malpractice suits. And physicians must learn to respect both the intelligence and the dignity of their patients. Doctors must lead patients to information and work with them, serving in the role of professional consultant. Only then can the patient exert a free and truly informed choice.

Your perceptions, your knowledge, and your judgment are intimately interrelated. In a real sense, knowledge is power, providing you with a sense of competence and giving you confidence in your own perceptions. You can and you should empower yourself by becoming educated about the way your body functions and about the array of current medical options for approaching dysfunction or disease.

Hysterectomy and ovariectomy are not mild procedures with no aftereffects. In fact, these surgeries have a profound impact on the well-being of a woman. If the benefits of the surgery are considered to outweigh the detriments it imposes, then it makes sense to go forward with it. The decision properly rests with the woman, who will be guided by her own knowledge and judgment, by the counsel she requests, by those who live with her and love her, and by a compassionate physician, whose diagnosis should always be reinforced by a second opinion from another doctor who has no stake in the first opinion.

Enabling yourself, empowering yourself to participate in these decisions, takes work. You may need to study, but the rewards are enormous. When faced with the possibility of either hysterectomy or its aftereffects, your choice will have a profound influence on the quality of your life, for the rest of your life.

# 2

# The Hormonal Symphony:
## How the Healthy Reproductive System Works

A healthy woman's body produces a marvelous symphony: a harmonious and interrelated flow of hormonal secretions. To offer a foundation for understanding how this nearly miraculous biological music is made, this chapter provides a basic overview of the ovaries, the uterus, and the hormones they produce. The information is detailed but will reward the reader with the knowledge she needs in order to participate intelligently in her own health care.

Hormones are substances that are produced in glands and then released into the bloodstream. They circulate through the body, within the arteries, capillaries, and veins, as the blood flows in a continual repumping and recycling process. Tiny enough to travel in the blood, hormones migrate to other parts of the body, leaving the bloodstream through the thin and porous walls of the capillaries to reach "receptor" molecules in various cells of the body, where they produce action often quite distant from the source of their production. In fact, hormones are the controlling substances that keep the body working.

The actions produced by the sex hormones are diverse and extraordinary. They influence the workings of cells throughout the body, affect the way we feel and think, cause glands to produce other hormones, make the skin smooth or pimply, increase energy or libido, and produce stronger muscles. While scientists are only beginning to understand their myriad effects on different body functions, a good deal of information is now available to show the profound importance of the sex hormones. They are vital to life.

In the body of a premenopausal woman whose uterus and ovaries are in place and who is enjoying the normal cycle of hormonal output from the ovaries, there is a dynamic interaction between the secretions of the uterus, the ovaries, the brain, and the pituitary gland. The ovarian sex hormones (the *estrogens, progesterone, androstenedione,* and *testosterone*) move into the bloodstream, circulate throughout the body, and cause the cells of the pituitary and the brain to respond with the secretion of their own hormones: the *luteinizing hormone* (LH), the *luteinizing hormone releasing hormone* (LH RH), the *follicle-stimulating hormone* (FSH), and the *beta endorphins*.[16, 176] These, in turn, circulate in the bloodstream and affect the release of hormones from the ovaries. Similarly, the hormones produced in the cervix (the *prostaglandins*) appear to provide "command signals" that control manufacture of hormones by the ovaries.[174] Ovarian hormones also exert command signals to the parathyroid glands, which control the secretions of bone hormones (*calcitonin* and *parathyroid hormone*) that affect bone metabolism and, indirectly, the development of osteoporosis.

In a design that is at once complex and elegant, the body performs a constant "cross talk" among the reproductive organs, the neuroendocrine system of the brain and the pituitary, and the parathyroid glands.[174, 793] As our knowledge continues to expand, we begin to discover further interactions between secretions of one part of the body and control of another part.

## THE OVARIES

The ovaries of a woman are among the most remarkable structures in nature. No other organ in the human body, male or female, undergoes a monthly cycle in which both size and content change from day to day, in a regular and repeating pattern. In addition to this repeating monthly pattern, the ovaries are in a state of almost constant change throughout life.

Our knowledge of these valuable body parts has grown considerably in the past thirty years, and the most recent data provide critical facts. Until the mid-1980s, the ovaries of women over age 40 were considered useless by many gynecologists, and this incorrect perspective was taught in many medical schools. Published research has now demonstrated that even older ovaries produce vital hormones. It is clear that both young and aging ovaries manufacture a variety of useful and important substances, and equally clear that some of the substances that ovaries manufacture remain to be identified. Clearly, if we don't yet know all that the ovaries produce, we cannot accurately assess the effects of removing them.

### The Hormones Produced by the Ovaries

One might think of the ovaries as miniature warehouse-factories, housing eggs and manufacturing hormones that enter the bloodstream through adjacent blood vessels and circulate throughout the body.

After menstruation begins, generally around the age of 12 or 13, it takes about seven years for the hormonal systems to mature. Until then, menstrual cycles are irregular and unpredictable. This adolescent phase is associated with surges and purges of hormone secretion. The levels of sex hormones can soar and they can plummet, producing the erratic patterns characteristic of adolescence. By about age 20, hormonal output from the ovary follows a generally predictable ebb-and-flow pattern each month.

Estrogen levels rise and fall twice during each monthly cycle. Working together, the three principal estrogens (*estradiol, estrone,* and *estriol*) begin each menstrual cycle at a low level and rise until ovulation approaches. After ovulation, an initial drop in ovarian output is followed by another slow and steady rise of hormone. On the seventh day before menstruation, estrogen reaches its second peak level of the month. During the last seven days before menstruation, estrogen levels continuously decline. When the menstrual flow begins, the estrogen cycle begins again.

(This cyclic variation in estrogen is shown in Figure 1. Note the two peaks during each monthly cycle: one at about day 12, the other at about day 22 of a typical 29-day cycle.) Many women experience a rise and fall in mood, a variation often timed to the rise and fall of estrogen. A lack of good cheer during premenstrual days can be explained by the cascading effects of the estrogen cycle.

Progesterone, the other major ovarian sex hormone, follows a rhythm of its own, with one peak each cycle. After ovulation, progesterone starts to rise significantly, reaching its highest level about seven days before menstruation. The progesterone peak level occurs at the same time as the second estrogen peak level of the menstrual cycle. Progesterone also plays a role in mood. As it rises, it has a narcotic effect, increasing the sense of pleasant sleepiness; as it falls, depression can occur. The ovaries make most of the estrogens and progesterone, but some portion of these hormones is also produced in the adrenal glands.

Androgens, including testosterone and the weaker androstenedione and dehydroepiandrosterone sulfate, are also manufactured by the ovaries. Androgens are usually referred to as male sex hormones, but women also have them, in about one-fortieth the concentration. Androgens play a major role in muscle strength, energy, and libido, but their pattern of secretion is less well studied.[174]

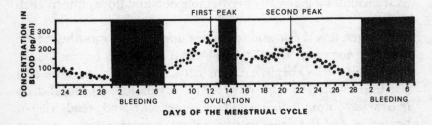

Figure 1. Estrogen changes during each menstrual cycle

## The Structure of the Ovary

Your understanding of ovarian production of the sex hormones will be helped by a close look at the structure of the ovary, which I sometimes think of as the concert hall in which the hormonal music is made. Although we have two ovaries, events occur rather randomly in one or the other and are therefore described as if there is only one. The ovary's structure changes as a woman grows older.

Figure 2 shows a magnified section, or light micrograph, of the ovary of a baby girl.* The ovary of a newborn baby contains her lifetime supply of 500,000 eggs. Around each egg *(ovum)* lies a flat sheet of cells. The entire structure of the egg with its covering sheet of cells is known as a *follicle.* Hundreds of follicles appear in this picture. Figure 3 shows one very large follicle (from a 30-year-old woman) that is almost ready to ovulate.

Figure 4 shows tissue from the ovary of a 30-year-old woman who experiences a regular 28- or 29-day menstrual cycle. In menopausal ovaries, further changes have taken place. Figure 5 shows a more mature ovary, with tissue in a different form than that of younger ovaries.

As these plates reveal, with increasing age the ovary changes. What had been a huge quantity of tightly ordered eggs housed within follicles gradually becomes the less-structured tissue of the older ovary. The unused eggs gradually disintegrate over the years; the follicular structure changes into an amorphous tissue, called *stroma,* that gradually makes up more and more of the ovary.

## The Ovarian Cycle During the Fertile Years

For a fertile woman between the ages of 20 and 40, a dependable, symphonic sequence of events takes place during the ovarian cycle. As menstruation begins (day 1 of the cycle), within the ovary eight to ten follicles are swelling as they absorb fluid

---

*A light micrograph is a photograph, magnified several hundred times, of a very thin slice of tissue that has been removed, usually during surgery.

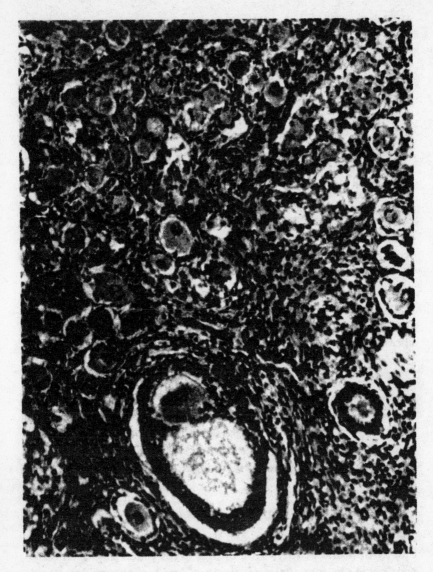

Figure 2. Light micrograph of a slice of an ovary of a baby girl. Figures 2–5 courtesy of Dr. Santo V. Nicosia, University of Southern Florida, College of Medicine, Pathology department.

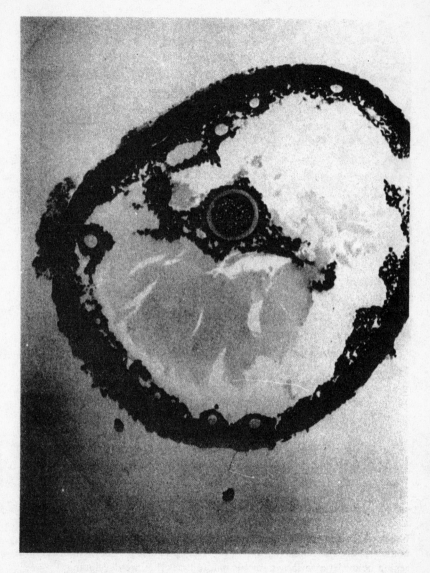

Figure 3. This picture shows one follicle that is very large and almost ready to ovulate. The circular structure toward the center is the egg that will leave the follicle and the ovary, and enter the fallopian tube.

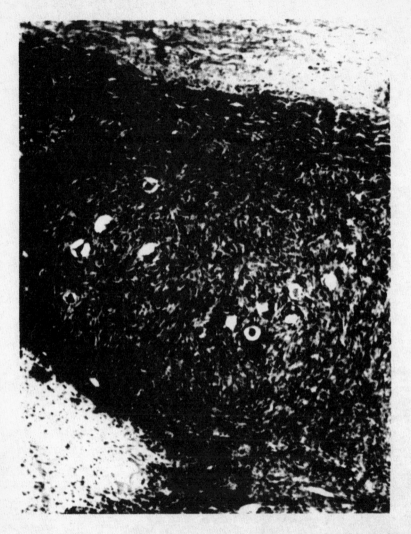

Figure 4. This magnified slice of an ovary from a woman in her thirties shows, at the top, the outer edge (cortex) of the ovary and also part of the more central region below. It also shows some small follicles that are developing.

Figure 5. This magnified slice of a menopausal ovary shows a part of the edge of the ovary along the right side. The straight edge at the top, bottom, and left side was formed from the edges of the glass slide on which the ovarian slice was mounted. Note the absence of large follicles.

laden with cholesterol from the surrounding ovary. (Figure 3 shows one such follicle, with its egg in the center. Although the massive density of follicular cells is not apparent from this picture, their orderly arrangement is.) Once absorbed, the cholesterol is converted into the steroid, or sex, hormones (predominantly estrogen), and some of these hormones leak back out of the follicle into the ovary.* The leaked estrogen works its way into the blood vessels that lie near the follicle and is carried into the rest of the body through the bloodstream.

Usually only one of each month's crop of follicles matures and keeps growing until ovulation, when the egg first is released from its follicle and then escapes from the outer surface of the ovary into the fallopian tube, also called the *oviduct* (see Figure 6). As it begins its journey down the fallopian tube toward the uterus, the egg is available for a rendezvous with a sperm; if the egg is fertilized (penetrated by a sperm), a pregnancy will usually result.

After ovulation, the exterior of the ovary resembles the surface of the moon, with craters where eggs have erupted during recent ovulations. Within the ovary, the cells that had formed the ruptured follicle reconnect to each other; multiplying and swelling, they assume a yellowish appearance. What has been a follicle becomes a *corpus luteum* (Latin for "yellow body"). By about seven days after ovulation, the corpus luteum gets so large that it can take up half of the ovary, crowding the thousands of remaining tiny follicles into the edges of the swelling ovary. The corpus luteum secretes estrogen and progesterone; as it continues to grow, the blood levels of these hormones rise. When the corpus luteum is at its largest, about seven days after ovulation, the progesterone level is at its highest. Then the corpus luteum begins a process of regression, shrinking in size as its cells die. Consequently, progesterone and estrogen levels in the blood de-

*The word "steroid" refers to the fact that steroids are made from chole*sterol.* Steroid hormones include estrogen, testosterone, and progesterone. The anabolic steroids, which have recently been outlawed for some athletic contestants, are composed of testosterone forms.

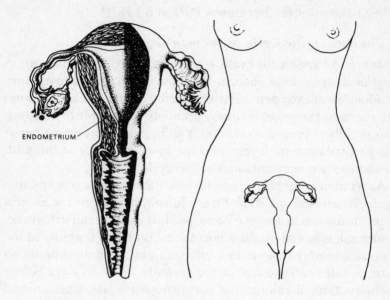

ENDOMETRIUM

Figure 6. The uterus and vagina in detail

cline. This "luteal regression" continues until the ovary is back once again to its smaller menstrual-phase size, and the next menstruation occurs.

This ovarian cycle—the swelling of the follicle, ovulation, the swelling of the corpus luteum, and its shrinking—repeats in a more or less regular fashion each month until menopause approaches. Follicle growth produces the estrogen in the preovulatory phase of the cycle; after ovulation, the corpus luteum is the main source of both estrogen and progesterone. Figure 7 shows the grand design of the various reproductive-system hormones, the changing appearance of the follicles in the ovary, and the appearance of the lining of the uterus (the *endometrium*) during the succeeding days of the repeating menstrual cycle. Notice how the changes in the follicle and corpus luteum control the levels of estrogen and progesterone, which stimulate the secretion of the pituitary hormones FSH and LH.[174]

### Changes in the Cycle as Women Grow Older

At around age 35, the cyclic estrogen and progesterone pattern begins to noticeably change. With the years, the preovulatory production of estrogen starts increasing, while as menstruation approaches, the postovulatory, premenstrual levels of estrogen continually decrease. As the years go by, the highs get higher at the preovulatory midcycle, and the lows get lower at the postovulatory, premenstrual end of the cycle.[174]

As women enter their early forties, the ovarian cycle changes again. At around age 40 to 43, the luteal phase begins to show a deterioration in function. The corpus luteum may fail to form or, if formed, may not produce hormones. With this inability of the corpus luteum to do its job, estrogen and progesterone levels start to fall precipitously in the seven to fourteen days before menstruation, heralding the perimenopause (the time around the menopause).

### The Aging Ovary

As early as 1951, studies showed that older ovaries have a distinct appearance when viewed through the microscope.[718, 872] (See Figure 5.) One major feature is the development of a layer of fatty tissue (the *stromal band*) that takes up increasing space within the maturing ovary.[202, 251] While the follicular and luteal tissue in an ovary (composed of follicles and corpora lutea) had long been known to produce estrogens and progesterone,[696] until relatively recently the stromal area was considered by some doctors to provide no hormone.[561]

In 1965 biomedical scientists suggested that menopausal ovaries (particularly the stromal area and another region) showed frequent evidence of biochemical activity.[646] Something was being manufactured that had not yet been identified. In 1970 two reports proposed that postmenopausal ovaries were often active in hormone production.[598, 645] Still, as late as 1973, challenges

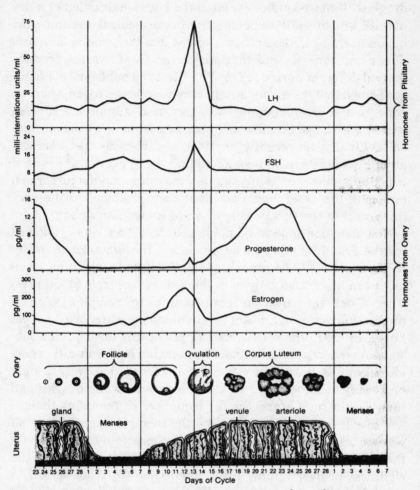

Figure 7. Cyclic variation in the reproductive system of a cycling woman

were published, suggesting that postmenopausal ovaries probably play no vital role in the hormonal milieu of a woman.[327]

Beginning in the mid-1970s, several studies resulted in a major breakthrough in our knowledge of the ovaries. In 1974 tests on blood collected from the ovaries of postmenopausal women proved that these "old" ovaries secrete both estrogens and androgens.[438] More studies explored the hormonal milieu of older ovaries, and by 1979 the perspective in the medical literature had begun to change. Researchers showed that the stromal area produces hormones[571] and that postmenopausal ovaries produce several different hormones.[123, 332, 716] In 1980 published evidence confirmed that the menopausal ovary supplies estrogen, testosterone, and androstenedione;[519] in fact, testosterone levels often increase with age because that hormone is made by the stromal cells. Finally, as recently as 1983, a consensus has emerged among scientists, who now agree that aging ovaries are indeed functioning tissue.[631] Although they may not manufacture much estrogen, the other hormones that they produce can be very important to the functioning of an older woman's body.

New data continue to be published. In 1986 a report showed for the first time that ovaries produce a hormonal *renin-angiotensin* system.[503] The renin-angiotensin system, which had usually been associated only with the kidney, controls blood pressure. Does this ovarian contribution to renin-angiotensin production play a significant role in blood pressure? We don't yet know. In 1987 other discoveries of previously unsuspected substances were reported.[455] Aside from its intrinsic value, this new knowledge is noteworthy because it means that we are only beginning to understand what happens within the ovaries and thus cannot fully assess the consequences of removing them.

While it is generally agreed by the medical community that women under age 40 who undergo a hysterectomy should retain their ovaries unless the ovaries are diseased, the question of the rightness of ovariectomy for women over 40 is not settled. A good deal of controversy has recently surrounded this topic (see page 345).

## Menopause

The word "menopause" describes the final "pause," or cessation, of menstruation. In this book, the word will most often refer to the events that lie behind the cessation of bleeding—the shutting down of the ovarian "egg factory" and the ovaries' diminished production of estrogen and progesterone. The sex hormone levels go *much* lower than those found at even the very lowest level within the fluctuating menstrual cycle.

The seven-year menopausal transition (perimenopause) stage, from about age 43 to 50, is characterized by hormonal, menstrual, physical, and emotional changes. Because of changes in estrogen and progesterone secretions as women grow older, the bleeding pattern at menstruation begins to change. For some women, the blood flow gets lighter; for others, it gets heavier. For an individual woman, the bleeding may be profuse at some times, scanty at others.[143, 210, 887, 889, 917] For the vast majority of perimenopausal women these changes in bleeding—which may at first appear to be abnormal bleeding—simply reflect normal changes in ovarian hormone secretion that are characteristic of the perimenopausal transition.

The early symptoms of menopause can include hot flashes, increased irritability, fatigue, headaches, depression, and emotional swings that are sometimes severe.[415, 570, 324, 605, 877] In a woman who has not had surgery, these early symptoms often appear six or seven years before the last menstrual flow. Since the last menstrual flow generally occurs at age 49 or 50, symptoms commonly begin at about age 43.

Hot flashes, or flushing, and night sweats, which are hot flashes that occur during sleep, are usually the first symptoms to appear. They are uncomfortable but certainly not dangerous.[604] Hot flashes are caused by the brain's response to the decline in estrogen level. It is as though the body's thermostat becomes confused, shooting up in spurts and causing flashes of intense heat. Flushing, which starts before the menopause in two out of three women, is initially infrequent and occurs on the face and neck only. By three to twelve months after their last menstrual period, 75 percent of the women report flashes and night sweats.[570] These symptoms may last only a few months, or many years. They may occur many times a day and affect the whole body, or may be felt just occasionally and on the face and neck only.[877] Each flash produces a host of physical effects (heat, sweating, temperature elevation) that last about eight minutes.[721] When the climate is hot or the temperature has increased, women suffering from hot flashes experience more of them.[145, 605] Flashes tend to continue for about seven years if no HRT is taken. Once the estrogen levels stabilize at a new lower value, hot flashes begin to diminish and eventually stop. HRT will stop them. But even five to ten years after the last menstrual period, 45 percent of women not using HRT still had hot flashes.[415]*

After the last menstrual period, muscle aches occur in 45 percent of women, and about 20 percent experience some tingling in the extremities.[415] Scientists don't know why, but androgen depletion is a good candidate for the cause of this muscular aching. The tingling may result from problems with either blood circulation or nerve firing.

These very apparent symptoms of menopause are important because of what they indicate about changes in body functions that are more difficult to perceive. Hot flashes and other early signs of "change of life" (such as aging of the skin, altered bleeding patterns, and emotional changes) herald a decline in estrogen and progesterone levels and as a consequence, potential changes in the functioning of bone metabolism, cardiovascular health, and sexual physiology.[365, 376, 579, 647]*

Although perhaps 20 percent of women do not suffer from the overt symptoms of perimenopausal distress, the silent, internal processes that accompany menopause are likely to be taking place to one degree or another.

Postmenopausal symptoms and changes, and ways of coping with them for maximum health, are discussed in detail in the book's later chapters.

---

*Men also can suffer hot flashes under certain circumstances in which their gonadal output of androgens is diminished.[306, 308, 377]

*For more detailed information about the change of life and the HRT options for women not undergoing surgery, you may want to consult *Menopause: A Guide for Women and the Men Who Love Them*, which I co-authored with Dr. Celso Ramón García and Dr. David Edwards.

## THE UTERUS

The uterus has no counterpart in the male body. All the other reproductive organs have male/female counterparts: the ovaries compare to the testes and the vagina to the penis, but the remarkable uterus is a uniquely feminine structure composed of a powerful outer muscle and an inner lining with glandular (hormone-producing) structures. An extraordinarily complex and rich contributor to the emotional and physical life of a woman, the uterus often plays a significant role in sexual lubrication, orgasmic contraction, and hormone production. The hormones and nerve impulses that it produces in turn affect hormone and neurochemical production in the spinal cord, the brain, the ovaries, and other glands.

### Structure and Functioning of the Uterus

The outer portion of the uterus, the *myometrium*, is formed of smooth muscle, the contraction of which is controlled by the involuntary nervous and endocrine (hormone) systems. When a woman's body has high blood levels of progesterone, such as during pregnancy or in the premenstrual part of each monthly cycle, the uterus contracts differently than when estrogen is dominant. When estrogen is dominant and the nerves impinging upon the uterus trigger directions for it to contract, the whole muscle contracts in synchrony with itself, forming a tight ball. In contrast, when progesterone is dominant, uterine contractions are lumpy, in discrete regions of the muscle.[174] For this reason, orgasm may be experienced differently in the various phases of the hormonal cycle.

The endometrial tissue (the lining of the uterus) is spongy, filling up with blood vessels during the premenstrual part of each cycle. As the corpus luteum in the ovary begins to shrink during the last seven days of the menstrual cycle (see Figure 7), there is a withdrawal of the estrogen and progesterone support that had been providing the impetus to maintain this spongy layer. As the hormones decline, the blood supply diminishes, and as that happens, the endometrial tissue becomes starved for the nutrients, particularly oxygen, and dies. The spongy tissue breaks off and sloughs away with the normal menstrual flow. The broken blood vessels that occur as a result of this sloughing off account for most of the bleeding of the menstrual flow.

The tip end of the uterus, the cervix, is structurally different from the uterine body. It has only about 20 percent as much muscle as the uterine body.[62] Instead, it is richly endowed with sensory nerve endings of the type that transmit electrical signals to the brain and spinal cord when stimulated by pressure.[174] It also serves as the opening from the vagina to the uterus.

Figure 6 shows the interconnection between the cervix and the vagina, as well as between the uterus and the fallopian tubes. Figure 8 focuses on the cervical region. Sperm enters the cervix, moves upward into the uterus, and from there into the fallopian tubes. Sperm can wait and live, in the tubes, for about two days. The fingerlike endings (the *fimbria*) of the fallopian tubes, like vacuum cleaners, suck the ovulating egg through the surface of the ovary and out into the fallopian tubes. When the egg finds a sperm waiting, fertilization can take place, and the fertilized egg then moves back into the endometrium. After embedding there, the egg can begin its nine-month gestation process.

### The Value of the Uterus

Women are often told that the uterus is not important after the childbearing years, but the facts prove this view to be incorrect. The uterus is not simply a baby-growing and baby-holding machine. This uniquely feminine organ performs multiple roles in promoting the health of a woman. Just as recent studies have revealed the important role of the ovaries, the many roles of the uterus are only beginning to be understood as scientists investigate specific potential interactions between the uterus and other body parts.

Information about the value of the uterus comes from two sources: planned studies of the organ and systematic analysis

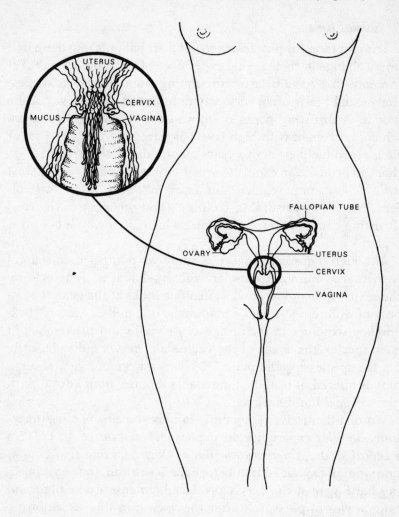

Figure 8. The uterus of a woman with a particular emphasis on the cervix.

of the complaints of women after hysterectomy, which often lead to conclusions about what the uterus must have contributed. From both types of studies we have learned that the uterus plays several roles in a woman's sexual life, in influencing the health of the ovaries, and in the functioning of the nervous system.

## Its Sexual Role

It is common for physicians to tell their patients that there will be no change in their sexual experience after hysterectomy. Yet the data that have been accumulating since the 1970s suggest that sexual life is often seriously diminished by removal of the uterus. A thrusting penis is stopped by the tip of the cervix, which, in women with high levels of estrogen (characteristic of their reproductively active years), is studded with nerve endings that can produce an exquisite sensitivity as the penis taps against it.[174, 974] For many women, this aspect of sexual intercourse offers intensely pleasurable feelings. (For others, too vigorous thrusting can be painful; and others have no awareness of this region.)

Although there is no rigorous study yet published, anecdotal reports are common from men who say that after hysterectomy the sexual fit is not as good. When one looks at the genital anatomy of different species of mammals, one finds a kind of lock-and-key structure in the design of the male and the female; in each species, the shape of the vagina and cervix quite elegantly fits the species-specific penis.[339] When a woman's genital anatomy is altered, it is almost inevitable that her male sexual partner will feel the difference.

Women themselves frequently lament the effects of hysterectomy on their experience during sexual intercourse. In 1981, in a report in the *American Journal of Obstetrics and Gynecology,* one woman explained that before the operation, the penis pushing hard against the cervix produced "intense excitement and huge waves of pleasure"; after the operation this sensation no longer existed and the absence was perceived as a real and saddening deficit.[974] Many, many other women have found the same thing.[174]

Through studies of a variety of mammals, we know that the body of the uterus is involved in sexual response, particularly in the orgasm. The large uterine muscle is smooth, somewhat like the heart muscle. Just as the heart muscle contracts regularly to produce a wave motion of blood, the uterus contracts at significant times in the reproductive life of a woman, under the control of both hormones and nerves. For example, a series of contractions permits expulsion of the fetus at childbirth. For many women, the uterus contracts at orgasm. This contraction is often perceived as intensely pleasurable and forms a significant part of their orgasmic response.[267, 459]

Lubrication during intercourse derives from two sources: cervical mucus and the vaginal transudate. Cervical mucus, produced at the tip of the uterus,[124] contributes a significant portion of the vaginal lubrication.[172, 174, 555] (See Figure 8.) The *vaginal transudate,* analogous to the beading of droplets of sweat on the skin, results from the pressure of increased blood flow to the pelvic region during sexual arousal; some of the blood fluid is squeezed across the vaginal walls. After a hysterectomy that removes the cervix, only half of the system that produces the lubrication of the vagina is left, and vaginal dryness can become a problem.

Fortunately, sexuality in humans is so much a composite of psychological, emotional, and spiritual dimensions that a great deal of sexual life should remain unchanged even when a hysterectomy is performed. Nevertheless, the removal of the uterus is likely to have notable effects on a woman's sexual life.

## *Effect on the Ovaries and Hormone Production*

Recent discoveries show that the uterus plays a pivotal role in keeping the ovaries healthy. Substances from the uterus appear to control hormonal secretions from the ovaries. Although researchers have not yet discovered all the reasons why, it is known that the ovaries stop cycling (that is, they stop producing a monthly variation in sex hormones) in about 50 percent of premenopausal hysterectomized women.

Many studies show relationships between hysterectomy and the subsequent onset of the symptoms of menopause. Within three days after surgery, temporary and sometimes permanent deficits occur in the hormones of the ovaries: estrogen, progesterone, androstenedione, and testosterone. The magnitude of these deficits varies according to the time of life when the surgery is performed.* Likewise, immediately after surgery there are changes in the hormones produced in the pituitary and brain: the luteinizing hormone, follicle-stimulating hormone, and the hormones known as the endogenous opiates, including the beta endorphins.

In 1984 the first scientific demonstration was published that showed that prostaglandins from the uterus enter the vein that connects the uterus and the ovary, and thus reach the ovary directly. It was shown, in experiments on sheep, that hormones of the ovary (estrogen and progesterone) in turn indirectly controlled prostaglandin production in the uterus.[568] This study is one of many to establish a clear interaction between the uterus and the ovaries. Other recent work has discovered an abundance of prostaglandins in human cervical mucus.[124] Because prostaglandins play a key role in maintaining the ovarian luteal phase,[174] their presence in the cervix may help explain why the ovaries stop cycling in about 50 percent of hysterectomized women.

But what of the 50 percent whose ovaries continue to cycle after hysterectomy? Where do they get their prostaglandin? Prostaglandins are abundant in semen. About 50 percent of women continue to be sexually active after hysterectomy; thus it is possible that those women get the necessary prostaglandins through sexual activity, and that they are the 50 percent whose ovaries continue to cycle.[174] This hypothesis has not yet been tested, but its logic offers a tentative answer.

Because hormonal deficits and imbalances follow hysterectomy even when the ovary is retained, surgery in a woman's reproductive system affects the whole person. Although the academic physicians who teach in medical schools agree that a

*Among the studies that document these changes are: 4, 40, 116, 117, 190, 209, 299, 402, 433, 469, 534, 793, 915, 967.

hysterectomy with bilateral ovariectomy (both ovaries removed) produces significant changes, they often do not teach the more recent findings, which have shown that the uterus plays a critically important role in keeping the ovaries healthy and that hysterectomy alone can profoundly change the hormonal output of the ovaries.

## Influence on the Nervous System

The uterus interconnects with the nervous system.[747] Hysterectomy frequently produces some predictable deficits in nervous system functioning, and these deficits, in turn, affect the whole person. Three main areas of nervous-system involvement have so far been identified:

1. *The beta endorphin contribution of the uterus.* The beta endorphins are associated with strong feelings of emotional well-being. The uterus influences the beta endorphins in two ways: first, it produces them in the glands of the endometrium; second, through its influence on ovarian cycling, the uterus affects the secretion of endorphins from the brain and pituitary gland. (See page 39.)
2. *The prostaglandin production of the cervix.* Prostaglandins have myriad affects on the nervous system of the body, and the cervix produces abundant quantities of this substance.[124] No studies of the effects of such deficits have yet been undertaken.
3. *The sensory nerve endings located in the cervix.* The cervical tip is richly endowed with nerve endings which, for many women, produce an extraordinary range of nerve impulse firings during deep rhythmic thrusting in intercourse. It has been demonstrated in studies of small mammals that there is a potential for this firing pattern to stimulate the areas of the brain that lead to the release of the hormones that influence the reproductive cycle.[12, 13] Physiological systems inevitably reveal, once adequate research has been done, that where

nerve fibers exist, so do physiological functions that make good use of them. The full range of use of these cervical nerve fibers remains to be investigated.

Five different sets of sensory nerves have been identified according to E.O. Lundberg, M.D., Ph.D., of the Department of Neurology, University Hospital, Uppsala, Sweden. Research being conducted there has confirmed the existence of nerves which carry sensory feeling from the female genital tissue into the central nervous system. No studies have yet been published to evaluate which of these five sets of nerves are altered by different forms of pelvic surgery.

## THE HORMONAL SYMPHONY

The uterus and the ovaries are together responsible for maintaining the hormonal cycles of estrogen, progesterone, androstenedione, testosterone, FSH and LH (the gonadotropins), and the beta endorphins. These hormones play important roles in the healthy functioning of the female body. Again, the evidence has emerged in two ways: from planned studies and from analysis of what happens after a hormonal deficit.

Radioimmunoassay (RIA), a laboratory technique that earned its inventors a Nobel prize in the late 1970s, allows the rapid testing of blood to determine hormone levels. Whereas before this technique was developed it was extremely difficult to evaluate the blood levels of hormones, RIA is now widely used to test most of the hormones mentioned in this book. More recently, saliva has been used, instead of blood, to analyze through RIA what the hormone levels are. This less onerous method of contributing body fluids to test hormone levels may someday replace blood sampling.

### Estrogen and Progesterone

Estrogen and progesterone work together, counterbalancing each other's force. One might think of estrogen as the hormone that distinguishes female from male, promoting full breasts, smooth skin, sexual wetness, the fat pattern of rounded hips and buttocks, and other yet-to-be researched "feminine" physiology. It also promotes the health of the bones and of the cardiovascular system. Progesterone is the necessary counterpoint to estrogen, helping to prevent the cancers of endometrium and breast that are thought to result from excesses of estrogen. Recently scientists have become aware that a woman's body needs both estrogen and progesterone in order to maximize health and minimize reproductive-system diseases. Beta endorphin secretion also requires the stimulation of both estrogen and progesterone.

The sex hormones directly affect the cells of physiologic systems throughout the body. Studies of skin tissue and bone thickness, cardiovascular health, sexual capacity, emotional wellness and depression, and immunity have revealed numerous ways in which the presence of these hormones, in intact women, predict relative good health. Studies of hormonal depletion and of reproductive-system surgeries consistently show the increased incidence of disease, discomfort, or lack of well-being when estrogen deprivation occurs. For example, because estrogen serves to promote growth, elasticity, and collagen synthesis in skin, and because it makes bones thick and strong, a woman who becomes estrogen depleted, at menopause or after surgery, shows it in her skin and her bones. Studies of the effects of these hormones are reported in chapters 6 through 12.

### Androstenedione

Androstenedione, a weak androgen hormone, undergoes a conversion within the fat cells of the body, where it is changed into estrone (one of the estrogen hormones). Estrone appears to be the principal hormone in protecting against osteoporosis in women.[424] Androstenedione is a very important hormone for maturing women, not only because it has been related to hot flashes after ovariectomy,[40] but more significantly because of its role (described in Chapter 8) in the prevention of osteoporosis. Menstruating women produce about half of this hormone in their ovaries and about half in their adrenal glands.[433] There appears to be a 25 percent to 40 percent loss of adrenal output of androstenedione in women between the ages of 50 and 55.[155]

Changes in the ovary as it ages can partially offset the loss of the adrenal output. As the ovary ages, there is less follicular tissue, and more and more ovarian tissue becomes part of the stromal band. This band of stroma appears to be the source of most of the ovarian supply of androstenedione. Not surprisingly, when ovarian function is interrupted through an ovariectomy and perhaps through a hysterectomy, there is a drop in the amount of circulating androstenedione.[4, 40, 433]

### Testosterone

Women circulate testosterone, an androgen hormone, just as men do but in much smaller quantities. Nonetheless, the effects of testosterone on a woman's body are probably profound. Testosterone is important in maintaining an adequate libido; as described in detail in Chapter 10, women frequently report a loss of sexual appetite after an ovariectomy and after hysterectomy. Postmenopausal ovaries secrete significant amounts of androgens. Some testosterone also derives from the conversion of androstenedione into testosterone; in both premenopausal and postmenopausal women, about 14 percent of the androstenedione circulating in the blood is converted into testosterone.[433] Because half of the testosterone in women is produced in the ovaries and half in another organ, most likely the adrenal glands, ovariectomy tends to reduce the circulating amount of the hormone by half.[432, 433]

Testosterone therapy appears to restore libido after ovariectomy.[805] Unfortunately, there are problems with this therapy. Few studies have yet been published to define the doses, forms, side effects, and risks for women who take this hormone. (See Chapters 6 and 7 on HRT and Chapter 10 on sexuality.)

### The Gonadotropins

The word "gonadotropin" has two parts: *tropin*, meaning "going to," and *gonad*, a gland that produces sex hormones. (A woman's gonads are her ovaries. A man's gonads are his testes.) In women, the two gonadotropins that are produced in the pituitary and travel to the gonads are the luteinizing hormone (LH) and the follicle-stimulating hormone (FSH). Although these two hormones have multiple functions, their names indicate the principal roles they play in a normal cycling ovary.

FSH stimulates the follicle cells to grow. Follicles (see Figure 3) are structures within the ovary; each one consists of an egg at the center and a large surrounding quantity of hormone-producing cells. These cells manufacture estrogen and a smaller amount of the other sex hormones. As the follicles enlarge, their output of sex hormones increases, as shown in Figure 7. LH plays a major role in the ovary. It stimulates ovulation and maintains the growth of the corpus luteum, which in turn manufactures sex hormones and causes the production and surge in both progesterone and estrogen in the second half of each menstrual cycle.

Beginning in the late twenties and increasing as women age, the amount of both gonadotropins increases. At menopause, the increase is even more pronounced. Then for about ten years after menopause, the gonadotropins begin to decline somewhat in quantity, although they never reach levels as low as they were during the cycling years. Why do the gonadotropins increase with age while the sex hormones decrease? Although there is speculation, there is yet no conclusive answer to this question.

Reproductive-system surgery alters the normal gonadotropin levels. Ovariectomy produces a tenfold increase in FSH and LH levels within three weeks after surgery,[967] an enormous magnification of the normal tendency with aging. Long-term studies of the effect of ovariectomy have shown that the level of gonadotropins stays high, unlike the condition in the natural menopause, when they begin to decline.[117] (Hysterectomy alone has not yet been studied to determine gonadotropin effects.) How do high levels of gonadotropins impact on the overall health and welfare of the body? We do not yet know, but hormonal changes invariably affect physiology.

## The Beta Endorphins

New research has recently been released on the endogenous (internal) opiates, or beta endorphins (the terms are used interchangeably here; "endorphin" is a contraction of *end*ogenous m*orphin*e). These tiny molecules sometimes act as hormones do; that is, they are produced in one region of the body, travel in the bloodstream, and affect cells in another part of the body. They were first discovered in the brain, but more recent studies show that they are manufactured in many locations throughout the body, including the spinal cord and the endometrium. The endorphins often relate to a strong feeling of emotional well-being. After exercise, endogenous opiates show large increases[106] that coincide with the exhilaration characteristic of the "runner's high." (Chapter 15 offers more detail.) Endorphins also appear to act as neurotransmitters (substances produced by nerve cells that cause adjacent nerve cells to either fire or stop firing).

Our understanding of the relationship between a woman's reproductive endocrine system and her endogenous opiate system is relatively new, and due in large part to the development of radioimmunoassay. Since the opiates affect the well-being of a woman, the issue is critical. The first reports of studies in mammals (pigtail monkeys) appeared in 1982, showing that normally menstruating monkeys produce beta endorphins in a particular area of the brain and that the hormone then trickles down into the pituitary gland. When monkeys were ovariectomized, their brain beta endorphin levels plummeted. Estrogen replacement therapy did not help, but when both estrogen and progesterone were given to mimic the normal cycle patterns, a full return of the natural beta endorphin level was detected.[249, 250, 929, 935]

Between 1983 and 1987 a number of studies were conducted on women with normal menstrual cycles, women with abnormal (infertile) cycles, women with premenstrual syndrome, and those who had undergone ovariectomy. All confirm the relationship found in the monkeys.

Women who show a normal menstrual cycle, with the normal pattern of estrogen and progesterone, show peak levels of beta endorphins (a fivefold increase) around the time of ovulation.[685, 911] Women with abnormal cycles, characteristic of a failure of the estrogen-progesterone rhythm, do not show the beta endorphin rise that is characteristic of a healthy cycle.[239] Women who suffer from premenstrual depression, in contrast to women who do not, show severe declines in blood levels of beta endorphin during the seven premenstrual days of their cycle.[239]

The opiates are also produced in areas of the body other than the brain. In 1986 the first report of endogenous opiates in uterine fluid appeared.[684] Only women with cycling ovaries or postmenopausal women taking HRT had them; the uterine fluid of estrogen-deficient women did not contain these opiates. This study provided the first data to suggest that the uterine glands also produce these endogenous opiates.

Blood levels of beta endorphins in ovariectomized women, as in postmenopausal women, are much lower than in intact menstruating women.[300, 685] A significant drop (of about 43 percent) was shown five days after surgery, with a sudden temporary increase immediately after hot flashes.[10] Although studies have not yet measured beta endorphin levels after hysterectomy, when the ovaries are retained, the disruption of the connection between the ovaries and the uterus may produce a postsurgical drop in beta endorphins, and thus explain the high incidence of posthysterectomy depression.

## Sexual Behavior Affects Hormones

While it is now clearly established that estrogen and progesterone affect the way the body functions, a recent set of studies has shown that behavior, particularly sexual behavior, affects hormones. Specifically, sexual behavior can affect your estrogen level. A series of research studies that I conducted with colleagues at the University of Pennsylvania, Monell Chemical Senses Center, and Stanford University, published from 1979 through 1987, has provided a new awareness about the effects of sexual activity within a woman's reproductive system. In these studies, which evaluated women in their early twenties, women in their late forties, and those in between, a consistent finding was demonstrated. Women who engaged in regular weekly sex with a man showed patterns of menstrual cycling and hormonal levels that reflected greater fertility (significant even if pregnancy is not desired because it reflects a better level of endocrine health). Their estrogen levels were about twice as high and in the normal ranges of optimal health. Their menstrual cycles were more regular than those of women who were celibate or who were sporadically active. Their basal body temperature graphs more commonly displayed patterns characteristic of fertility.

The critical component in the behavior turned out to be the regularity with which the sexual activity occurred. Weekly activity—that is, never missing a nonmenstruating week—was the critical component in producing these hormone and fertility responses. Sporadic behavior, a kind of feast-or-famine approach, seemed to have a negative effect on the endocrine system.[158–171, 177] Women who had a stable occurrence of sexual behavior did best in tests for estrogen and fertility. Celibate women did next best. Sporadically active women were the ones most likely to show extremely low estrogen levels.[177] Perimenopausal women who had regular weekly sexual activity also showed higher estrogen and fewer hot flashes than age-matched women who did not.[167, 171]

The definition of sexual behavior also proved relevant. Whether sex was defined as sexual intercourse or merely genital play in the presence of a man did not seem to matter; the two were just about equally effective. However, self-stimulation did not produce changes in hormonal level or fertility.[168, 169] In 1987 researchers at the Kinsey Institute reported preliminary results to show that lesbians who engaged in regular three-times-weekly sex showed the same tendency to experience regular 29-day menstrual cycles as heterosexuals who engaged in minimum once-per-week sex; they have not yet tested the other measures of hormones or fertility.

Because it was known that regular weekly patterns of heterosexual activity might influence menstrual cycle length and that women who lived together tended to cycle together, and in light of the studies on nonhuman mammalian species suggesting that chemical signals from other same-species animals might be involved, an investigation was undertaken to evaluate whether an extract from the secretions of the underarm region of men and women could offer a sufficient stimulus to induce changes in the menstrual cycle pattern of recipient women. The preliminary studies have provided evidence indicating that both men's and women's secretions are effective. These substances, called *phero-mones* (chemical substances produced by the body of one person or animal that affect the endocrine system of another person or animal), are in the preliminary stages of research.[173, 698, 699] They hold the promise that someday they may be useful for promoting the health care of women. For now, human phero-mone extracts remain unavailable for purchase by the public, and it is unknown whether they, like sexual behavior, will increase estrogen levels. I suspect that they will, once the dosages are resolved.

Taken together, these studies provide evidence that hormonal systems are responsive to external influences. The sex hormones respond to sexual behavior. (What probably happens is that testosterone stimulates libido, the drive and desire for sexual activity, and as counterpoint, sexual activity, when patterned in a way that provides stability, serves to promote estrogen secretion.) Sexual behavior, then, can serve to enhance or to disrupt a woman's endocrine system. If she does not have access to a regular, stable sexual relationship, the current evidence suggests that it may be better for her to be celibate. Sporadic sexual behavior frequently disrupts ovarian hormonal production.

The delicate hormonal balance of an intact woman is like a dynamic piece of music, changing daily within the rhythm of the monthly cycle and moving into a new refrain with the onset of the menopausal years.

Hormonal milieu is seriously altered by ovariectomy and probably by hysterectomy as well. While HRT is currently available and extremely helpful for women who have had pelvic surgery, we still lack full knowledge about dosages that will provide levels of hormonal stimulation exactly equivalent to those of cycling and aging ovaries. And because we do not yet know all the substances that the uterus and the ovary produce, nor their many effects, we cannot hope to completely replace them after surgery.

The ovaries and the uterus are organs that are important for the good health of women. Knowledge about these organs and the hormones they produce should help women recognize the pattern of their bodies' functioning and feel confident about participating in the decisions surrounding their own health care.

# 3

# When Disease Strikes:
## Symptoms and Diagnosis

When a woman's body signals that something may be wrong, or when she is troubled by a known condition or disease, she wants relief and a satisfactory resolution of the problem. All too often, doctors and patients choose hysterectomy to resolve problems, incorrectly assuming that pelvic surgery has no negative consequences. But surgery to remove the uterus is not a mild or innocuous procedure.

If the uterus is perceived as having no health value, then whenever it becomes troublesome, it would be logical to think of removing it. But the uterus does have value, as described in Chapter 2. Its removal can damage your physical health by accelerating aging, bone deterioration, and cardiovascular disease, and your psychological health by causing depression.

There are times when a hysterectomy is appropriate, when it will enhance your health, and there are times when it is unnecessary. If a doctor tells you that a hysterectomy seems the best course of action, you need to know how to evaluate that suggestion.

This chapter has three sections. The first provides advice on responding to symptoms: the time factor, the importance of accurate diagnosis, and the need for information about treatment options. The second section discusses bleeding, the symptom that most commonly sends women to their doctors. The third section, on getting a diagnosis, discusses the question of who should do the diagnosis and reviews current diagnostic techniques. The chapter that follows, "Some Common Uterine Diseases," can be referred to for more detailed discussions of specific problems, their causes, and treatment options.

## THE BODY'S SIGNALS

Disease can strike from several directions. Bleeding or pain might prompt you to visit your physician. As a candidate for hormonal replacement therapy, you may be tested and be told that there is a problem with your uterus. You might be taking HRT and begin to experience abnormal bleeding. A Pap smear may indicate the presence of cervical disease. Any of these conditions, and many others, can lead to a prescription for a hysterectomy. *But they don't have to.*

In order to maximize her health care options, a woman must be alert to the body's signals of possible disease. Pain in the pelvic area or abnormal (that is, unexpected) bleeding is definitely a sign that a woman should see her doctor for evaluation. Yet bleeding and pain do not necessarily reflect disease, and many diseases can be successfully treated by nonsurgical means. In very few cases does a woman need to rush into surgery.

### The Question of Time

Abnormal bleeding, pain, or any other indication of possible disease must be addressed—but how quickly, with what degree of urgency? Three facts about uterine disease are important in thinking about timing: First, diseases are often progressive—that is, they progress to ever greater pathology until some action is taken to reverse the condition. Second, the early stages are relatively easy to remedy while preserving the uterus. Third, most diseases have a long, slowly developing process. Thus, women should be quick to consult a doctor for early detection, but they should not be rash in hurrying to a diagnosis.

You may be frightened and want an immediate solution. Although it can be frightening when you discover a symptom or suspect the presence of disease, the best thing you can do is to stifle the sense of panic and instead start a systematic search for an accurate diagnosis. Fortunately, a large body of research data shows that there is rarely any need to rush.

A beautifully detailed study, published in 1974, reported on the results of almost 2,000 evaluations of endometrial tissue, performed because of suspicion of disease. The evaluated women either were in pain, were bleeding heavily, or had had an abnormal Pap smear.[358] Two facts about the study are relevant here:

- The authors were slow and careful in establishing a diagnosis before considering that hysterectomy might be appropriate.
- They said, "We're convinced that in no case was the therapy outcome compromised by waiting, but in many, many cases [the women] were able to avoid an unnecessary hysterectomy by thorough examination and evaluation."

Other scientists and physicians have reported the same results.[960] It seems that, even in the most serious cases of reproductive-system disease, the general outcome is almost never compromised by taking the necessary time to thoroughly investigate and diagnose. Time spent searching for the cause of a symptom can prevent unnecessary hysterectomy.

### Finding the Cause and Choosing the Right Treatment

The first task with unexplained bleeding or pelvic pain is to determine its cause. A number of studies that evaluated uterine tissue after a hysterectomy found no disease or pathology that could have justified the surgery. It seems likely that those hysterectomies were performed for one or both of the following reasons: (1) The uterus was not considered to be of any value. (2) A sense of urgency caused the woman and her doctor to proceed with a hysterectomy before thoroughly and carefully considering whether a less drastic measure may have been suitable.

A look at the results of a typical study provides an idea of the range of possible diagnoses of abnormal bleeding among premenopausal women. One report studied 204 women whose endometrial tissue was removed and analyzed. Of the 204, only

5 women showed a disease that was serious enough to mandate a hysterectomy; 4 of these had cancer of either the cervix or the uterus.[937] For the rest, diagnoses worked out as follows:

Normal preovulatory endometrium 114
Normal postovulatory endometrium 37
Inflamed endometrium (but no serious disease) 5
Inactive tissue (characteristic of aging) 11
Menstrual tissue (normal) 11
Endometrial polyp (see Chapter 4) 4
Decidua (pregnant tissue) 6
Mixed healthy tissue 2
Hyperplasia (see Chapter 4) 9

By virtue of a careful diagnostic evaluation, 98 percent of the women were able to avoid a hysterectomy.

Just as important as a correct diagnosis is the ability to successfully treat a problem or disease. Hysterectomy will treat a wide range of problems, but most often at great risk to a woman's overall health. Many uterine problems can now be treated hormonally and through reconstructive surgical techniques that leave the uterus in place or that at least spare the cervix and/or ovaries.

## If You Are Bleeding Abnormally

Most commonly, gynecologic disease first appears as abnormal (that is, unexpected) bleeding. Usually not at all dangerous in and of itself, such bleeding does need to be investigated and stopped. Because abnormal bleeding can result from a variety of conditions, it is very important to define the condition in order to know how to treat it.

First, be sure that the bleeding is actually abnormal, rather than simply a change in your personal pattern that falls within the range of normal bleeding for women at your stage of life. (See "Bleeding—When It Is a Symptom and When It Is Not," page 51.)

Second, rule out systemic diseases that may be causing the bleeding.[590] You might be suffering from hypothyroidism, anemia, vitamin deficiency, or inadequate food intake.[262] If you find and correct these conditions, the bleeding may stop.

Third, rule out psychological problems that may be reflected in abnormal bleeding. Such serious emotional problems may require the attention of a psychotherapist as well as a physician who provides an early medical evaluation.

Fourth, rule out behavioral problems that may be causing the bleeding. Unfavorable, hostile, or shocking kinds of living conditions can upset the endocrine system and produce unexpected bleeding. For example, if you live with a physically or emotionally abusive person, your reproductive endocrine system can reflect this stress. It is important to consider whether such is the case, and if so, to address that problem first.

It is unwise to remove the uterus simply because there is unexpected and unwanted bleeding. Very often the bleeding can be stopped with less drastic treatment. (For a review of treatment options for particular diseases, see Chapter 4.)

### If You Have Pain

Although pain can be overwhelming and can send a woman to the surgeon, research on pain is very limited. Ethical constraints prevent any responsible investigator from creating double-blind studies to identify the different kinds of pain and what they reflect.* We do know that sexually transmitted infectious organisms, endometriosis, fibroid tumors, polyps, and cancer can all cause pain as the diseased tissue presses against or strangles vital organs and nerves.

If you suffer from pelvic pain, your doctor should perform a physical examination to localize its source. But pain does not always reflect disease. Sometimes a person feels pain that is emotionally driven or that cannot be localized. In other cases,

---

*In a double-blind study, neither the experimenter nor the subject knows who is getting what treatment until all the results are in.

pain is "referred," meaning that the place in which the pain is sharpest is not the source of it. When the source is found, a diagnosis can be made and the cause can be treated. If the true cause of pain is not found beforehand, there is no guarantee that surgery will fix it—so a woman could end up with pain still continuing *and* posthysterectomy problems as well.

### Disease Without Overt Signals

Disease does not always manifest itself through bleeding or pain. In fact, studies have suggested that in 20 percent of the cases of cancer and hyperplasia (overgrowth of the uterine lining), there are no overt symptoms.[629]

Several published studies have shown that 20 to 30 percent of women who were evaluated by their physicians for HRT had some form of an endometrial disease but no accompanying symptoms.[96, 385] Other studies show much lower percentages.[80] Among 208 women who came to their doctors for HRT and had no abnormal symptoms, 6 (3 percent) showed severely abnormal tissue cancer; another 16 percent showed hyperplasia.

As the menopausal transition approaches, ovaries can develop cysts. These cysts are generally formed of preovulatory follicles that fail to ovulate but continue to secrete estrogen (but not progesterone). Often these cysts are painless and become apparent only when medical evaluations are performed.

One team of investigators examined bodies after death (from all causes) to determine the incidence of endometrial disease.[397] They studied two groups: one at Yale New Haven Hospital, the other at Massachusetts General Hospital. These women had died of causes not related to uterine disease, but some had uterine disease, growing silently. At Yale the investigators found that 67 percent of the endometrial cancers had been unsuspected before death and at Massachusetts General, 52 percent. Vaginal bleeding had not occurred in any of the cases that were first diagnosed after death. These findings are important because they prove the silent nature of some conditions, and hence the importance of the Progestin Challenge Test and other examinations that will be discussed later. Ideally, women should have health checkups twice a year during menopausal transition years. These will help to isolate small problems before they have a chance to loom large.

### Depression and Hysterectomy

Women who have psychological problems of depression and neurotic illness are at a much greater risk of having a hysterectomy than is the general population;[18, 34] several reports have shown that there are twice as many hysterectomies among women with psychological problems. Among noncancer hysterectomy patients, "the most striking finding was the high frequency of psychiatric illness in general (57%) and hysteria in particular (27%)."[552] Another study of 540 women found that 49 percent of the psychiatric cases versus 23 percent of the nonpsychiatric cases reported excessive bleeding.[34] The question emerges as to whether a psychological problem can produce either a misperception of or the reality of excessive bleeding; either is possible. A psychologically disturbed woman probably ought to have her psychological problem addressed before opting for a hysterectomy unless there is an urgent requirement to have the uterus removed. Hysterectomy will not make a psychological problem disappear.[609, 730]

## BLEEDING—WHEN IT IS A SYMPTOM AND WHEN IT IS NOT

Consider a statement that appeared in 1981 in the journal *Surgery, Gynecology & Obstetrics:* "Dysfunctional uterine bleeding has been a common waste-basket diagnosis for many condi tions in which the true anatomic cause has not been detect and many unnecessary hysterectomies may be performe cause of persistent uterine bleeding without pathologi ings."[904]

Women should not permit the label "dysfunctional uterine bleeding" to short-circuit their search for an accurate diagnosis. There is an understandable tendency for a woman to panic when she is bleeding unexpectedly. If the physician she consults says, "Let's just remove this offending organ," she may agree to an unnecessary hysterectomy. However, if she can muster the patience to undertake a thorough diagnostic process, she has a good chance of finding a healthful resolution to her problem that does not include hysterectomy.

You need to know what normal bleeding is in order to distinguish it from bleeding that needs medical treatment. As described in Chapter 2, the different stages of life have different normal characteristics. In the perimenopausal, or transition, years (beginning in the late thirties or early forties), many women experience changes in their bleeding pattern. While most often the changing pattern is a normal occurrence, it may be difficult not to be anxious. Be sure to discuss your transition cycles with your physician so that you can confirm their normality.

Table 1, reprinted from a classic textbook on menstruation,[254] lists and defines types of "dysfunctional uterine bleeding." While some require medical attention, most of the types of bleeding are not at all dangerous and require no treatment.

In the table, abnormal bleeding is grouped in three basic categories: ovulatory cycles, anovulatory cycles, and noncyclic (arrhythmic) bleeding. The term "cycle" refers to the time span between the first day of one menses (menstrual flow) and the first day of the next menses. It does not refer to the number of days during which bleeding takes place. For example, a woman with a 28-day cycle who gets her period on a Monday will get her next period on a Monday, four weeks later. She may bleed for 3 days, or 6 or 10, but she has a 28-day cycle. An *ovulatory* cycle is one in which ovulation took place. An *anovulatory* cycle reflects the absence of ovulation in that cycle, a condition that occurs in about 15 percent of menstrual cycles.

**Table 1.** *Disorders of Menstruation and Abnormal Uterine Bleeding*

---

I. Ovulatory Cycles
   A. Disorders of Incidence of Menstruation
      1. Polymenorrhea (cycles are shorter, and therefore bleeding is more frequent)
      2. Oligomenorrhea (lengthened cycles, therefore less frequent bleeding)
      3. Amenorrhea (absence of menstrual flow)
         a. Physiologic amenorrhea (normal; absence of bleeding at menopause or during pregnancy)
         b. Cryptomenorrhea (normal cycles; mechanical blockage of blood due to abnormalities of the lining of the uterus)
         c. Amenorrhea of uterus (normal hormonal cycles; absence of endometrial bleeding)
         d. Postcastration (organs are missing)
         e. Functional (all organs present; no flow)
   B. Disorders in Amount of Menstrual Flow
      1. Hypomenorrhea (scanty flow)
      2. Hypermenorrhea or menorrhagia (profuse flow)
   C. Periodic Intermenstrual Bleeding (bleeding between normal monthly flow, most common at ovulation)
II. Anovulatory Uterine Bleeding
   A. Anovulatory menstruation (normal type bleeding, but no ovarian ovulation)
   B. Hyperplasia of the endometrium (cellular overgrowth of the lining of the uterus)
III. Arrhythmic Uterine Bleeding
   A. Continuous bleeding starting at time of expected menses, which does not end at the expected time
   B. Acyclic interval bleeding (occurring repetitively without a rhythmic cyclic pattern)
   C. Intermenstrual spotting
   D. Bleeding after a period of time with amenorrhea
   E. Atypical irregular bleeding

---

### Bleeding Before Menopause

There are three categories of unexpected premenopausal bleeding that a woman may experience: extended bleeding after the menstrual flow should have stopped; bleeding between menstrual flows; and the irregular bleeding characteristic of the menopausal transition.

*Extended Bleeding After the Menstrual Flow Should Have Stopped*

A premenopausal woman who continues to bleed after her normal menstrual flow should have stopped should see a physician for diagnosis. A normal length of flow can be anywhere from two to eleven days, and most women have a flow length that is pretty consistent from one cycle to the next. If you always bleed for ten days, this flow length is normal for you, and you do not require medical attention. However, if you are a four-day bleeder and suddenly shift to ten, this signal may indicate a problem, and you should seek medical evaluation.

Several conditions can account for this continuing bleeding. One frequent cause is infection, often of a type that is transmitted sexually; persistent pain, malaise, or fever should signal the need for immediate medical evaluation. An ectopic pregnancy also causes continuous bleeding and demands immediate medical attention. Another frequent cause is *cystic glandular hyperplasia*, a common condition in which the lining *(endometrium)* of the uterus becomes overgrown with excess tissue. Though generally not serious once it is recognized and treated, if not treated, hyperplasia can develop into precancerous disease, and this potential should be prevented through medical treatment to reverse the overgrowth.

Many other problems can interfere with the proper healing of the endometrium after menstruation and thus account for the unexplained bleeding.[256] Sometimes a physical mass interferes with the normal regrowth of the lining of the endometrial tissue after menstruation. Such an obstruction can be caused by fibroid tumors, by polyps, or, very rarely, by cancer. Tumors and polyps usually can be removed without harming the uterus.

Seven different causes of bleeding that occurs after a menstrual flow should have stopped are well known by the gynecologic community:[256, 257]

*Gross pelvic lesions* is a term used to describe large (gross) lesions in the pelvis. (A lesion is an abnormal change in a tissue or organ due to injury or disease.) In about 25 percent of cases, these lesions are accompanied by fibroid tumors (lumps of tissue growing under the influence of estrogen) and in an equal number of cases, by pelvic inflammatory disease (infection that may involve inflammation and pain). The bleeding seems to come from interference with the ability of the uterus to control blood flow. For example, a fibroid tumor may block healing or produce pressure that breaks the tiny blood vessels of the endometrial glands. Also, many blood vessels with thick walls develop in response to local diseases, compounding the interference.

*Endometrial diseases* (such as hyperplasia, polyps, and fibroids) can cause bleeding by interfering with the healing of the uterine lining after the menstrual flow is completed. Extended bleeding that takes place as part of the menstrual cycle is generally not related to endometrial cancer, which is usually characterized by arrhythmic, or irregular, bleeding.

*Hormone imbalances* can stimulate blood flow.

*Irregular shedding of the endometrium* is generally reflected in a long flow (nine to twelve days) with a normal (26- to 33-day) cycle length. This condition occurs most often in women who have had more than one child and who had infrequent cycling as adolescents. It does not seem to be dangerous. Medical evaluation will be able to reassure you.

*Blood disease,* such as anemia, can cause abnormal bleeding. Since anemia of nongynecologic origin can coexist with other diseases, such as fibroid tumors, a thorough diagnosis of the bleeding should be sought even if anemia is identified.

*Systemic diseases* such as diabetes and hypo- or hyperthyroidism only rarely cause abnormal bleeding, but sometimes they do. Regulating the disease stops the bleeding.

*Psychogenic bleeding* (bleeding that is psychologically and emotionally induced) has been poorly documented. There is a widespread understanding that severe shocks can either stop or start blood flow, but very little is known about this. For example, the death of a loved one is said to start or stop blood flow. Neither the scientific nor the medical literature has provided documented studies.

For any of these seven diagnoses, immediate hysterectomy is too drastic. Ask your doctor for help in overcoming the specific problem by seeking medical, not surgical, cures first. For example, uterine tumors can be treated with progestins first.* If tumors remain troublesome, ask your physician if you are a candidate for a myomectomy, which removes the tumor while sparing the uterus. (See "Uterine Fibroid Tumors," page 89, and "Consider Myemectomy," page 101.) Diseases such as anemia, diabetes, and thyroid dysfunction can usually be treated by an internist. If you have psychogenic problems, it makes sense to try to deal with them through psychotherapy or counseling, not through surgery or gynecologic intervention.

## Bleeding Between Menstrual Flows

Pink or brown spotting between menstrual flows can suggest ovulation if it occurs at about day 13 of the cycle.[263] It is not dangerous. Spotting other than at the presumed time of ovulation may suggest that the endometrium is simply slow in repairing itself. Alternatively, it could reflect a real disease problem: uterine cancer, an endometrial polyp, hyperplasia, fibroid tumors, or some other condition that demands a medical diagnosis. Thus it is important that spotting be evaluated.

*The distinction between "progesterone," "progestin," and "progestagen" is biochemical and not important here. It is explained on page 163. For our purposes, the terms can be used interchangeably to indicate a progesterone substance.

Injuries can cause either heavy or slight bleeding. Sometimes a physical trauma, such as excessively vigorous sexual intercourse, a pelvic exam, or an attempted abortion, can produce bleeding, especially if these traumas occur in the second (post-ovulatory) half of the menstrual cycle. Severe injuries cause bleeding, shock, and nausea. But any injury requires medical evaluation since the injured person does not know how severe the injury is.

More serious conditions include the twisting of a fallopian tube or a pedical (the "foot" of a fibroid tumor, which looks like the stalk of a mushroom) and the presence of a benign ovarian cyst. If they are causing bleeding, severe pain will probably coexist. These problems demand surgical intervention. Bleeding can also reflect the interruption of a pregnancy, which requires medical attention.

## The Menopausal Transition

The irregular bleeding characteristic of the seven years before menopause can mislead you into believing that you are experiencing abnormal bleeding. As described in Chapter 2, the menopausal transition has a characteristic pattern of irregular bleeding lengths and timing; that is, irregular bleeding can be normal then.

If you have become irregular in your menstrual cycle but are getting periods at least once a year, then you probably have not reached menopause. In order to define abnormal post-menopausal bleeding, one generally counts bleeding that occurs more than one year after there has been a "clear span," a period of time without any bleeding. If you are past 40, have not had a period in more than twelve months, and then start bleeding, you should consider this as abnormal and seek a medical evaluation.

### Bleeding After Menopause

Unexpected postmenopausal bleeding is defined as bleeding that occurs more than one year after the final menstrual flow characteristic of menopause.[73]

For women who have passed menopause and are not taking HRT, abnormal bleeding must be treated extremely seriously.[541, 585]* With increasing age after the menopause, the risk for abnormal bleeding to be related to uterine cancer becomes greater. In one study, 3 percent of the women with abnormal postmenopausal bleeding who had experienced menopause within the previous two years were diagnosed to have uterine cancer; in contrast, the group with abnormal postmenopausal bleeding who were more than twenty years past their menopause had a 27 percent incidence of uterine cancer.[449] The relationship also holds up when investigators measure the length of the clear span. Three different studies showed that the longer the clear span before postmenopausal bleeding occurred, the greater was the incidence of cancer.[108, 674, 707]

Studies published before 1970 reported more cancer associated with abnormal bleeding than more recent studies have.[73, 128, 674] In recent years, perhaps with the capacity for early detection or perhaps through our understanding that hyperplasia can be reversed to normal endometrial tissue by progesterone therapy, fewer than 15 percent of the women who have abnormal postmenopausal bleeding are found to have cancer.[288, 358, 588, 937] Yet cancer in the postmenopausal period is much rarer than other diseases. According to the vital statistics records of the U.S. Government, deaths from selected causes among women in 1980 were cardiovascular disease (485,000), hypertension (12,225), diabetes mellitus (20,525), breast cancer (38,400), cervical cancer (6,800), uterine cancer (2,900), and ovarian cancer (11,600). The total for the three pelvic cancers is 21,300.

Although cancer is a most serious disease that usually mandates hysterectomy, the side effects of hysterectomy—including an increased risk of cardiovascular disease—are so powerful that a woman should make sure that a condition that is sus-

*Bleeding patterns of women who take HRT are discussed on page 60.

pected to be cancer is in fact cancer. In other words it would be rash, and health-threatening, to agree to an unnecessary hysterectomy that could put you at a three- to sevenfold greater risk of cardiovascular disease.

Studies have investigated whether the amount of bleeding provides information about either the likelihood of cancer or other serious pathologies. The answer is no. *A single spot that is unexpected should be investigated just as rigorously as a heavy flow.* Although some investigators believe that malignancy is more common in postmenopausal bleeding that is profuse,[449] others have provided data to show that a few spots of blood can be just as reflective of malignancy.[73, 128, 588] The amount of bleeding is not informative.

Common causes of postmenopausal bleeding include the following:[212]

*Cervical polyps* can be benign or malignant. A polyp on a broad stalk is harder to remove than one on a narrow stalk.

*Fibroid tumors* need treatment only when they are growing or when they are pressing against adjacent structures and causing related difficulties such as pressure on the bladder or pain in the pelvis. Otherwise, they are relatively harmless. Nonsurgical treatment options are discussed later in Chapter 4.

*Endometrial hyperplasia* is a cellular overgrowth that can be treated with progestin hormones (see the box on page 77).

*HRT-induced withdrawal bleeding* is healthy and normal. See page 62.

*Cervical erosion* (deterioration of the cervical tissue) is generally treated by destroying with heat or cold the velvety soft-textured tissue.

*Ovarian tumors,* if malignant, mandate removal of the ovary. However, any enlarged ovary must be evaluated for malignancy.

*Viral warts* should be evaluated to be sure that they are benign. The warts can be removed by a variety of means: cryosurgery (freezing), laser, cautery, or with a topical drug (podophyllin when used outside the vagina, other topical drugs inside the vagina or on the cervix).

*Vaginal endometriosis* is very rare. This disease is caused by the growth of endometrial tissue in nonendometrial locations, in this case the vagina. It produces pain and can cause bleeding.

*Atrophic vaginitis,* in which the vaginal walls deteriorate, can generally be cured within two weeks through the use of estrogen creams.

Among women with postmenopausal bleeding, atrophy (deterioration caused by estrogen deficiency) of either the vagina or the endometrium is very common. In one study of 1,100 women with abnormal postmenopausal bleeding, 28 percent of the cases were attributed to atrophic (deteriorating) endometrium;[707] in another study, it was 82 percent;[133] and in another study, 25 percent.[288] Fortunately this condition can be effectively treated with HRT.

More than 75 percent of women with abnormal postmenopausal bleeding do not show a recurrence of the abnormality after seeing their physician.[674, 960] The bleeding often stops of its own accord. If you seek a medical evaluation for postmenopausal bleeding and the bleeding subsequently stops, your physician may suggest waiting and seeing, particularly if no disease is found in an initial battery of tests.

Even if the bleeding returns there should be no urgent rush to remove the uterus.[960] Instead, a woman and her doctor should search for the most appropriate cure, which very well may not include hysterectomy. Depending on the diagnosis of the cause, the cure may include progestin, estrogen, combination HRT, polyp removal, or myomectomy.

### Hormonal Replacement Therapy and Bleeding

In addition to abnormal bleeding from the causes just reviewed, there is a characteristic range of bleeding responses among pre- and postmenopausal women who take HRT. Most of this bleeding reflects normal healthy functioning, but women need to know how to gauge it.

Although there has been a great deal of scare publicity suggesting that HRT causes endometrial cancer, that conclusion is a misleading and dangerous oversimplification. High doses of unopposed estrogen increase the risk of endometrial cancer, but estrogen with progestin opposition (see "The Bleeding Day Test," page 65) decreases the risk.[285, 290, 437] Moreover, among endometrial cancer patients, generally less than 25 percent ever used HRT,[937] indicating that other causes of endometrial cancer are more significant than the known relationship to high doses of unopposed estrogen therapy.

### Before Menopause

Most premenopausal women take HRT because they experience luteal phase deficiencies (low estrogen and progesterone) during the last seven to fourteen days of their menstrual cycle as they approach menopause, resulting in hot flashes and other symptoms (see page 27). HRT during this time of the month may be helpful in delaying the effects of menopause, including hot flashes and bone deterioration. Commonly, in the first two weeks of the cycle (the follicular phase), the ovaries do produce adequate estrogen and HRT may be unnecessary then.

If you are a premenopausal woman on HRT and experience patterns of bleeding that differ from a normal repeated cycle akin to menstruation, then that bleeding needs to be diagnosed and the hormones you are taking better balanced. Abnormal bleeding in a premenopausal woman who is taking HRT generally reflects a cystic glandular hyperplasia, caused by an imbalance in the estrogen/progesterone ratio (see "Hyperplasia," page 75). Not particularly dangerous once discovered and treated, it is corrected by increasing the progesterone level.[937] Premenopausal women can, even on HRT, experience the causes of bleeding (lesions, polyps, fibroids) that a premenopausal woman not on HRT can experience. Abnormal bleeding should always be medically evaluated.

Endometrial cancer is relatively uncommon among premenopausal women on HRT. The average yearly incidence of this cancer is less than 1 woman per 1,000 among those who are not using HRT,[434] and for those using appropriately balanced HRT the incidence is even lower.

When HRT was initiated in the 1960s, many women were given doses of unopposed estrogen that are now seen to have been excessive. This dosing increased the uterine cancer incidence to about 4 women per 1,000.[174] Women were overdosed because radioimmunoassay techniques that measure blood levels of estrogen had not yet been invented. Women felt great when they took estrogen, and a physician could not tell if he or she was overdosing the patient. Happily this situation no longer exists.

It is now well appreciated by the academic medical community that estrogen should never be given to a woman who has a uterus without either a monthly thirteen-day prescription of progestin in opposition to the estrogen, a Progestin Challenge Test (see page 63), or other annual evaluation of the endometrium.

### After Menopause

One kind of postmenopausal bleeding is normal: the "withdrawal bleed" associated with HRT. The term "withdrawal" comes from the awareness that in a fertile menstrual cycle about seven days before menstruation there is a withdrawal of the estrogen and progesterone support that had nourished the growing endometrial "nest" (see Figure 7, page 25). The withdrawal of this hormonal support produces endometrial cell death as the blood supply dries up. As a result, the endometrium breaks off, producing cuts in the blood vessels, bleeding, and sloughing of tissue. In other words, the normal monthly process of menstruation is a direct consequence of hormonal withdrawal. The term "withdrawal bleeding" describes a uterine bleeding that mimics this process after either the administration of progestin hormones or the withdrawal of estrogen. The labeling is somewhat misleading and confusing since "withdrawal bleeding" often oc-

## The Progestin Challenge Test

First reported in the literature in 1980,[290] the Progestin Challenge Test has now become an established, wise practice. Used to insure the health of the endometrium by causing it to shed as in menstruation, the test has been developed by Dr. R. Don Gambrell, at the Medical College of Georgia, who now recommends that it be given to all nonhysterectomized perimenopausal (menstruating) women and to postmenopausal nonmenstruating women who are taking estrogen replacement therapy without a progestin opposition.[285] It is also helpful as an annual checkup and therapeutic for postmenopausal women not taking hormones.

In the test, progestin is taken for thirteen days. If the woman is either postmenopausal or a daily user of estrogen, the time to begin can be established according to convenience. If the woman is still menstruating, day 13 of the menstrual cycle is probably ideal, because this timing will mimic the normal cyclic hormonal pattern. Bleeding that occurs after the course of progestin has begun indicates that the endometrial lining of the uterus has been building up (developing hyperplasia) and needed the progestin in order to stimulate the shedding. If withdrawal bleeding does occur for an HRT user, then continued monthly use of a thirteen-day course of progestin is called for in order to promote a monthly shedding. Although Dr. Gambrell has not defined when the bleeding should occur, the Bleeding Day Test (page 65) refines that concept. Withdrawal bleeding is safe. The absence of bleeding indicates that the endometrium did not need to shed; that is, it was not overgrown.

Dr. Gambrell gives all mature women the Progestin Challenge Test at annual intervals, beginning at the time when regular menstruation stops.* The incidence of endometrial cancer has been drastically lowered in his medical practice as well as in other medical practices that use the test. According to Dr. Gambrell, it can be used in place of the more uncomfortable process of an endometrial biopsy (see page 69). It appears to be effective in protecting women against endometrial disease that could go on to become endometrial cancer.

*Dr. Gambrell uses either a 10 mg/day dose of Provera® (medroxyprogesterone acetate) or a 5 mg/day dose of Aygestin ®, but that dose sometimes produces severe uterine cramping. If cramping occurs, a lower (5 mg-Provera®) dose may work equally well. (See The HRT Bleeding Day Test" for a discussion of dosing estrogen and progesterone.)

curs during the days in which estrogen and progesterone are being taken.

If you are taking HRT that includes both estrogens and progestins and experience a regular pattern of bleeding after beginning the progestin, you have a clue that the bleeding is healthy. By the time most women reach age 60, HRT fails to produce a bleed.

Since each woman and her metabolic interactions are unique, it is helpful for a woman to have a way to figure out the dose of progestin that works best for her. Although averages can be determined through scientific studies, rarely is any individual right on the line of average. Using the Bleeding Day Test, you should be able to gauge your endometrial health.

HRT doses should be individualized. It now is most sensible, given the body of our knowledge, for an HRT regimen in a postmenopausal woman who has her uterus to work this way:

Whatever the particular estrogen dosage is, it should be taken every day. (There are exceptions, cases in which when a day or two off each week may be wise; chapters 6 and 7 review these subtleties.) The amount of estrogen that is appropriate is generally determined by bone studies (described in Chapter 8), as well as by relief from hot flashes and vaginal atrophy, and by the sense of well-being. Some scientists suggest that dosage levels should change across the month, to mimic the hormonal pattern of the premenopausal years, but this approach has not yet been rigorously studied.

The progestin dosage generally begins on the first day of each month. It is probably best to take it for thirteen days, but at least ten days per month are necessary.[672] The lowest daily dose of progestin that will produce a withdrawal bleed on day 11 or later seems to be the ideal amount for preventing hyperplasia (see "The HRT Bleeding Day Test"). Therefore, if you are taking a low-dose progestin for thirteen days per month and experience a withdrawal bleeding on day 10 or sooner, it would make sense to increase the dosage to whatever dose it takes to produce bleeding on day 11 or later.

In their exhaustive clinical studies of the pathology of post-

## The HRT Bleeding Day Test

In 1986 a team of investigators clarified how the timing of the first day of bleeding could help evaluate endometrial health, specifically in gauging whether the endometrium is becoming overgrown, or hyperplastic. They had noticed that when progestin was given in an HRT regimen, the number of days between the start of progestin therapy and the onset of withdrawal bleeding was significant in defining what was going on in the endometrium.

Under normal circumstances, estrogen causes a proliferation, or buildup, of the endometrial lining, as shown in Figure 7 (page 25). The addition of progestin causes a transformation from a proliferative state to a secretory state, characterized by active secretion of fluids by large glands. These studies showed that if the withdrawal bleeding occurred before day 11, the endometrium was in a proliferative state rather than a secretory state. Organs with too much proliferation are at risk for developing cystic glandular hyperplasia.

The investigators reported "a simple method for determining the optimal dosage of progestin in postmenopausal women receiving estrogens." They showed that when a woman was on the correct progestin dose, regardless of which form or route estrogen and progestin she might be taking, her withdrawal bleed began on day 11 (counting the beginning of progestin as day 1) or later.* The latest that the bleeds began was seventeen days after the onset of progestin therapy. If the bleeding occurred before day 11, the progestin dose could be increased to postpone the bleeding onset into the correct range.[659] Because the Bleeding Day Test prevents hyperplasia by refining daily dosages of hormones, there is no longer any benefit in a woman going off HRT entirely for several days each month to avoid endometrial buildup.

Remember: an absence of bleeding is also healthy, indicating that your endometrium does not create sufficient buildup to produce shedding.

*For a description of the available forms and routes (such as pills, creams, injections), see page 148.

menopausal bleeding, Dr. R. Don Gambrell and his colleagues established that when properly balanced doses of estrogen and progesterone are taken, HRT reduces the incidence of endometrial disease below that of women taking no hormones. When improper doses are taken, such as too much estrogen and not enough progestin, an increased incidence of endometrial hyperplasia emerges.[289] Other biomedical investigators confirm this finding.[672]

With this information, you can monitor the use of HRT while keeping your endometrium healthy. Correctly balanced dosages of HRT maximize your endometrial health, providing a lower likelihood of disease than if no hormones were taken. For more details on hormonal therapy regimens, see chapters 6 and 7.

## GETTING A DIAGNOSIS

Abnormal bleeding or pelvic pain quite appropriately triggers the search for a cause. You should consult a doctor as soon as you become aware of a symptom.

Because diseases of the endometrium—such as polyps, hyperplasia, and cancer—can exist simultaneously, the diagnostic process must rule out as well as home in on specific diseases.

### Who Should Make the Diagnosis?

Your choice of diagnostician is an important one. In an ideal world, your doctor would:
- be willing to take a conservative approach when appropriate;
- bring to your relationship reasonable amounts of time, patience, and goodwill;
- be capable of listening to you and reflecting about your problem and your overall health needs;
- have the proper training to deal with your problem;
- be frank about the limitations of his or her training or skills, and be willing to recommend another doctor when appropriate.

You should search for someone who is familiar with the information and attitudes contained in this book, because such an individual will be best able to help you. Postgraduate courses and journal articles can be studied by doctors in many of the medical specialties, and you want someone who studies because so much has happened in biomedical science during the past few years.

If you already have a good relationship with a physician, particularly a reproductive endocrinologist, fertility specialist, gynecologist, internist, general practitioner, or other doctor in whom you have developed confidence, it makes sense to begin there. Sometimes it is the pelvic surgeon who is best equipped to diagnose pelvic diseases, but there is a kind of catch-22 here. Surgeons, who naturally regard surgery as a suitable option, may be less inclined than others to search for a nonsurgical cure. What can you do? Be informed and alert, use your common sense, and find the best diagnostician available.

The process of searching out the cause of a particular disease takes time, patience, and goodwill. Ask your doctor questions that reflect your understanding both of the normal functioning of your body and of the kinds of problems your symptoms suggest.

By taking the time and following the approaches suggested in this chapter, you may solve the problem with your doctor and never need to find a surgeon. However, if you conclude that you need to explore surgical options, Chapter 5 offers detailed advice on finding a surgeon, including ways to check a surgeon's credentials and track record, and questions to ask when interviewing surgeons.

### The First Step

When your physician starts to work with you to discover the source of a disease, he or she will first establish your medical history through conversation and then will conduct a complete physical examination.

During the exam, your doctor will work to rule out the variety of problems that can cause uterine pathology. Blood tests may be done in order to evaluate for anemia, diabetes, and other systemic disorders. The blood may also be tested to define your reproductive endocrine status; levels of FSH (follicle-stimulating hormone) and estrogens, in combination, might provide information to indicate whether you are pre- or postmenopausal. Using touch, the doctor will palpate your uterus, breasts, and ovaries, searching for lumps that might indicate tumors. Using a speculum to dilate the vagina, the doctor will visually examine your vagina and cervix. A Pap test is essential before any intervention; cervical smear samples will be taken from the cervix with a cotton swab and a small wooden spatula. The test investigates cervical health and screens for hyperplasia and cancer (see pages 75 and 78). The Progestin Challenge Test or the Bleeding Day Test can provide assurance of your endometrial condition. This would be prescribed with subsequent follow-up scheduled.

### Endometrial Assessment

If office examinations and preliminary laboratory tests fail to uncover a cause for your symptoms and you continue to have abnormal bleeding or pain, the second step involves direct assessment of the endometrium. If your symptoms suggest a need to sample tissue from the uterus, then a D & C or an endometrial biopsy may be performed.

### Sampling the Tissue

Various methods have been used to take tissue out of the endometrium in order to examine it under the microscope.

*Dilation* (or dilatation) *and curettage* (D & C), also known as surgical curettage, involves dilating (enlarging the opening of) the cervix and scraping away the soft lining of the uterus. Although it is not generally understood why, a D & C is often curative as well as diagnostic;[531] that is, abnormal bleeding is frequently halted by a D & C. The general assumption has been that the removal of the endometrial lining somehow resets the stage for a new buildup of healthier lining.[670]

The published complication rate after a D & C is about the same as the complication rate after hysterectomy: 1.7 percent of women who undergo either procedure have significant complications from it.[531] These include significant loss of blood and, extremely rarely, death.

Through various methods of *endometrial biopsy,* pieces of endometrial tissue are removed for study in the laboratory. In endometrial suction, pieces of tissue are sucked out by a pumping procedure. Endometrial scrapings (without suction) involve a scraping of samples. The advantage of the biopsy approach is speed: biopsy takes 3 to 5 minutes, compared to about 15 minutes for D & C. According to some physicians who have used it, biopsy rarely requires drugs or anesthesia.[201] Other studies indicate that the need for anesthesia during an endometrial assessment is probably a function of the patient's stage of life, as the cervix loses its nerve endings during the times of life when estrogen is very low.[174, 974] If you are postmenopausal and without estrogen therapy, the procedure would probably not be painful because of cervical and vaginal wall atrophy. If you are still menstruating or are taking HRT, it probably could cause some discomfort; this can easily be decreased with a medically supervised drug.

For one study, doctors performed endometrial suction biopsy on 141 women and then did a D & C on each as well. A comparison of the diagnoses of the two tests revealed that they correlated 98 percent of the time. Because endometrial biopsy is less traumatic, it is probably a better way to test for diseased tissue. However, because a D & C can of itself halt abnormal bleeding, it may make sense to undergo that procedure if you are bleeding abnormally. However, as refined approaches have been developed for performing biopsies and evaluating the tissue in the laboratory, the procedure of choice has changed from D & C to biopsy of endometrial tissue.[386, 405, 407] In large part, this may be due to the recent discoveries that progestin therapy can reverse endometrial hyperplasia. Since the progestin is a less invasive approach, the D & C's curative power becomes less valuable.

Each way in which tissue is evaluated has its limitations. If a biopsy of tissue is taken randomly or if it is blindly removed from different regions, the diseased section may be missed and the diagnosis may be incorrect. Likewise, when a D & C is performed, it is possible to incompletely remove endometrial tissue, leaving behind some that could contain disease.[904] One way doctors avoid these problems is to use hysteroscopy and laparoscopy while doing either a D & C or an endometrial biopsy.

It is useful to understand the variety of options available, but it is important to remember that not every physician is skilled in every option. Likewise, the laboratory personnel who will evaluate the tissue may have specific skills that mandate using a specific procedure. Almost all of them appear to be very effective.[358, 386]

### Hysteroscopy and Laparoscopy

The effective use of a hysteroscopic evaluation of the endometrium significantly decreases the need for hysterectomy by accurately defining the uterine condition.[194, 641]

*Hysteroscopy* is a "scoping," or viewing, of the inner walls of the "hyster," or uterus. A long, hollow stem serves as a periscope, with lights (fiberoptics) and lenses for visualizing built into the equipment. Surgical tools can also be passed through the hollow tube, and these tools can be used to cut, grasp, and remove tissue. In the hospital, or in an adequately equipped office, with the woman under anesthesia, the uterus is distended with fluids or gas. Then the hysteroscope is inserted through the vagina and through the cervical opening into the center of the uterus. Special lighting techniques permit this dark region of the body to be visualized completely.

*Laparoscopy*, a similar viewing procedure that lets the physician look within the abdominal region and thus view the outer walls of the uterus, is also performed with a kind of periscope, usually through the navel. After a tiny incision is made, a tube is inserted and gas is blown into the belly region, inflating the middle region of the body so that the tissues are separated from each other in order to prevent inappropriate puncturing of healthy tissue. With the aid of fiberoptics, the physician can then look inside the body and see the outside walls of the uterus and the adjacent anatomical structures.

The major risk associated with hysteroscopy is the potential that the examiner will insert the instrument too deeply and puncture the uterine wall. By using a laparoscope simultaneously with the hysteroscope, an assistant can watch the uterus from the outside and see light (coming from the hysteroscope as it shines across the uterine wall) that would indicate that a puncture is imminent. This process serves to protect the patient against the danger of puncture wounds to her uterus.

Hysteroscopy should not be done under certain conditions. For example, the insertion of this equipment could drive a uterine infection up the fallopian tubes. Likewise, if there is profuse uterine bleeding, cervical malignancy, or suspicion of pregnancy, one would not undergo a hysteroscopy.[905]

These procedures produce discomfort afterward, particularly from gas pains. (The body must rid itself of the gasses that were blown in to separate and protect the internal organs.) Physicians have reported that this discomfort lasts about 36 hours,[853] but the potential of avoiding a hysterectomy may make it worth enduring.

The removal of tissue for biopsy in conjunction with a hysteroscopic viewing of the entire endometrial lining provides the greatest accuracy for diagnosis.[194, 641, 905] This combined procedure, which is considered simple,[641] has been in existence for more than thirty years.

## Ultrasound and Computerized Tomography

New instrumentation has allowed the development of two diagnostic techniques that have the advantage of requiring no surgery. Ultrasound uses sound waves that are beamed at a fluid-filled section of the body; the echoes are automatically tabulated. Computerized tomography (CT) refers to the computer-driven analysis of information taken from different angles in order to produce a "visual cross-section" of the body. The ultrasound procedure is safe and, except for the bladder distension that is sometimes required, painless. The CT requires significant X-ray exposure and, therefore, should not be used routinely.

These procedures have some limited value in the detection of gynecologic disease, but until recently did not appear to be useful in diagnosing unexplained bleeding. Neither of the techniques was very helpful in detecting the most curable problems, those with minimal disease. For example, in one study, with computerized tomography misleading results occurred in 33 percent of cases; with ultrasound, in 27 percent.[451] In other words, about 30 percent of the time these techniques would say nothing was wrong when something was. Not good enough! In one evaluation of ultrasonography, the results were poor for the capacity to detect most pelvic problems, although the test was helpful in detecting ovarian cysts.[649] Therefore, these techniques have limited use; while they will not find all conditions, they probably are helpful in certain diagnoses. In March 1988, the journal *Maturitas* published what appears to be the first report showing that ultrasound can be useful for diagnosing post-menopausal bleeding. In the case cited there, a vaginal wand (something like an elongated tampon, inserted vaginally, with a round end which sits at the cervix) was used to "read" endometrial condition. Former ultrasound methods had tested from the skin surface of the belly after a woman filled her bladder with a great deal of fluid. The results of the transvaginal approach appeared to produce a breakthrough in the ability of the ultrasound method to detect endometrial health versus pathology.[808a] Replication and further studies will be needed before this method can be confirmed as useful. It does appear promising for the future because it is relatively noninvasive (equivalent to a speculum), comfortable (it does not require a distended bladder), and apparently informative.

Magnetic resonance imaging (MRI) is likely to become a new tool in pelvic disease evaluation, but currently it is very expensive and not thoroughly studied. MRI uses a radiofrequency pulse beamed across (and through) the body to disturb the magnetic field in such a way that will permit magnetic "readings" of the alteration. The method appears safe and informative.

### If You Are Advised to Have a Hysterectomy

If your doctor recommends a hysterectomy, you should take the following steps:

*Have a thorough examination of the tissue in question to rule out cancer.* It is uterine cancer, which is extremely rare, that currently mandates a hysterectomy. (Uterine cancer is responsible for fewer than 3,000 deaths per year in the U.S., a figure that is about 0.5 percent of the yearly 485,000 female deaths from cardiovascular disease.)

*Having obtained a diagnosis, get a second opinion from an objective physician.* You will get the most objective diagnosis possible when the second evaluation is from a doctor who does not have any stake in the outcome. That is, the second physician should be from a different institution and should not have access to the first diagnosis until after having rendered an independent judgment. Sometimes women feel timid about requesting such rigorous objectivity. Remember, you have every right. It is your body and your life.

*Consider the alternatives to hysterectomy that may effectively treat the problem.* If you will hold hysterectomy as an option to be turned to only after all other treatments have been tried and have failed, your chances of needing a hysterectomy will be greatly reduced.

If it becomes clear that some offensive tissue needs to be removed, such as a noncancerous tumor or an abnormal cervical area, *consider removing only that tissue rather than the entire organ.* Generally, greater surgical skill is required to remove a diseased part while conserving the healthy tissue. Therefore you will need to locate a surgeon who has expertise in "conservative," or reconstructive, surgery (see Chapter 5).

# Some Common Uterine Diseases:
## Their Causes and Treatment Options

The diseases described in this chapter were selected because of their potential to lead to a recommendation of hysterectomy. Although some diseases are more common among young women (cervical dysplasias, endometriosis, infections), all of them can strike at any age.

By finding the cause of a problem as well as what can be done to cure it, a woman prevents further development of the disease process.

Fortunately, the news is good and getting better. Treatment approaches developed in the past ten years can overcome most problems in ways that save the uterus.

### ENDOMETRIAL POLYPS

A polyp, any protruding growth attached by a stem, can form in the cervix, in the endometrium, and in any other structure in the body that contains a mucous membrane lining. Polyps are common and usually benign, although they can coexist with hyperplasia or cancer. Endometrial or cervical polyps can cause abnormal bleeding, but usually they provide no symptoms; generally one remains unaware of them until an examination reveals their presence. Most of these diseases (hyperplasias, cancers) can also be present without abnormal bleeding.

Most endometrial polyps are not dangerous in younger women, although in women over age 60 they are said to have an increased likelihood of developing into a cancerous environment.[670] For this reason, if your physician finds polyps, tissue samples will be microscopically evaluated by a histopathologist, a medical expert on the tissue changes that accompany disease. Sometimes performed during hysteroscopy, polyp removal is usually a simple procedure unless the structure of the polyp causes heavy bleeding when it is cut off. Polyps do not contain nerves, so removing them, from the cervix for example, is painless.

Whenever cancer is found, the likelihood is high that surgery to remove all traces will be recommended. This may lead your doctor to suggest hysterectomy. Unfortunately, because data have not yet been published to determine the potential safety of saving the uterus when the polyp is cancerous, no clear recommendation can be made.

## HYPERPLASIA

When estrogen is too high, either naturally or because hormone replacement therapy is creating an imbalance, there is a tendency for the endometrial lining to become overgrown with excess tissue, or *hyperplastic*.[945] An overgrowth of the uterine lining can exist with or without bleeding to signal it, but it is the most frequent cause of abnormal bleeding in women.[255] If untreated, hyperplasia can progress from *cystic glandular hyperplasia,* a mild hyperplastic condition that requires no surgery and can be effectively treated with progesterone; through *adenomatous hyperplasia,* which can overgrow and invaginate (push into) the uterine wall; to *atypical hyperplasia,* also known as *anaplasia,* in which the individual cells show abnormalities although not actually cancer.[777] Fewer than 1 percent of patients with cystic glandular (endometrial) hyperplasia will subsequently develop endometrial cancer.[565]

It appears that estrogen and progesterone have profound influences on the development of hyperplasia and the subsequent capacity of anaplasia to progress into cancers.[333, 400, 520] Progestin has proved to be curative for most women (see "The Role of Progestin Opposition in Reversing Hyperplasia," page 77).

### Adenomatous Hyperplasia

The more serious and more developed adenomatous hyperplasia is characterized by more advanced overgrowth but no cancer. Studies have shown that it, too, responds when sufficient doses of progestin are given.[802] Table 2, produced by Dr. W. Budd Wentz in 1974, shows that all of the patients who took progestational therapy for six weeks had a complete reversal of their hyperplasias;[941] that is, *they prevented a hysterectomy through the use of progestins.* In 1985, Dr. Wentz published further details and refinements of this treatment, which he developed at Case Western Reserve University School of Medicine.[941a] Confirmation comes from other investigators as well. In one study of 105 women who developed hyperplasia, 101 showed a complete reversal within six months after the initiation of progestin treatment for ten days each cycle.[288]

Unfortunately, adenomatous hyperplasia that is untreated has a high risk of developing into a cancer. In one study of women with adenomatous hyperplasia who were not receiving treatment, 30 percent developed endometrial cancer within ten years.[335] The cumulative risk begins to accelerate five years after adenomatous hyperplasia is discovered and not treated.[336] This kind of evidence confirms the slow developmental pattern of uterine disease and emphasizes the importance of early detection and aggressive action.

### Preventing Endometrial Hyperplasia

Although it has not been common medical practice to evaluate the endometrium unless HRT is about to be prescribed or a disease symptom is present, the incidence of endometrial disease is so high that such an evaluation probably should be standard practice as soon as the menstrual cycles become irregular at the menopausal transition. Either an annual Progestin Challenge Test (page 63) or an annual Bleeding Day Test (page 65) should be given for this purpose.

### The Role of Progestin Opposition in Reversing Hyperplasia

Endometrial hyperplasia, the most frequent cause of abnormal bleeding in women over 40 years old,[255] appears to be reversible with appropriate hormonal intervention.

The makeup of an HRT regimen can have a profound influence on the endometrium. Unopposed estrogen (that is, estrogen alone, without a counterbalancing progestin) will increase the likelihood of endometrial hyperplasia when the dose is too high. Studies have shown that cyclic unopposed estrogen (a week off each month) and constant estrogen are equally unsafe in relation to the risk of endometrial hyperplasia.[862] Although doctors commonly prescribe HRT regimens that call for a week without hormones and three weeks with hormones, there is no demonstrated advantage to endometrial health in taking a week off.

In contrast, women who also take progestin for thirteen days each month can almost always prevent the development of cystic glandular hyperplasia.[27, 100, 347, 860, 907] As the studies continue to be published, an interesting pattern has emerged. Scientists now know that high doses of progestin given for a few days are much less helpful than low doses of progestin given for many days each cycle.[521] What constitutes a high dose varies among individual women, as described in "The HRT Bleeding Day Test," page 65.

Progestin therapy has been established as an effective treatment to overcome endometrial hyperplasia. For example, Dr. John Studd and his coworkers showed that endometrial pathology was reversed to normal in twenty-eight out of twenty-nine cases of cystic glandular hyperplasia within two cycles of treatment with progestins.[860] In this study, 5 milligrams per day of norethisterone was given for fifteen to twenty-one days each cycle. Three out of five cases of adenomatous hyperplasia were also reversed. Other studies confirm that hyperplasia can be reversed back to normal endometrial tissue through progestin therapy.[521, 941]

Doses vary according to the degree of disease and the perception of the investigator. Progestin can feel unpleasant when the doses get too high, producing irritability and uterine cramping. Inappropriate progestin doses can produce adverse lipid changes (detailed in Chapter 9). For these reasons women should take the lowest effective dose to overcome the problem. Chapter 7 discusses the relationship between progestin brand, progestin dose, and emotional affect.

Dr. Don Gambrell has been studying the use of progestin to prevent and reverse endometrial diseases at the U. S. Air Force Medical Center at Wilford Hall;[285] in 1975 he began a prospective study of 5,500 postmenopausal women, and his group continued the investigation through 1986. Among those women, 325 identified as having endometrial hyperplasia were treated with progestins. In the early years, progestin was given for seven to ten days and a reversal rate of 95 percent was found. More recently, with advanced understanding, progestin was given for a minimum of ten days monthly, and this dosage increased the reversal rate to 99 percent.

## ENDOMETRIAL CANCER

Most of the problems that have a potential for uterine (noncervical) cancer occur in women between the ages of 46 and 55.[358] In fact, 75 percent of the reports of uterine cancers and precancerous reports seem to occur in the age span from 46 to 60.[358] It is precisely at this time of life—the transition years from the menstruating to the postmenopausal state—that the hormonal environment of a woman is undergoing enormous changes, in terms of reductions of progesterone and alterations in estrogen. But even in these years, the "disease" is generally not cancer.

Endometrial cancer, which requires a microscopic diagnosis to confirm, is a very serious matter.[802] Cancer grows when it is not stopped, and it can kill if it invades the rest of the body,

**Table 2.** *Reversal of Persistent Endometrial Hyperplasia by Oral Progestin Therapy*
*(Megesterol Acetate 20 mg per day for 6 weeks)*

|  | No. of patients | Length of follow-up (number of years) | | | Recurrence |
|---|---|---|---|---|---|
|  |  | 1 | 3 | 5 |  |
| Adenomatous hyperplasia | 80 (27–53)* | 10 | 38 | 32 | 0 |
| Atypical hyperplasia | 30 (5–25)* | 5 | 8 | 17 | 0 |

*Numbers in parentheses indicate pre- and postmenopausal patients, respectively.

destroying cells and tissues in its path. If a woman has endometrial cancer, the best medical judgment is that she should undergo a hysterectomy.[670]

While invasive cancer of the endometrium now accounts for half of all the new genital cancers in women,[539] cancer of the uterus has been declining since 1930.[496] The decline appears to be attributable to three factors: earlier detection and aborting of the cancer's growth; the use of progestins to prevent the cancer; and the appropriate balancing of HRT regimens. The probability that a nonhormonally treated postmenopausal woman will develop cancer of the endometrium is very low: less than 1 per 1,000 per year.[386, 940] For HRT users, the likelihood is even lower when the HRT provides sufficient progesterone.

The risk factors for endometrial cancer, in order of importance, are obesity, nulliparity, and hypertension.

*Obesity* increases the risk for endometrial cancer;[532, 597] in one study, 51 percent of the cancer patients were obese.[628] Obesity is a tough problem to correct (see Chapter 14 for a discussion of recent research). If you are obese, it would be wise to try to lose weight, under a doctor's care if you are very overweight. The question of whether HRT can be safely used by women at risk for endometrial carcinoma because they are obese is not settled because the information available is meager. In one study, estrogen replacement therapy did not increase the risk of endometrial cancer among obese women;[774] it appeared that if a woman was obese, whether or not she took estrogen was not going to affect the likelihood of her developing endometrial cancer.

*Nulliparity* (never having given birth), although a risk factor, has not been systematically studied. Scientists don't know why it is a risk factor and therefore don't know how to prevent the risk. If you have never given birth, you may want to consider the evaluative approaches described on pages 63 and 65.

*Hypertension* is also a risk factor. Again, researchers do not yet know why, but they do see an association with endometrial cancer.[597] (See Chapter 9 for a discussion of ways to promote cardiovascular health.)

Once endometrial cancer is diagnosed, the survival rate seems to be the same for women who use HRT as for those who do not.[539] And the survival rate is highest when the cancer is discovered at its earliest stages.[539, 628, 629] Although most endometrial cancers (80 percent) do show abnormal bleeding, 20 percent have no symptoms at all.[629] For this reason the progestin regimens discussed on pages 63 and 65 are important measures for detecting possible problems.

Although progestational agents (progesterone, medroxyprogesterone acetate, megesterol acetate) have been somewhat helpful in slowing down the course of the progression of endometrial cancer, the results are not good enough. Only six of the twenty-one patients so tested showed objective (clear-cut) regressions of advanced endometrial cancer.[450] Once the disease has reached the cancerous state, hysterectomy is your safest choice.[777]

## CERVICAL ABNORMALITIES

In contrast to the endometrial diseases, which occur most often after age 40, diseases of the cervix are most common among women in their twenties.[486] Perhaps because of the desirability of saving the uterus in women of childbearing age, medical treatment of younger women tends to be more conservative. Cervical diseases susceptible of progressing to cancer, such as dysplasia and viral warts, often exist without telltale bleeding. Abnormalities are usually discovered through routine pelvic exams and Pap smears. Similar to the process with endometrial hyperplasia, an abnormal growth of cervical cells (called *dysplasia* in the early stage) can progress. The terminology associated with cervical dysplasia is confusing because several different medical naming systems are currently in common usage. Table 3 lists the various labels used to describe the five classes, or stages, of dysplasia.

The disease process is progressive, and if the dysplasia is untreated, it has a high likelihood of leading to cancer. By the time the cervix has become cancerous, an offensively smelly dis-

**Table 3.** *Pap Smear Classifications*[853]

| Common Terms | Class | Other Terms |
|---|---|---|
| Normal | I | Benign, normal<br>Metaplasia<br>Squamous metaplasia |
| Inflammatory | II | Inflammation |
|  |  | Inflammation with atypia<br>Koilocytotic warty atypia |
| Mild CIN* | III | Mild dysplasia<br>Atypia<br>Warty atypia |
| Moderate CIN* |  | Moderate dysplasia |
| Severe CIN* | IV | Severe dysplasia<br>Carcinoma in situ |
| Cancer | V | Invasive cancer |

*Cervical intraepithelial neoplasia
Table 3 used courtesy Dr. Felicia Stewart

charge is produced.[873] If the cancer is untreated, it can then invade the rest of the body.

Several behavioral conditions are associated with the disease process that leads to cervical cancer. Deficiencies of vitamins C and A are common among women with cervical cancer.[748, 749, 964]

Dietary habits can have a significant effect on the likelihood of cervical abnormalities. In one study of dietary vitamin C and uterine cervical dysplasia, the investigators found dietary habit differences when comparing eighty-seven women with cervical abnormalities to a control group. Those who had the cervical abnormalities had much lower intakes of dietary vitamin C than those that were in the healthy control group. They concluded that deficiency of vitamin C is an independent risk factor for severe dysplasia when age and other known concomitants of the disease are controlled.[932] Other investigators have also shown that vitamin C circulating in the bloodstream is in lower concentration among women with uterine cancer than among control subjects without uterine cancer.[748, 749] (See the discussion of vitamin C in Chapter 13.)

*Viral warts* in the genital region are also a potential transmitter of cervical cancer and therefore must be treated whenever you or your sexual partner experience them. A genital wart generally has a lumpy, ugly appearance, although flat, nearly invisible (to the naked eye) ones also exist. On men, they may emerge anywhere on the penis or surrounding skin. On women, genital warts are common on the labia (the lips around the vagina), in the vagina, and on the cervix.

Sexual habits also appear to play some role in cervical disease. Women with cervical cancer are more likely to have begun their sexual life young and to have experienced more sexual partners than age-matched women who are free of this disease.[748, 964] One study suggests that cervical cancer might sometimes be the result of a virus sexually transmitted from an infected man.[873]

Annual Pap tests and the use of condoms are advisable if you are in a high-risk group, that is, if you have poor vitamin habits and are not sexually monogamous. If you are not in a high-risk group and can be sure that your partner is also sexually monogamous, it is probably sufficient to have your cervix tested every three years, because cervical cancer is a very slow-growing disease process. To enhance the accuracy of your Pap smear, avoid intercourse, tampons, or any vaginal intrusion for forty-eight hours before the test.[853]

An abnormal Pap smear that indicates the presence of precancerous cells (dysplasia or CIN) often leads to removal of the abnormal region without hysterectomy.[853] Cure rates are good when the disease is caught early, and happily most women who discover a cervical disease can save their uterus and most of the cervical tissue.

Now that colposcopy (magnified viewing through the vaginally inserted speculum) is available to precisely localize and assess the abnormality, in most cases a cone biopsy is not needed. Sometimes, however, a cone biopsy is needed—both as a diagnosis and as a cure. This is wise when the lab tests don't match, when visual viewing is limited by internal body changes, or if severe disease returns after less invasive treatments were attempted.

In a cone biopsy, a cone-shaped piece of tissue is removed from the cervix and tested in a laboratory to confirm the presence of cancerous cells. If the test is positive, the depth of the growth of cancer cells is then measured. The cone biopsy, unlike the endometrial biopsy discussed earlier, can mean removing enough tissue to scar the cervix and reduce the potential for fertility. (A healthy intact cervix helps fertility in several ways, including production of fluids that enable sperm to function, providing an inviting entrance for the sperm, production of prostaglandins, and sexual lubrication.) Even so, if a cone biopsy will help you gain knowledge that may save your uterus, it would be wise to have it done.

Good management of true cancer (invasive cancer as opposed to in situ or CIN) is much more complex and requires a specialist in cancer management.

Try your best to locate medical professionals with a reputation for conserving rather than removing the uterus when Pap smears are abnormal. If you undergo a biopsy to remove tissue, your physician will want you to repeat the Pap smear test of your cervical cells at least yearly to ensure that all the diseased tissue was removed. If it was not, then a second and possibly a third biopsy should complete the job.

For true invasive cancer, more drastic treatment approaches (radiation therapy or hysterectomy) are currently the best available options.

## *PROLAPSED UTERUS*

The pelvic floor, a sheet of muscular structure that supports the pelvic organs, connects the coccyx bone at the base of the spine to the pubic bone. Figure 9 shows this anatomical arrangement. Sometimes the muscular sheet becomes weak and sags, causing incontinence and discomfort. This is a common condition among women who have borne many children and who have not done pelvic muscle exercises to strengthen this support system. If the muscles become sufficiently weak, and especially if estrogen levels become deficient, the uterus can drop down, sagging into the vagina. Your pelvic exam can detect this condition in its early stages, so be sure to ask your doctor if your uterus is starting to show any signs of sagging. In cases of extreme prolapse, the uterus can hang so far down that it emerges between the legs.

A prolapsed uterus must be corrected because it is a progressive condition. It is uncomfortable, it pulls other organs with it, and it will get worse unless it is treated. A prolapsed uterus can also weaken the bladder and lead to urinary incontinence, the inability to contain the urine.

The least invasive alternative should be attempted before going to any more drastic treatment. Since the problem comes from muscular weakness, the most logical approach is to strengthen the weak muscles through exercise. Often successful, this therapy requires the care of a specialist in biofeedback muscle training of the pubococcygeal (PC) muscle system. (PC muscle exercises are discussed in detail in chapters 10 and 12.) HRT also helps to build the muscle mass. Estrogen deficiency leads to the wasting of genital muscle, and the replacement of estrogen can correct some of the muscle weakness. Surgery to "resuspend" the organ is sometimes reported with some success.

Surgeons who do not realize how valuable the uterus is may suggest simply removing a prolapsed uterus. If you seek professional help among medical experts who will try to help you keep your uterus, you may be able to overcome the problem medically and thereby avoid a hysterectomy. The sooner you seek a remedy, the better are your chances of correcting a prolapse through noninvasive treatments.

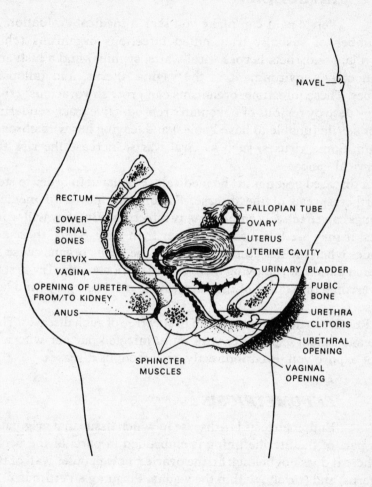

RECTUM

LOWER
SPINAL
BONES

CERVIX

VAGINA

OPENING OF URETER
FROM/TO KIDNEY

ANUS

FALLOPIAN TUBE

OVARY

UTERUS

UTERINE CAVITY

URINARY BLADDER

PUBIC
BONE

URETHRA

CLITORIS

URETHRAL
OPENING

VAGINAL
OPENING

SPHINCTER
MUSCLES

NAVEL

Figure 9. Sagittal section of female pelvis

## INFECTIONS

Pelvic pain can make you seek a medical evaluation. A number of sexually transmitted infectious organisms (chlamydia, gonorrhea, herpes, viral warts, syphilis) find a lush and supportive environment in the vagina, uterus, and fallopian tubes. These infectious organisms can grow so voraciously that they destroy regions of a woman's reproductive tract, rendering her sterile (unable to have babies) and leaving her with chronic pain. Some viruses, such as viral warts, increase the risk for cervical cancer.

A diseased organ must be medically evaluated in order to stop further spread of the disease. Fortunately, powerful medical drugs can effectively combat many infections. But they will work best if they are taken sooner rather than later. Sadly, there are times when the diseased remnants of the pelvic organs cause so much pain that removing them is actually a blessing. Try first to overcome the source of the pain, saving pelvic surgery for a last resort.

Resolve to do all that you can to stay free of such diseases. This means sexual exclusivity with an uninfected partner who will not expose you, even indirectly, to infectious diseases.

## ENDOMETRIOSIS

Endometriosis is a disease in which tissue that originates as part of the uterine lining is embedded in parts of the pelvis where it does not belong: on the ovaries, bowel, outer wall of the uterus, and (rarely) within the vagina. Plaguing an estimated 15 percent of women, endometriosis varies in degree from minor to pervasive involvement. Wherever it locates, the tissue behaves like the normal endometrial lining, proliferating, secreting, and then bleeding in response to the normal hormonal variation in estrogen and progesterone. Endometriosis can be very painful, usually during the menstruating days of the cycle.[218] It tends to diminish with menopause for those women who are estrogen-deficient. According to Dr. Felicia Stewart, HRT rarely causes any problems for such women.[853]

The cause of endometriosis is unknown, although it has been suspected to result from "retrograde" menstruation, that is, menstrual tissue moving up the fallopian tubes and out through the fimbria (the ends of the tubes), which provide access to the body cavity, rather than the normal route down through the vagina and out of the body. I have suspected that uterine contractions at orgasm could drive the sloughing menstrual tissue in this retrograde direction, but no research on this hypothesis has yet been published.

A number of investigators are actively studying endometriosis and trying to figure out how best to treat it.[969] When hormones are given to reduce the relative balance of estrogen, the endometriotic tissue shrinks and sometimes disappears. Various doses of progesterone, danazol (an androgen-type synthetic hormone) and LH RH analogs (see page 91) have proved helpful for many women. Unfortunately, because the treatment of the disease usually produces an estrogen deficiency, the "cure" can produce a host of menopausal symptoms.

Women certainly should attempt a course of treatment with hormones before considering surgical intervention. Laser surgery, as well as more conventional surgery, is sometimes successful in eliminating the individual pockets of disease. Such surgery, which leaves the uterus in place, can be performed through the laparascope or by opening the abdomen. The choice will depend on the particular skills of the surgeon you select. Either is appropriate in competent hands. Hysterectomy is sometimes prescribed but is not always effective. Even if the uterus is removed, the diseased tissue has already usually seeded itself throughout the pelvic region. These seeds of endometrial tissue often can't all be removed.

If you have endometriosis, you should seek a specialist in its treatment. The American Fertility Society (2131 Magnolia Avenue, Suite 201, Birmingham, AL 35282) has recently focused a great deal of attention on the search for cures; members of this society will be knowledgeable about the most recent discoveries. You might also want to contact the Endometriosis Association (U.S.-Canada Headquarters, P. O. Box 92187, Milwaukee, WI 53202). This women's support group provides information on the latest research discoveries and offers help in locating competent medical people who specialize in conservative treatment.

## PREMENSTRUAL SYNDROME

*Premenstrual syndrome* describes a regular, repeating cycle of distress (depression, irritability, bloating) that usually occurs each month during the seven to ten days that precede menstruation. Although most women are aware of a cyclic variation in mood that coincides with the estrogen and progesterone cycle, the decline of spirits is more severe with PMS. For women plagued with severe PMS, doctors sometimes suggest a hysterectomy with ovariectomy in order to do away with the cyclic variation in hormonal milieu. However, hysterectomy is *not* recommended for premenstrual syndrome problems. Such a drastic action hardly makes sense because the removal of a source of hormones will almost certainly require their replacement through HRT.[24]

Psychotherapy alone has proved ineffective in the treatment of PMS, suggesting that the syndrome has a physiologic origin for many women. Recent studies showing that PMS sufferers experience a drastic reduction in beta endorphins during their PMS days offer the beginnings of an objective hormonal approach to its cure. Until sophisticated methods of diagnosis and hormone therapy are developed, women should seek PMS programs that demonstrate a positive record of helping their patients. Current treatment options include progesterone, nutritional changes, and exercise regimens that will improve the endorphin balance. These nutritional and exercise regimens are discussed in chapters 13 and 15.

I suspect that when estrogen and progesterone are properly

balanced, improved beta endorphin levels will provide emotional harmony. In order to balance them, one would need frequent radioimmunoassay testing through several cycles to define one's cyclic variation. Only then could a prescription of progesterone and/or estrogen be sensibly defined to meet an individual's needs. Future research in this area is likely to significantly help the women who suffer from PMS. For now, the idea remains theoretical.

## UTERINE FIBROID TUMORS

Fibroid tumors, also called *uterine myoma,* are common, occurring in 20 percent of women. Often the uterus contains a number of these tumors, and when a tumor does not cause any problem, it often makes sense to just live with it. Fortunately, they are benign (noncancerous) more than 99 percent of the time.[853] Very often cystic glandular hyperplasia exists at the edges of the tumor.[799] While these tumors are usually not cancerous or dangerous in themselves, their growth can cause problems. Pressing against the endometrial lining, they can distort and elongate the tissue and lead to dilatation (stretching or expanding) or atrophy of the glands. Their bulk can interfere with the necessary monthly healing of the endometrium after menses, thereby causing abnormal bleeding. Extending out of the uterus, they can exert pressure on the bladder and other organs.

While it is generally accepted that fibroid tumors originate from intramural tissue (muscle tissue of the uterine wall), the cause of their growth and development remains unknown. As the tumors grow, they gradually push muscle aside in the direction of either the outer wall or the endometrial wall.[670] Although estrogen appears to stimulate their growth, a more complex and as yet unresolved hormonal mechanism may be responsible.[807, 856, 870] By the time menopause arrives, the fibroid tumor will probably have shrunk to a much smaller size. HRT may affect the tumor, but estrogen coupled to appropriate progestin can probably be balanced on the low side to prevent estrogen-stimulated growth.

According to some doctors, fibroid tumors that coexist with excessive bleeding may require hysterectomy if they do not respond to hormonal treatment.[670] Fortunately, others differ. Myomectomy, the surgical removal of the tumors while sparing the uterus, generally cures the bleeding: moreover, 60 to 97 percent of the time patients need no further treatment.[294] Progestin therapy has been somewhat successful for some women, and the newer uses of luteinizing hormone releasing hormone (LH RH) analogs (also called Gn RH analogs) in conjunction with myomectomy should also be considered (see "LH RH Analogs," page 91).

If a fibroid tumor is pushing against other vital tissue and causing pain or bleeding, a myomectomy may be a preferable choice. If you have a fibroid tumor that is causing you problems, and if you can find a surgeon who is skilled in this technique, you may want to consider myomectomy. Surgical skills more advanced than those of hysterectomy are required for reconstructive surgery.

Two studies evaluated the ability of a myomectomy to prevent further regrowth of the fibroid tumor.[720, 792] More than half of the time, the myomas do not regrow, and when they do, a repeat myomectomy can be performed. The prevention of regrowth depends on two things: the surgical skill in completely removing all parts of each tumor, and the ability to locate all the seedlings.[294] Because myomas that are near the outer surface of the uterus or within the wall have a lower regrowth rate than those in other uterine locations, you may want to ask whether your fibroid tumor falls into this group. If it does, then myomectomy would seem to be a viable option for you.

Timing of a myomectomy may be critical. Dr. Celso Ramón García, an expert in endocrinology and surgery at the University of Pennsylvania Hospital, notes that because of the hormonal cycle and its influence on endometrial growth, the first eight

## LH RH Analogs

**The LH RH analogs** are synthetic hormones that mimic the natural gonadotropin hormone LH RH (luteinizing hormone releasing hormone), which is produced in the brain and travels into the pituitary. In the pituitary, the normal action of the LH RH is to stimulate the production and release of the two hormones that go to the ovaries, the luteinizing hormone (LH) and the follicle-stimulating hormone (FSH), described in Chapter 2. The synthetic analogs are frequently more potent than the natural form.

LH RH analogs are the most impressive medically effective treatment in reducing the volume of fibroid tumors in the uterus. The LH RH analogs are also used for several diseases that respond to the production of hormones in the ovary, including endometriosis, breast cancer, and polycystic ovary disease.

In the case of fibroids, the value of the LH RH analogs rests in their ability to shrink a tumor that will then be removed surgically. Some surgeons state that myomectomy can more easily be performed on a small tumor than on a large tumor. In skilled hands, laparascopic myomectomy, a procedure in which surgery is performed through the laparascope, may be possible, avoiding the need to open the abdomen in order to remove these tumors.

In 1987 the first series of research studies to show the remarkable use of these agents for fibroid tumors were published. Because the treatment is so new, it absolutely mandates caution. In fact, along with the five reports of their effectiveness came another report showing one case of severe allergic reaction (anaphylactic shock) in a 28-year-old woman on her third treatment.[528] Because of this reaction, the authors of the report recommend that every treatment be started under medical supervision, with the patient being observed for the first hour within a hospital setting. Yet the treatment is potentially so beneficial that this one case of shock, while mandating caution, should not prevent the use of the agent when it is appropriate.

The mechanism by which the LH RH analogs work involves a two-step process. In step one, usually complete within the first two weeks of treatment, the pituitary is hyperstimulated to secrete excess amounts of LH and FSH. This action commonly produces a surge of estrogen and sometimes progesterone from the gonads. Testosterone may also increase.[828] In the second stage the pituitary slows down, in a process called "down-regulation." As a consequence, the ovaries severely reduce their output of estrogen and progesterone. This second stage generally lasts for as long as the hormones are administered. As the tumors shrink, the pain and bleeding they were causing will diminish; menses will also cease. Side effects tend to be similar to those of the initial stage of menopause; hot flashes, sometimes quite severe, can last as long as the treatment lasts.[537, 676] These drugs should not be taken for extended periods because they will ultimately induce the whole panoply of estrogen deficiency symptoms (osteoporosis, sexual systems deficiencies, loss of menstruation, depression, and so on). The treatment was initially tested for a six-month period. Since it subsequently became apparent that good results are generally obtained within two months, there seems to be no extra benefit to taking the hormone for a longer period, particularly in view of the significant negative effects.[537, 676, 942]

The route of administration must not be oral because the drug is rapidly degraded in the digestive system and therefore will not get into the bloodstream. LH RH treatments are generally given either as regular injections every eight hours or so, as tiny implants that can be injected once a month, or as a spray that is inhaled at the nose.

The results of this treatment have been quite remarkable. Most women who take this hormone have between a 40 and an 80 percent reduction in the size of their tumors within two months.[495, 537, 676, 942] Each woman is different, and on rare occasions tumors will actually get larger. But for the most part, LH RH treatments lower the estrogen and lower the tumor mass. Unfortunately, when a woman goes off this treatment, the tumors return to their original size. When the treatment ends, women who were menstruating before it began tend to resume menstruation within thirty-five to sixty-five days.[676]

days of the menstrual cycle offer the best potential for preventing surgical aftereffects such as the implanting of endometrial tissue into the muscular portion of the uterus.[295]

Vaginal myomectomy (surgery that is done through the vagina, avoiding opening the abdomen) has been shown to be able to stop hemorrhage (bleeding) and help control infections that had been exacerbated by fibroids, but it often fails to prevent the regrowth of myomas.[720]

According to a 1987 report by Dr. Ana Murphy, the use of the laparascope, fiberoptics, and related instrumentation has advanced to the point where a number of surgical procedures that formerly required opening the abdomen (laparotomy) can now be performed through the laparascope.[617] The benefits of this procedure, in skilled hands, are a shortened hospital stay, less trauma, faster recovery, and a return to full activity at a much faster rate (seven to ten days as opposed to four to six weeks). Hospital costs are about 50 percent less because of the shorter hospital stay, although the actual time in the operating room is no different.

Dr. Millicent Zacher, a highly trained infertility surgeon at Albert Einstein Medical Center, Philadelphia, comments that even in "skilled hands" two other relevant considerations include *physical factors* (size and location of the tumor) and *hemostasis* (the ability for surgically induced bleeding to be controllable during the operation). A competent surgeon will assess these factors before considering laparoscopic myomectomy.

The removal of fibroid tumors that have been made small enough through the LH RH analogs (see page 91) should be feasible in the hands of a skilled laparascopic surgeon. However, there is medical controversy on this topic. Dr. García comments that in abdominal surgery a large fibroid tumor is easy to see and that in skilled hands, its large size need not make the surgery more difficult. Dr. García suggests that a tumor that is not shrunken by the LH RH analogs presents the surgeon with very clear "cleavage" lines that provide a neat cutting edge for removal. His concern is that the removal of shrunken tumors may not be so accurate or complete because their cleavage lines are less clear. Furthermore, he notes that the LH RH analogs may shrink tiny tumors so much that the surgeon may not see them and may leave them behind.[295] Fibroid tissue that is inadvertently left behind can regrow.

(See "Consider Myomectomy," page 101.)

If you have searched to cure a uterine disease but still suffer—from bleeding that leaves you weak, from pain, or from the threat of a deadly cancer—then you may conclude that your best option is to have a hysterectomy. If so, you have a number of very significant choices to make. You need to *very carefully* select your surgeon and the type of surgery you will have. You should consider whether the cervix should be retained and negotiate to keep your ovaries if they are healthy and if you have no cancer. You need to prepare yourself by building up your immune system and by planning for the immediate aftereffects. These and other aspects of preparing for surgery are discussed in Chapter 5.

# 5

# *Planning for Surgery:*
## *Choices for Optimal Health*

If you and your physician have concluded that a hysterectomy is appropriate in order to optimize your health, several decisions must be made. Your choices and attitudes in preparing for surgery can increase your control over your health. You do have choices, which are best addressed in sequence:

1. You can select a surgeon who is right for you. Because you will want a competent surgeon with whom you can discuss all your concerns and who can help in your thorough preparation for surgery, read through this chapter, and the preceding ones, before you start your search.
2. With your surgeon, you can decide on the type of surgery you will have, including whether you can preserve important parts of your reproductive anatomy, and by what route the surgery will take place.
3. Before surgery, you can build up your strength (that is, your immune system) so that you will heal faster afterward. Sound habits of nutrition and rest, as well as spiritual preparation, can have an important impact on your health.
4. You can prepare yourself, mentally and physically, for the illness that many women experience after surgery. If you do so, the illness will loom less large if and when it occurs. Before the surgery, you should plan for postoperative hormonal therapy, both to ease short-term hormonal shock and to begin to address your long-term needs.

5. Recognizing that a slow recovery process is normal, you can prepare to be patient with yourself during that period.

## SELECTING THE SURGEON WHO IS RIGHT FOR YOU

If women always sought unbiased second opinions, the incidence of hysterectomy would be drastically reduced, probably by half or more. Ideally, a woman should undergo the appropriate diagnostic procedures outlined in chapters 3 and 4 with the expert help of a gynecological specialist in fertility, because this specialty is particularly attuned to saving the ovaries and uterus, even in the face of disease, or with a competent internal medicine specialist, because these specialists do not usually favor surgery unless it is dramatically indicated. Other physicians, such as family doctors and general practitioners who attend postgraduate courses and study pelvic problems, may also be competent to help you. Unfortunately, reality is often less than ideal.

If you trust the doctor who is suggesting surgery, you may feel inclined to go with this person as your surgeon. Even so, you should rigorously require a confirming second opinion from another expert, one who is not "down the hall." Avoid the temptation to let your physician find someone to render the second opinion.

Even people of goodwill and competent training make mistakes. You should insure against the normal existence of human error by asserting your healthright to an objective, unbiased second opinion. As scientists well know, even among honest colleagues who employ rigorous quality-control techniques (such as double-blind research design, in which the theorist does not manipulate the data), there is a proven tendency to interpret results according to preconceived expectations. For this reason, competent scientists welcome the process in which other scientists (not friends or close associates) replicate the analysis of data. Give your body and your health at least as much respect and consideration as you give your home or car when you seek a second estimate before committing to expensive repairs.

Because your diagnosing physician may not be a surgeon, you may need to seek one out. You should approach the search for a surgeon as a very important process that demands your intelligent participation. Ask everywhere for suggestions. Ask women who have had surgery. Ask internists you already know. Ask hospital surgical nurses for the names of surgeons they consider particularly competent—just call a hospital and ask to speak to the head surgical nurse. Check with university teaching hospitals for their recommendation by calling the department of obstetrics and gynecology. Seek out women's resource groups such as HERS (the Hysterectomy Educational Resource Service, 422 Bryn Mawr Avenue, Bala Cynwyd, PA 19004; 215-667-7757). And use the community services pages of your telephone book to find others. Focus your energy on compiling a list, and from that list select your candidate surgeons.

The surgeon you select should have your well-considered approval in at least four areas:

- The surgeon's competence, including medical training and experience, and the ability to communicate on a personal level.
- The surgeon's attitude about conservative surgery.
- The rapport you feel with the surgeon, including your emotional reaction to the penetration into your body by this person.
- Finances.

When you call to make an appointment, state that you are searching for a surgeon with whom you will feel comfortable. Ask if he or she would be willing to explore the possibility with you. The response you receive by phone (from either the doctor or the secretary) may help you to sense whether this person is likely to be respectful of women who are considering hysterectomy. If not, you have saved the time and the expense of a wasteful appointment.

The interpretation of competence is complex. First, there are the academic degrees and the training that the surgeon has obtained. You might ask for information about the special skills this person has. To determine surgical skill, you will need medical references; you can contact hospitals and other physicians on the phone or in person. When you speak with the surgeon after he or she examines you, ask questions such as: What procedure do you recommend? How much experience do you have with this procedure? What kinds of complications have you encountered? You should ask the surgeon for the names of three or four women who have undergone similar surgery and who might be willing to discuss their experience. You want a person competent both in surgical skill and in "bedside manner" (the ability to communicate) because both are necessary for your well-being. Find someone with sufficient competence that you can sense it, apart from the existence of qualifying credentials.

The attitude of the surgeon toward conserving healthy tissue should be an important consideration. You will be best served if your surgeon has a tendency to conserve rather than remove healthy tissue. By asking whether he or she usually prefers to retain or to remove healthy ovaries when performing a hysterectomy, you will learn what to expect for your own circumstance. By finding out whether the surgeon understands the value of the uterus, particularly the cervix, you will increase the likelihood of receiving supportive surgery. Try to discern whether he or she is willing to discuss your disease problem with you in detail, providing a defensible rationale for removing any of your body parts.

Equally important, seek to establish a mutually respectful and comfortable relationship with the doctor under consideration. Both give and look for courtesy. Does the surgeon respect the importance of your time by honoring appointments, or are you usually kept waiting without apology? Are you spoken to in a respectful way?

It is necessary that you find a patient and understanding surgeon who can help you deal with the stress that you will inevitably feel before surgery. And because rapport is built during time spent together in quiet conversation, you should look for a doctor who is willing to give you that time. Consider that quality of generosity of time as one of your criteria in the selection process.

The surgical penetration of your body is an intensely intimate exposure, and you must be able to receive this intimacy with as little resistance as possible. By finding someone who can pass your test—call it a penetration test—you will be enhancing your potential for healing. If anything about the surgeon makes you feel uneasy, trust your intuition.

Finally, be sure to discuss the financial aspects of the surgery. Check that the surgeon will accept your insurance as full payment. If not, or if the costs are simply more than you can afford, you should not hesitate to explain that because of the cost you will have to go elsewhere. Often when surgeons hear this, in spite of having quoted a fee that entailed additional cost, they find a way to avoid these additional fees. Don't be shy in discussing money. The subject is relevant to your well-being.

When you have found one surgeon who meets your needs, repeat the process. Locate another doctor, discuss the procedure he or she would recommend, speak to former patients, gauge your sense of his or her competence, sense the rapport between the two of you. The economic and time costs involved are real, but they are trivial compared to the costs of not taking the trouble to find the surgeon who is right for you. Your diligence will pay off.

Once you have made your final selection, you and your surgeon will address two important considerations: what will the surgery remove, and what will be the route of your surgery.

### DECIDING ON THE SURGERY YOU WILL HAVE

Depending on the disease or condition that is being addressed, a woman and her surgeon can explore together the several surgical options available:

*Myomectomy,* sometimes referred to as "reconstructive" surgery, which removes only the diseased portion of the uterus, preserving most of the organ.

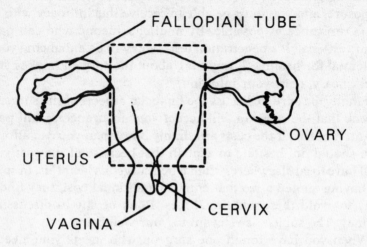

Figure 10. Subtotal hysterectomy

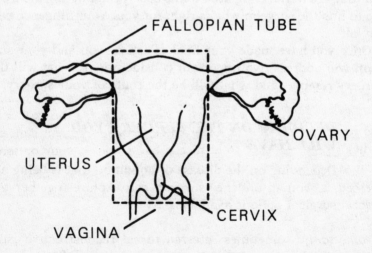

Figure 11. Total hysterectomy

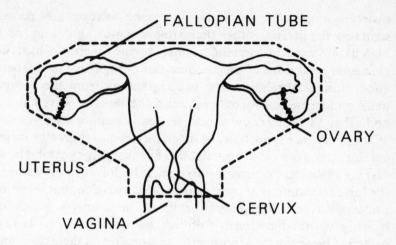

FALLOPIAN TUBE

OVARY

UTERUS

CERVIX

VAGINA

Figure 12. Total hysterectomy with bilateral salpingo-ovariectomy

*Subtotal hysterectomy,* or supravaginal hysterectomy, in which the cervix is retained within the body (see Figure 10).

*Total hysterectomy,* which removes the entire uterus, including the cervix, but retains the ovaries (see Figure 11).

*Total hysterectomy plus tubes and ovaries,* technically known as hysterectomy with bilateral salpingo-ovariectomy (see Figure 12).

In a *radical hysterectomy,* which is performed for certain cancers of the reproductive organs, a wide margin of the vagina is also removed in order to lower the risk of subsequent cancer. Radical hysterectomy is not discussed as one of your options because it is often mandated by current medical opinion about the treatment of cancer.

### *Consider Myomectomy*

A myomectomy removes the diseased portion of the uterus, usually a fibroid tumor, a group of fibroids, or other growths. The surgeon then reconstructs the remaining uterus into as nearly normal a uterine tissue as can be salvaged. By reconstructing the uterus, rather than simply removing it, one has a high likelihood of preserving normal uterine function. Thus, the glandular secretions of the endometrial lining (such as the beta endorphins), lubrication and prostaglandins from the cervix, neuroendocrine control of the ovaries, the ability to have babies, and other as yet unknown functions can continue as before.

The procedure is not new, but because it requires greater surgical skill, it has not often been applied by most surgeons who treat uterine diseases. Perhaps in large part the infrequency reflects the false assumption in the past that the uterus does not serve an important role in the general health of the woman once childbearing wishes have been fulfilled. Myomectomy can be expected to be performed more often as women and their surgeons increase their sophistication about its value in promoting a woman's healthrights.

The surgeon's fees are generally higher for myomectomy than for other surgical methods because of the added skill required. And, unfortunately, most third-party insurers reimburse less, apparently because less tissue is removed. As understanding increases, it is hoped that this unreasonable policy will change.

### Try to Retain the Cervix

Retaining the cervix at hysterectomy (subtotal hysterectomy) offers three advantages:

- It minimizes the potential for a loss in capacity for orgasm during intercourse.[174, 459]
- It reduces the incidence of painful coitus after the surgery.
- It reduces the common posthysterectomy problem of unduly frequent urination.

Classic scientific work published in 1973 established that the cervix of premenopausal women has nerve endings heavily localized within the tissue.[747] In contrast to younger, nonhysterectomized women, postmenopausal women did not seem to have any of these nerve endings in the cervix.[747] Why should this matter? Because nerve endings transmit feelings to the nervous system and brain, often setting in motion physical reflex reactions, such as the knee-jerk reflex and vaginal (and uterine) contractions at orgasm. One investigator in Scandinavia recently compared sexual response in women who had a subtotal hysterectomy to those who had a total hysterectomy.[459] There was a significant loss in the capacity to experience orgasm during intercourse in the group of one hundred women who had the total hysterectomy. Among the one hundred women who retained the cervix, there was no significant loss in capacity for orgasm at coitus.[459] This was the first scientific study to consider in a systematic way the role of the cervix in sexual response in women.

Because it appears to be likely that the cervix plays an important role in sexual response during intercourse,[174] as well as in the release of beta endorphins during intercourse, it makes sense to retain the cervix unless there is some clear reason to remove it.

A comparison of subtotal and total hysterectomy patients showed that women who retained the cervix had less than half the incidence of coital pain (6 percent as opposed to 16 percent).[458] Presumably the reason relates to the anatomical changes caused by the surgeries. Whereas total hysterectomy shortens the length of the vagina, subtotal hysterectomy can avoid altering the vaginal anatomy.

Urinary control problems also seem to occur less frequently after hysterectomy that retains the cervix. Dr. P. Kilkku suggests that the support provided by the remaining structure helps to reduce the urinary symptoms because the bladder is less extensively manipulated when the cervix is not cut away.[457]

No studies have yet evaluated the substances that a retained cervix produces after hysterectomy, or whether keeping the cervix enhances the ovarian secretion of hormones.

If you are considering a hysterectomy for a reason other than cancer, there appears to be no increased risk of cancer to the cervix by keeping it.[456, 559] In one Scandinavian study, one hundred women who underwent hysterectomy with removal of their cervix were compared with another one hundred women who retained the cervix. With the second group, the investigators took the protective measure of using electrical current to melt down cervical tissue (to prevent cancer growth when precancerous cells exist), forming scar tissue in its place. They later examined the incidence of subsequent cancer of the cervix. Their study showed that subsequent cervical cancer incidence was even lower among the women who retained the cervix at hysterectomy than among the population at large.[456] Therefore, if you are considering a hysterectomy and have no cancer, retaining your cervix seems a perfectly safe health choice and perhaps even an optimal decision.[456, 559]

Subtotal hysterectomy requires greater surgical skill than a hysterectomy that does not retain the cervix. The physician who is untrained in this procedure is unlikely to express enthusiasm for it. If you decide to have this kind of an operation, you will have to search carefully for a competent surgeon trained in this technique.

### Keep Your Ovaries Unless They Are Diseased

Even "old" ovaries are vital sex hormone producers; at any age, their loss produces a significant physiologic deficit. You should try to keep your ovaries, regardless of your age. Pelvic cancer (in the uterus, tubes, or ovaries) still appropriately leads to a hysterectomy that removes the tubes and ovaries as well, but until recently it was also considered good medical practice to remove the ovaries of the vast majority (80 to 95 percent) of women without pelvic cancer. They were routinely removed whenever a hysterectomy was performed on a woman over the age of 40 or 45. Much of the decision to remove healthy ovaries was based on two incorrect assumptions: first, that once the uterus was removed, the ovaries no longer contributed hormones necessary to a woman's well-being; and second, that retained ovaries might become cancerous.

It is true that the ovaries stop cycling in 50 percent of hysterectomized women. It appears that the uterus may contribute something to the ovary that allows it to continue to cycle—for example, that prostaglandins secreted from the cervix are needed by the ovary. Yet the evidence from five different studies supports the idea that about half of the women who retain their ovaries continue to show a normal ovarian cycle for some substantial amount of time after the hysterectomy, if the hysterectomy occurs before menopause.[30, 50, 199, 220, 719] If, as I think most wise, the ovaries are retained, a woman has a 50 percent chance of maintaining ovarian functioning. Since, as discussed below, there are no benefits in removing healthy ovaries, this is definitely an option worth pursuing.

The second assumption is simply based on an error. Dr. Richard Grogan in 1967 published a paper in the *American Journal of Obstetrics and Gynecology* in which he said that 4 percent of the time, women who retain their ovaries at hysterectomy will go on to develop ovarian cancer.[327] His work was widely cited as a reason to routinely remove ovaries. Dr. Grogan supported his conclusion by citing the work of Dr. George Smith, published in 1958.[824] Dr. Smith had cited the work of Dr. Virgil Counseller, who had published a study in 1955.[151, 824] When I went back to the original 1955 study by Dr. Counseller, I found that a subtle but powerful error had been made. Counseller's finding was not that 4 or 4.5 percent of women who have a hysterectomy can be expected to develop ovarian cancer if they keep their ovaries, but that 4 to 4.5 percent of the women who have ovarian cancer have previously had a hysterectomy. The true fact tells us nothing that would guide any sensible decision to remove ovaries to prevent cancer.

Keeping the ovaries does not increase the risk of ovarian cancer.[21] One 1979 study reported in the journal *Cancer* showed that when 116 patients with ovarian cancer were compared with four times as many controls, matched for age, the hysterectomy rate in the women without cancer (23 percent) was five times higher than the hysterectomy rate (5 percent) in the group who did have cancer. Among women who had kept their ovaries at hysterectomy, there was no increased risk for ovarian cancer.

In fact, removing healthy ovaries is of questionable value even in addressing a specific risk factor. Although preventive ovariectomy was performed in twenty-eight women who were at very high risk for ovarian cancer because of a family history of this disease, the surgery did not prevent the development of cancer in the abdominal region.[884] Therefore, even when a woman is at a high risk because of her family history, "preventive" ovariectomy does not seem able to stop the cancer "seeds" from dispersing into the pelvic region.

The subject of keeping healthy ovaries has been discussed and debated at length in the very recent literature,[195, 292, 293] and many medical schools have changed their teaching to recommend that surgeons retain healthy ovaries. While we can now say with quite clear assurance that there is no logical reason to remove ovaries in an attempt to prevent some disease that does not exist, we can also say that the aftereffects of ovariectomy on bones, cardiovascular health, and hormonal milieu are so profound that an awful lot of danger would have to be involved in keeping ovaries before it would make any sense to increase the risk of heart attack and hip or spine fracture through ovariectomy. And since we know that old ovaries produce useful substances and do not yet know all of the useful substances they manufacture, it seems good judgment to keep the ovaries unless they are diseased.

If your physician does not agree, you might wish to change physicians or at least to ask for powerful arguments that can convince you of the rightness of ovariectomy in your case. Physicians (and perhaps lay readers as well) might find it interesting to read Appendix A, which reprints an article, published in 1984, in which Dr. Celso Ramón García and I argue for the retention of healthy ovaries at hysterectomy; the subsequent disagreement by Dr. Alan DeCherney, written as a letter to the editor; and the subsequent reply to Dr. DeCherney in favor of retaining the ovaries. Compelled by these arguments, your physician may experience a change in perspective, as have many who have read this paper.

If one of your ovaries shows serious disease but the other is healthy, you should discuss with your surgeon the benefits of keeping the healthy ovary. A rather extensive literature on studies of other animals shows that when only one ovary is removed there is generally a compensatory response in the remaining ovary. Very likely, a remaining ovary will adequately supply hormones and compensate for the one that was lost.[538] However, women who have had one ovary removed should maintain an awareness about what is happening to their bone mass and their cardiovascular health.

### Total Hysterectomy Plus Tubes and Ovaries

This procedure, more formally called a total hysterectomy with bilateral salpingo-ovariectomy, is depicted in Figure 12. The woman who must undergo it will experience a complete deprivation of the hormones normally supplied by the removed organs. Depending upon the age at which such surgery is performed, the shock to the body will be relatively more or less severe. The older the woman, the less severe will be the reduction of hormones because presumably her own sex hormone levels will already have started to diminish. At any age, this form of surgery will produce an immediate postoperative hormonal shock and an inevitable requirement for adequate replacement hormones to protect the bones, cardiovascular health, sexual response systems, and the beta endorphin levels that promote well-being. Although no studies have yet been published to compare the recovery time from this surgery with those for the less extensive hysterectomies, the likelihood is high that recovery will be slower. Nutritional and exercise planning will offer some help in overcoming the negative effects, but hormonal replacement therapy will be a very valuable adjunct to the recovery.

### The Route of Surgery

A hysterectomy or myomectomy can be performed by traditional means through the vagina or the abdomen or by using the newer technique of laparoscopy.

*Abdominal Versus Vaginal Hysterectomy*

Between 1970 and 1978, 3.5 million women in the United States between the ages of 15 and 44 underwent a hysterectomy that was not for major cancer. Of these, 72 percent had the operation through the abdominal route and 28 percent through the vagina.[214] Several studies have compared issues involved in the two surgical routes, including:

*The removal of small endometrial and cervical tumors,* which is effectively performed using the vaginal route.[559]

*Total sickness after surgery,* which is about the same for the two routes, occurring in about 30 to 45 percent of patients although the particular kinds of sickness are different for each.[219, 483]

*Bleeding,* which according to some surgeons is easier to control with an abdominal hysterectomy.[559]

*The need for blood transfusions,* which is at a higher rate with abdominal hysterectomy.[944]

*Fever,* which has about a 50 percent higher incidence after surgery via the vaginal route.[483, 944]

*The use of antibiotics,* which when given before abdominal surgery did not seem to improve the overall postoperative complication from infection. However, preoperative antibiotics were effective in vaginal surgery in preventing postoperative complications.[214] If you are having the vaginal route, you should probably plan on antibiotics as a preventive measure.

Our growing understanding of sexual physiology leads to an awareness that vaginal surgery may interrupt the G Spot reflexes (see Chapter 10) as well as the capacity for vaginal "ballooning" that immediately precedes orgasm. (As with a yawn, just before the orgasm the back part of the vaginal barrel balloons outward, producing a tightening of the musculature and precipitating its release.) Cutting into this musculature may interfere with these reflexes.

### Laparoscopic Hysterectomy

Techniques involving the use of the laparoscope, fiberoptics (lighting instruments), and related instrumentation have advanced to the point where a number of surgical procedures that formerly required opening the abdomen can now be performed through the laparoscope (see page 70). The benefits of such procedures, performed by skilled surgeons, are a shortened hospital stay, less trauma, faster recovery, and a return to full activity at a much faster rate (seven to ten days as compared to four to six weeks). Hospital costs are about 50 percent less because of the shorter stay, although the actual time in the operating room is no different. (Laparoscopic surgery is slow and tedious since the uterus must be minced into pieces small enough to pass out through the scoping tube.) However, because not every surgeon is an expert in this technique, laparoscopic hysterectomy may not be one of your options.

The particular skills of your surgeon will be a determining factor in the decision whether to remove the uterus through a surgical opening in the abdomen, by the insertion of the laparoscope into the closed, gas-inflated abdomen, or through the vagina. A surgeon who is especially skilled in one technique will probably prefer to use that technique, and rightly so. If you have not selected a surgeon and are also considering these procedural options, it is probably wisest to choose the surgeon first and then decide on the particular route of surgery with him or her.

## PREPARING YOURSELF FOR SURGERY

All the types of hysterectomy and even myomectomy are serious surgical procedures, involving the entering of your body and the removal of tissue or organs. Your careful selection of a surgeon and your decision about the type of surgery you will have are part of your preparation for this important event. Knowing that you have done your best in making these decisions should to some degree lessen your anxiety in facing surgery.

Your surgery may be scheduled relatively quickly, or you may have several weeks before going into the hospital. During the time you have available, try to prepare yourself with knowledge, with sound nutrition, and with the kind of rest that will help you feel emotionally and spiritually centered.

### Questions for Your Doctor

In interviewing potential surgeons and in your conversations with the surgeon you choose, you should refer to a written list of questions, the answers to which will enhance your understanding of what to expect after surgery. The more clearly you understand what to expect, the less traumatic the experience is likely to be. You and your physician should have an open dialogue in which you are comfortable asking questions and clearly understand the answers that are given. When you are confused, you should not hesitate to continue the discussion until your confusion has been cleared up. Ask questions like these:

When will the surgery be scheduled?

How long will the surgery last?

Should I store some of my blood in the weeks before surgery, to avoid anxiety about the possible transmission of diseases, especially hepatitis and AIDS, through blood transfusion?

How long will I be in the hospital?

What kinds of complications can you foresee and how would you deal with them?

What kind of anesthesia will be used?

Will I be in pain after surgery?

Where will it hurt, and for how long? What can we do to lessen the pain?

When will I be able to eat normally?

Will I have bowel and bladder problems after surgery? What kinds? For how long? What can we do about them?

Will there be stitches? For how long? How can we lessen their discomfort?

Will there be tubes in me (such as a catheter or IV)? Why? For
how long?
How long will the recovery process take?
When can I return to work? Sex? Exercise?

Through the dialogue on these subjects, you should be able to
develop a respectful, adult relationship with your surgeon. You
will be able to prepare yourself because you will know what to
expect.

### Building Up Your Immune System

The field of nutrition with respect to immunology is in its
infancy; nevertheless, there is a compelling case for a relationship between several vitamins and good immunity. While the
relationship between reduced immune strength and feelings of
weakness and vulnerability is less well understood, recently published studies suggest that people who feel helpless don't have
strong immune systems, and a new scientific field called psy-
choimmunology is forming. Taking action—that is, taking control of your life—is likely to build your sense of empowerment
and to enhance your immune strength.

Personal power comes not from demanding it but from ac-
quiring knowledge and skills, such as ways to courteously and
competently assert your healthrights as you interact with medical professionals. With respect to your surgery, the active role
you take in learning what is happening and in making informed
choices will probably enhance your immune strength. One of the
many benefits of carefully selecting a compassionate surgeon is
that respectful treatment from your surgeon will enhance your
feelings of control.

Good nutritional information is now available. Adequate levels of vitamin A, vitamin $B_{12}$, pantothenic acid, folacin, and vitamin C are particularly important for your immune system.[673] It
appears that vitamin C has the most significant influence on
priming the immune system. One investigator studied a group of
British research workers isolated in an Antarctic research sta-

tion. Those who had an increased intake of vitamin C showed an increased production of immunoglobulins, the antibody molecules that fight diseases.[902] In another study, twenty-five healthy male students were given 1 gram of vitamin C per day while twenty comparable university students were given a placebo (blank) pill. Investigators found that after seventy-five days, there was a significant increase in the blood levels of three of the immunoglobulins (IgA, IgG, and IgM[699b]) among those students who took the vitamin C. There may be value in strengthening the immune system this way, and fortunately there are no substantiated side effects from taking even 6 grams of vitamin C per day.[673]

Individual needs for vitamin C vary considerably from one person to the next, and there are no clear data to tell us exactly how much is an optimal daily dose when you are preparing for surgery. Dr. Linus Pauling suggests that in general one way to determine the healthy amount of vitamin C for you is to slowly increase the daily amount you take until it exceeds your "bowel tolerance" level.[673] When you begin to take too much vitamin C, a mild diarrhea ensues. If this happens, cut back from that daily dose. At one time there was some controversy in the literature about the possibility that vitamin C might destroy the vitamin $B_{12}$ content of meals. Don't worry about it! That controversy has been resolved, and there appears to be no such danger.

Vitamin A, like vitamin C, appears to be related to cervical dysplasia and cancer.[748, 964] A higher proportion of women with cervical diseases than without disease showed a lower intake of vitamin A and the related molecule beta-carotene.[384] But be cautioned here: high doses of vitamin A are not recommended. Although the recommended daily amount (RDA) for vitamin A in adults is 5,000 International Units (IU's), a single dose 1,000 times that amount has been shown to be dangerous. Since there are no clear studies to define an optimal dose of vitamin A, it seems sensible to be certain that before your surgery you get at least the RDA of 5,000 IU's and that you consider increasing that dosage mildly to 25,000 IU per day.[673]

In order to arm yourself before surgery (ideally as far ahead as you can), you might want to consider taking a daily multivitamin (one that contains 5,000 IU of vitamin A) or its equivalent in separate tablets and capsules, and increasing your vitamin C content to at least 2 grams per day, up to perhaps 10 grams per day depending on your bowel reaction. (Spread the doses of vitamin C apart so that you get about four servings a day.) If you do increase your vitamin C content, it is very important that you continue at these doses while you are in the hospital and in the first weeks of your at-home convalescence. A sudden shift in vitamin dose shocks the body; gradual changes are better tolerated and can be more helpful in strengthening your body. Also recommended once a day are one or two vitamin B tablets to supply $B_{12}$, pantothenic acid, and folacin. For a more detailed discussion of nutrition, see Chapter 13.

If you are a smoker and are contemplating surgery, it would be extremely wise to stop smoking before you enter surgery. Because smoking inhibits the capacity of the body's immune system, by eliminating smoke from your system you give yourself the best chance for a healthy recovery. (See Chapter 14 for help in stopping smoking.)

Rest is an important component for building your immune strength. Be certain both to nap during the day and to get as much sleep as you need at night so that your strength will be at a maximum.

### Rest—For Emotional and Spiritual Strength

Having prepared your physical strength for the surgery, the next consideration is your preparation of spirit and emotion—a benefit that derives from the nonactivity called rest. Most people allow themselves at least enough rest to maintain the physical stamina they need day by day, and this type of rest is especially important in the preparation for surgery. Even more significant, however, is the rest that has an emotional or a spiritual dimension.

Calm and a sense of quiet peacefulness come from the deliberate decision to stop doing things. To achieve this, you will need to set aside a time and a place for renewing your energies. If you will reserve three twenty-minute periods a day for rest and renewal, and then use these minutes to sit or lie down quietly— simply becoming absorbed in the world around you without trying to control that world—your body and spirit will reap great rewards. If you have a religious background, you might use one of these periods for prayer or spiritual reading. The individual way in which you rest can differ from what works for other people, but the underlying discipline of setting aside a time and a place is very important. Your overall strength will increase when you learn how to rest well.

Because the life of the spirit is not the subject of scientific research, there are no data to guide us. But when you must put yourself into the care of another—in this case, your surgeon— you are drawing on a greater power than your own. If you can submit to it gracefully, after doing all you can to prepare, your body will cooperate with your surgeon, and this cooperation provides a positive force.

## POSTOPERATIVE ILLNESS

It helps to know what the recovery period will be like. If you know what to watch out for, you are better equipped to cope.

Postoperative illnesses fall into four classes:

- Fever, resulting from an infection
- Bleeding and wound healing
- Sudden hormonal shock
- Loss of energy and slow recovery process

### Fever

According to Dr. Russell Laros, fever and pelvic inflammation more often follow vaginal hysterectomy, although they can occur after abdominal surgery. The fever is generally short-term and may be accompanied by a urinary tract infection.[483] Thirty to 40 percent of women experience a temperature above 100.4

degrees Fahrenheit, most commonly caused by a normally harmless intestinal bacterium that works its way into the surgical wound or vaginal area.[559]

About 40 percent of women who do not receive preventive antibiotics experience sickness and fever in the first days after their hysterectomy. The cost of postoperative infection is high. Recent studies have shown that for a vaginal hysterectomy, the cost to the patient or insurer averages $1,777, based upon excess days in the hospital, the laboratory tests necessary to define the disease, and the appropriate antibiotics. For women who undergo an abdominal hysterectomy, the excess cost is less ($716).[797]

Some discussion has emerged in the recent medical literature about whether women should take a preoperative antibiotic. In general, the conclusion is that there is a dollar saving as well a reduction in discomfort when antibiotics are taken before a vaginal hysterectomy.[214] The strength of your own immune system should also play a significant role in your ability to withstand infection.

### Bleeding and Wound Healing

Most frequently postoperative bleeding begins between seven and fourteen days after surgery, as the stitches dissolve and slough off.[559] A bit of bloody, foul-smelling discharge may be expected on about days ten to fourteen. (If your surgeon uses a method other than stitches to close the wound, you may not experience these problems.) A hemorrhage can be life-threatening if the patient has left the hospital. One eminent surgeon, Dr. Richard Mattingly, strongly believes that patients should stay in the hospital longer than two or three days after their surgery in order to prevent such a potentially tragic situation.[559] However, your insurance policy will probably limit your hospital stay. If you begin to bleed heavily on day ten or later, you should immediately call your surgeon for treatment.

Wound healing will be greatly accelerated if you take vitamin C. There is now strong evidence to show that whenever you have a wound—and surgery most certainly produces a wound—vitamin C can double the rate of healing. One research team concluded that daily doses of 500 to 3,000 milligrams (0.5 to 3 grams) of vitamin C "significantly accelerate healing for persons recovering from surgery."[735] To reduce your wound-healing time, as well as to increase your immune strength, it is strongly recommended that you take vitamin C before your surgery, arrange to have it in the hospital, and continue with it until you are healed.

### Sudden Hormonal Shock

If you undergo a hysterectomy and keep your ovaries, it is highly likely that you will experience an acute, but possibly temporary, drop in estrogen on the second day after your surgery.[854] Some experts suggest that a local interruption of the ovarian blood supply is responsible for the temporary alteration in hormonal milieu.[414]

This hormonal shock can produce menopause symptoms, which will disappear if and when the ovaries return to normal. As many as 70 percent of patients might experience hot flashes, night sweats, headaches, dizzy spells, sleeplessness, palpitations, and depression.[570, 731] If you have kept your ovaries and experience these symptoms, it may be a temporary condition that will last only a few days. As part of your presurgery discussions with your surgeon, you might want to consider taking some estrogen for the duration of this shock period, because it will help.

About half of retained ovaries do not resume a normal cycle after hysterectomy. They fail to produce the symphony of hormonal secretions that is characteristic of an intact cycling woman. If you experience this ovarian failure, you may have begun your menopause. You will need to consider ways to prevent the effects of hormonal deficiencies and to maintain your well-being, including HRT.

If you undergo a hysterectomy with removal of your ovaries, you can be sure of experiencing a sudden hormonal deprivation. Ovariectomy predictably leads to a rapid decline in sex hormones and an immediate menopause.[25] The reduction in estrogen and progesterone generally produces hot flashes and the other symptoms of menopause, including a dramatic loss of bone mass in the first three years. About 20 percent of the spinal bone can be lost in the first two years if no HRT is taken. Chapters 6 and 7 discuss HRT, and the following chapters take up, in detail, the several problems associated with the loss of hormones caused by hysterectomy.

Regardless of the type of hysterectomy you have had, HRT is entirely appropriate for preventing or reversing postoperative hot flashes and for helping your body to function normally during the recovery period, beginning as soon as you emerge from anesthesia.

## THE SLOW RECOVERY PROCESS

Lying in bed and recovering from major surgery is bound to affect a person psychologically. Although the biomedical literature has paid very little serious attention to the subject and studies of the immediate postoperative period are not easily available,[560] many women have described their personal experiences during that period. Two typical comments are given here.

> After my hysterectomy, I had the usual postoperation discomfort. About one week after the surgery I became very depressed and cried all the time. My feelings reminded me of how I felt after I had childbirth. I really had no reason for feeling so blue. My family and friends had been very supportive and loving. I had my tubes tied seven years ago, so it wasn't that I was upset about not being able to have children.
>
> I remember when I was taking a shower one day, I was crying so hard I thought I was drowning in my emotions. I talked to my doctor and he said that it would pass, that probably there was a shock to my ovaries, that they had stopped producing estrogen, and that it was a change in my chemistry that was causing my depression. He was right. About a week later I felt much better. I have felt

better all the time, and the fact that I don't have to worry about heavy periods draining me every month is such a relief.

I don't remember too much about how I felt after the surgery (which was four years ago), except for this. . . . I spent only two nights in the hospital. I was sent home much too soon. I don't recall much pain in the hospital, but I was so doped up I don't recall much of anything then. When I came home I did have pain.

But other than the pain, it was the weakness. I felt an incredible weakness. My poor husband and daughter didn't know what to do with me. I could hardly navigate. I was so weak that the only thing I could do was to lay there. It lasted a good week. I think I needed hospital care and shouldn't have been sent home so soon. After all, a hysterectomy is major surgery. The year before I had had a much more trivial operation (a double hernia), and they kept me eight days. The hysterectomy had much less pain than the hernia repair but the weakness . . .

The recovery from hysterectomy is usually slower than with other surgeries. Although some women seem to bounce back right after surgery, they are in the minority. For most, recovery is slow, and it often involves depression. One study compared hysterectomized women with age-matched control women who were undergoing a variety of other surgical operations (removal of the appendix, thyroid, breast, gallbladder). Hysterectomy entailed the slowest convalescence of all: on the average it took about thirteen months for a woman to feel as if she were her old self again, compared with four months for recovery from the other operations.[731] If you understand that it will take time, perhaps even a long time, you can better prepare. Perhaps this is a time to lower your aspirations, to do less, and to wait out the recovery. HRT may be profoundly helpful during this period.

Even assuming that you have an excellent surgeon, you can expect that the abdomen may feel easily bruised; it may be three to four months before coital pressure can be enjoyed rather than merely tolerated.[15] Temporary shrinkage of the vagina occurs. This shrinkage results in a short and narrow vault.[15] Adhesions (scar tissue) are also a common result of surgery and occur in about half of women who undergo pelvic surgery.[213] They can be painful, and sometimes further surgery is necessary to remove them.

On occasion, after an ovariectomy some pieces of ovarian tissue are left behind. This problem occurs rarely, but when it does happen, most frequently it is after endometriosis or pelvic adhesion surgery. It is intensely painful, with the pain tending to be cyclic.[868] Surgery to remove the remnants relieves the problem.

For many women the immediate postoperative effects rapidly fade from memory, and while total recovery may take about a year, healing from surgery is generally complete within a few months. More serious, however, are the threats that the surgery produces to the overall long-term health of the woman. The rest of this book describes the things you can do to help maintain your optimum health after surgery.

It is best to plan ahead, but it is never too late to start.

# 6

# Hormonal Replacement Therapy:
## Benefits, Side Effects, and Contraindications

After a hysterectomy or ovariectomy, many changes inevitably occur in a woman's body, some of them for the better. The disease process that precipitated the need for a hysterectomy will probably have ended. If you had been bleeding, once healing is complete the bleeding will not recur, and your energy is likely to increase when there is no longer a continual loss of blood. However, other changes are not so good. Hot flashes are usually the first signal of hormonal declines. Later, more serious effects of hormonal deficiencies include loss of bone mass, an increased risk for cardiovascular disease, deterioration of the urinary and genital tissues, depression, and general acceleration of the aging process.

For women who enter a natural menopause, deficiencies of estrogen occur gradually. But for women who undergo pelvic surgery and thereby lose either their ovaries or the hormonal functioning of their ovaries (the case for 50 percent of women whose ovaries are retained), the effect of estrogen deficiency is much more shocking and profound. For both groups, hormonal replacement therapy (HRT) has profound life-enhancing benefits. Bones become stronger, and the devastation of osteoporosis can be prevented or halted. Cardiovascular health improves, and the likelihood of death from cardiovascular disease can be vastly reduced. The sense of well-being and joy in life will improve, and sexual life is enhanced. HRT can make an important contribution to the quality, the energy, and the strength of a woman's physical and emotional health, and all women should explore the possibility of HRT after pelvic surgery.

The growth of knowledge about hormones is an exciting new phenomenon in biomedical science. Because of the recently developed capability to test hormone levels and to manufacture natural forms of hormones, the usefulness of HRT has tremendously increased. Safety has also improved as we have come to understand which doses are too high and which too low, which forms are dangerous and which safe. The technique called radioimmunoassay will permit your doctor to take a sample of your blood, send it to a laboratory, and within several days have a measurement of your blood levels of estrogen, progesterone, luteinizing hormone (LH), and follicle-stimulating hormone (FSH). The tests are relatively inexpensive compared to their value in helping determine your need for and dose of HRT.

This chapter reviews the benefits as well as the side effects and known risks of HRT. A review of contraindications to hormones is included, and alternatives to HRT are discussed. Chapter 7 provides detailed advice about types of hormone dosages.

In the early days of HRT, doctors had relatively unrefined information on which to base their prescriptions, and some women* were given HRT dosages that were too high, with results that were damaging to the health of their uterus. Likewise, awareness of some of the side effects of oral contraceptives, which contain much higher concentrations of hormones (synthetic estrogens and progestins) than does HRT, have made some women and their doctors skeptical about the safety of HRT. Our knowledge has improved significantly in the past twenty years. While certain hormones carry with them risks that are best avoided, others are extremely beneficial and safe. The information and techniques that are available today make it possible for women to have full confidence in competently prescribed HRT.

Since the mid-1980s, a vast number of studies have been published about different kinds of hormones and their effects and

*Perhaps 3 to 7 out of each 1,000.

side effects. It is entirely possible that a lay reader of this book will receive this information before her physician has had an opportunity to receive it. Doctors are generally very busy people. The more compassionate the physician, the greater the number of patients who will line up in the waiting room. By the end of a day filled with seeing patients, most physicians are tired, and many have very little energy left for disciplined study. Thus it is especially significant that you can exert control and help shape your treatment through an informed and respectful two-way dialogue with your doctor.

Not every woman needs HRT.[579] A small proportion of women who have undergone hysterectomy continue to produce adequate hormones throughout their lives. Since the sex hormones—estrogen, progesterone, and testosterone—are manufactured in both the ovary and the adrenal glands, surgery that alters ovarian output changes only one of the hormonal factories. And the ovaries continue to cycle (produce hormones) for a variable length of time in 50 percent of the women who retain them. But for the vast majority of women, probably 85 percent,[172, 174] HRT offers a number of very relevant and important benefits to physical health and emotional well-being.

## THE BENEFITS OF HORMONAL REPLACEMENT THERAPY

You can expect at least ten different benefits from taking HRT. And unless you have contraindications (see page 130), it makes sense to start HRT as soon as you emerge from an ovariectomy or as soon as tests or symptoms produce evidence of hormonal decline after a hysterectomy. HRT, when judiciously prescribed, provides the following benefits:
• Relief of menopausal symptoms
• Preservation of bone mass
• Prevention of cardiovascular disease
• Prevention of sexual problems
• Improvements in the sense of emotional well-being

- Prevention of atrophy in the urinary system
- Slowing of the aging of skin
- Maintenance of muscle tone and strength
- Improvements in the quality of sleep and dream states
- Potential for an increased immunological capacity
- Reduction in the death rate from all causes

If you have contraindications, you must balance the risks against the benefits and make an informed judgment about which negative effects you would rather accept—those posed by the loss of hormones or those made possible by HRT. Whichever course you choose will entail some risk and some benefit.

### Menopausal Symptoms and Relief

Menopausal symptoms associated with hormonal deficiencies diminish or disappear with appropriately dosed HRT.[489] Women who are having menopausal distress tend to be thinner than women without menopausal distress because of the nature of fat cells, which act as factories for the conversion of the androgens (produced in both the ovaries and the adrenals) into estrogens. This is just one example of the many factors determining dosage. You can score your personal degree of menopausal distress by following the instructions in "Calculations of Menopausal Distress," page 124.

Hot flashes are described on page 27.

Headaches and sex hormones have shown some relationship. One study showed that after ovariectomy headaches were more common in the one week of each month when hormone users were off hormones,[208] but another study did not confirm this.[899] However, conjugated equine estrogen (discussed in Chapter 7) relieved headaches in twenty-two of twenty-eight women who had frequent headaches before taking the estrogen therapy.[118] High levels of testosterone are associated with headaches.[209] Testosterone is created by the adrenals as well as the ovaries; if you become very stressed, your adrenal glands may secrete extra androgen and trigger headaches. Progestagen

## Calculation of Menopausal Distress

Each menopausal symptom is listed with a given "factor." In the column headed "Severity," enter the number that reflects the severity of your current experience: 0 for none, 1 for slight, 2 for moderate, and 3 for heavy. Then multiply your severity score by the listed factor to fill in the numerical conversion.

When you add up the numerical conversion column, you will have a score known as the Kupperman Menopausal Index. If your score is more than 35, you have severe menopausal symptoms. If your score is less than 20, your symptoms are mild.[474]

| Symptom | Factor | × | Severity (0–3) | = | Numerical Conversion |
|---|---|---|---|---|---|
| Hot flashes/night sweats | 4 | × | ———— | = | ———— |
| Prickling/burning | 2 | | ———— | | ———— |
| Insomnia | 2 | | ———— | | ———— |
| Nervousness | 2 | | ———— | | ———— |
| Melancholia (depression) | 1 | | ———— | | ———— |
| Vertigo (dizziness) | 1 | | ———— | | ———— |
| Weakness (fatigue) | 1 | | ———— | | ———— |
| Muscle/joint pain | 1 | | ———— | | ———— |
| Headache | 1 | | ———— | | ———— |
| Palpitation | 1 | | ———— | | ———— |
| Formication (itchy feeling on the skin) | 1 | | ———— | | ———— |

*Kupperman Menopausal Index (Total)*          ————

dosages, when given without estrogen, have been implicated in causing headaches in about 7 percent of women.[83] Thus, estrogen seems to prevent and reverse headaches for many women while excess progestins and testosterone may sometimes trigger them.

Women with menopausal symptoms show low sex hormone levels. Most experience significant or complete relief of symptoms on all forms of estrogen and progesterone replacement therapy that have been tested, provided that the dose is adjusted to each woman's particular requirement.* Estrogen with testosterone also effectively relieves the menopausal symptoms.[404]

### Preservation of Bone

In the 1970s and 1980s, a vast world-wide research effort led to the publication of hundreds of individual studies on bone in relation to hormones. Loss of bone mass was revealed to be a major problem for women once their estrogen levels decline. HRT in combination with adequate calcium, vitamin D, and exercise can usually prevent or halt the deterioration of bone. (See Chapter 8.)

### Prevention of Cardiovascular Disease

Hysterectomy and ovariectomy greatly increase the risk for cardiovascular disease, the major killer of postmenopausal women. You will be wise to take aggressive action to protect yourself. Appropriately selected HRT helps enormously, in combination with proper nutrition and adequate exercise. (See Chapter 9.)

### Prevention of Sexual Problems

Vaginal dryness and painful intercourse, but not loss of libido, are relieved by estrogen therapies.[99, 118, 206, 207, 485] Genital tract infections, which are common, are usually reversed with estro-

---

*Many studies demonstrate such relief, among them 118, 204, 340, 373, 382, 485, 504, 892, 920.

gen therapy.[908] Libidinal deficiencies are overcome with testosterone therapy. (See Chapter 10.)

### Improvements in the Sense of Well-Being

A woman's sense of well-being—that is, her emotional health, her sense of the joy in life—is affected by hormonal deficiencies and HRT. Estrogen helps.[118] Although progestagen during the early stages of therapy temporarily reduces these estrogen benefits, once three months have passed the sense of well-being is usually good.[99, 205] (See Chapter 11.)

### Prevention of Atrophy in the Urinary System

Estrogen deficiency also leads to atrophic changes in the urethra and in the urinary bladder. The cells deteriorate, dry out, and produce an easily bruised surface. Urinary tract infections are common but are usually reversed when estrogen therapy is administered.[908]

### Slowing Down Aging of the Skin

Pelvic surgery will probably accelerate the aging of your skin. After ovariectomy, without HRT a continual thinning of the epidermis (the outer layer of skin cells) becomes more pronounced as the time since the surgery increases.[711, 712] Several different studies have revealed that HRT stops the deterioration.[74, 544]

The first demonstration of the influence of estrogen on skin at a molecular level was published in 1980. Scientists showed that the facial skin of a woman is the most responsive area of her skin surface to the amount of estrogen in her blood.[356] This is probably why the face shows aging long before other skin surfaces look old. Although you might be tempted to apply estrogen cream to the face, the question of skin cancer has not been adequately studied. For now, it is wise to avoid direct hormone application on the face.

### Maintaining Muscle Tone and Strength

Both women who take HRT after a period of hormonal deficiency and sports fitness personnel are well aware of the profound influence of the sex hormones on maintaining muscle tone and muscle strength. HRT will permit and promote a better muscle tone. Appropriately dosed HRT will allow women to feel a greater muscular strength.

### Improving Sleep and Dreams

When we sleep, our brains emit electrical waves. Scientists have investigated the brain waves of people during sleep. One of the major discoveries was that one of the stages of sleep, the rapid eye movement (REM) stage, is characteristic of dreaming. When we REM dream, although our eyelids are shut, the eyeballs move rapidly. Deprivation of REM sleep increases irritability and makes people unhappy.[198] Since the amount of REM sleep that we get appears to be related to our overall physical and emotional health, it is noteworthy that studies of women after ovariectomy showed that HRT substantially increased their REM sleep.[773]

### Increased Immunity

In the late 1970s and early 1980s, Dr. George Feigen, working with others at Stanford University, showed that when a female guinea pig was ovariectomized, its blood levels of antibodies decreased significantly.[245, 246] When it was given estrogen replacement therapy, the antibody production improved.[246] A later study showed that the castration effect, wherein blood levels of antibodies are reduced, could be corrected either by estrogen or by large doses of vitamin C.[245] Further studies provided more details to show the beneficial effects of either estrogen or vitamin C on an ovariectomized mammal with respect to her immune defense system.[247, 270]

We can conclude that in some mammals, ovarian hormones contribute to the general health of the immune system and that there is a synergy (a working together) that takes place between vitamin C and estrogen. Are humans the same? Probably yes. It appears to be optimal to have adequate levels of both traveling in the blood. Estrogen appears to be a useful hormone for general health and satisfactory immunity.

### Reduction in the Death Rate

The results are very clear: for women who have had a hysterectomy, HRT reduces the death rate from all causes. For example, one study followed 1,000 women with more than five years HRT use after hysterectomy and revealed that there was an 80 percent drop in death from all causes compared to what was expected for that size sample. Deaths not related to hormones, such as automobile accidents, were equivalent to the population norms.[86, 95]

A different investigating team followed more than 2,200 white women, subdividing their data into hysterectomy, ovariectomy, and intact groups.[93] In that study, estrogen replacement therapy reduced the "all-cause mortality" in all groups.

If you have a hysterectomy or an ovariectomy, it seems to be very important for your overall health that you consider taking HRT. As you weigh your decision, these beneficial results should be considered.

## SIDE EFFECTS

There are two kinds of possible side effects from HRT. The short-term discomforts, such as fluid retention or nausea, generally self-correct within three months.[157, 373] When progestins are part of the prescription in addition to estrogen, about 15 percent of women report some irritability and tension.[920] Others experience a pleasant hypnotic effect.[820] There has been some implication that the synthetic progestins are responsible for the bad feelings and that natural progesterone therapy promotes the hypnotic effect, but more research is needed to be sure.[203] HRT is most commonly taken orally in the United States, and it is good to know that recent (1987) studies of many different oral HRT regimens showed no negative effect on either thyroid or liver function.[3, 608]

The more substantial side effects, such as those that produce a dry vagina or dangerous cholesterol increase, generally reflect a relative deficiency of estrogen, either because it is too low or because the progestin opposition is disproportionately high. Correcting the balance should correct the problem.

Breast tenderness is a common side effect that investigators consider a result of excessively high doses of estrogen. [67, 99, 908] Another symptom that suggests the estrogen dose is too high is leg cramps, which occur in about one out of five women who are on high doses of conjugated equine estrogen.[99]

Estrogen-androgen combinations also have been reported to produce side effects for some women. These side effects include virilization (a tendency to masculinize), hirsutism (the growth of facial and body hair in a male pattern), and deepening of the voice.[489] These symptoms probably reflect too much androgen hormone. Because androgens improve libido, you may want to take them if libidinal deficits are a problem for you. You can work with your prescribing physician and lower the dose of androgen if you experience negative effects.

### Adjusting the Dose to Relieve Side Effects

If you take HRT incorrectly, side effects are your signal that the dosage needs to be changed. Since your body is different from anyone else's, the amount of hormone that you need to maximize your hormonal balance will be unique to you. Once you understand how hormones influence your body, you will become sensitive to your own dosage options. Set up a diary and record your reactions each day. You also need to establish a relationship with a physician or health center in which your reactions are respected as appropriate signals in the process of defining the right dose of hormone. Your prescription should be adjusted in response to your reactions in the following areas: symptom relief, side effects, sexual responses, bone measurements, cardiovascular health parameters, and your sense of well-being.

As you come to understand the relationship between HRT and the different body systems, you will be able to tell whether you are getting enough, too much, or too little. It is rather like the situation with calories and weight control. Although a physician may tell you that a certain number of calories is ideal for you, you will know whether that number is correct by any one of several tests: looking in the mirror, stepping on a scale, noting how your clothes fit. Hormones work the same way. The prescriptions that are commonly given are based on averages. But you are not average; you are unique. Chapter 7 provides more detailed discussion of dosage levels.

### Interpreting Manufacturers' Warnings

Because law requires that any negative effect be mentioned, package inserts that come with hormonal regimens can be frightening, and women should be cautioned against taking out of proportion what is written there. The inserts rarely give a full and complete disclosure of all the value of the agent, while they do give a full and complete disclosure of all the negative effects that have ever occurred. In most cases, the relative balance between negative and positive is so profoundly in favor of the value of HRT that a woman can take comfort that if she is not in a group for which hormones are specifically contraindicated, she will probably find major benefits in taking them after surgery.

## CONTRAINDICATIONS TO HORMONAL REPLACEMENT THERAPY

Out of the desire to prevent giving HRT to anyone who might be at any risk respective to a particular disease, the federal Food and Drug Administration (FDA) has developed a list of contraindications to HRT, which appears on packaging inserts and in medical textbooks. Contraindications differ depending on the hormone in question, but among those most often cited are conditions related to:

- Venous thrombosis (clots in veins)
- Breast cancer and benign breast disease
- Effects on the liver
- Gallbladder disease

There are four problems with the contraindications that the FDA publicizes. First, they derive from side effects that some women experienced when they took oral contraceptives, which are made up largely of synthetic hormones and much higher dosages than those in HRT prescriptions. Second, there are no data to support the contentions that these contraindications are valid for HRT. Third, a simple listing of (supposed) containdica- tions does not reflect the relative risks imposed by the conditions and HRT. Fourth, this list places physicians in the unfortunate position of being reluctant to prescribe HRT for women with any of the contraindications even though HRT may produce a pro- found benefit. Malpractice suits, which cripple the medical pro- fession, have mandated that physicians defend themselves against this potential devastation to their economic solvency. The medical community is faced with a very difficult problem. Since knowledge about treatment efficacy comes from prospec- tive double-blind research studies, until such studies are done there is no rational way in which decisions can be made about whether women with contraindications should have HRT.*

The existence of the list from the FDA makes physicians, even those who understand that there are very few valid contraindica-

*The terms *prospective, double blind, retrospective,* and *epidemiologic* have very important distinctions.

Epidemiologic studies use data collected retrospectively (from memory) after a condition has emerged. Such investigations ask whether people with a certain condi- tion have a different incidence of use of a drug or other agent than people (from a selected population) without the condition. Epidemiologic results cannot assert cause and effect; they can only pinpoint associations between conditions. Those epidemi- ologic publications using the term *risk-ratio* can be very misleading if one interprets the words *risk* and *ratio* according to common English usage. In scientific writings, the terms have a specific meaning that does not indicate either risk or causal relation- ship. The real value of a good epidemiologic study is that it can light a beacon that will allow for the subsequent planning of a proper prospective research study under double-blind conditions, in which neither the experimenter nor the research subject knows what treatment is being given.

In a prospective study, a treatment group and a control group are formed by in- dividuals being randomly assigned treatment or placebo. After a period of time has passed, the investigator measures whether the treatment group performed differently than the control group. If they did, and if the study is subsequently replicated, then biomedical conclusions about cause and effect can be drawn.

tions to HRT, reluctant to prescribe HRT for women with these conditions; the fear of malpractice suits is heightened by the FDA list. This situation puts the burden for getting HRT on the women who want it.

Even in the face of our meager knowledge, there are women with contraindicating diseases who discuss with their physicians the risks of taking hormones versus the risks in not taking hormones. They make a choice in favor of what they perceive to be the greater gain for their overall health. What is needed is a central registry to tabulate data that emerge from the experience of these women, allowing scientists to understand the results of HRT and to thus help women make better-informed decisions. Until such data are available, women continue to take uninformed risks. The very limited set of published studies on HRT use among women with diseases are discussed next.

### Venous Thrombosis (Clots in Veins)

The ability of your blood to clot or coagulate is an essential health requirement. Studies have been conducted to evaluate whether HRT interferes with this process, and the results are essentially consistent in finding safety. One exception, published in 1976, reported on an increased tendency to clot among a subgroup of menopausal women who were given conjugated equine estrogens in doses of 1.25 milligrams per day.[844] It was particularly the young women who took estrogen that seemed to be the group at risk. None of the other investigations have agreed with that result. For example, the Boston Collaborative Drug Surveillance Program has concluded that estrogen replacement therapy does not affect thromboembolic events (those caused by clotting).[68] Others have provided data in agreement that HRT is safe.[28, 644, 770]

It has long been noted that clots have been associated with oral contraceptive use in young women (albeit rarely) but not with estrogen replacement therapy.[642] In fact, one study showed that the stronger oral contraceptive doses led to increases in a specific blood globulin, "clotting factor VII," that leads to an increased risk of thrombosis.[573] This risk appears to exist for some users of oral contraceptive estrogens; it does not appear to be a concern for users of ERT.

Dr. John Studd and his colleagues, after investigating six different estrogen preparations, some of which were opposed by norethisterone or testosterone, concluded, "This study does not reveal any change towards hypercoaguability [increased clotting] in any of the parameters with the treatment regimens studied." In 1986 investigators reporting in the *New England Journal of Medicine* also concluded that there were no clotting factor changes on any dose of any preparation when they compared oral estrogen in the conjugated equine form to transdermal estrogen (skin cream contained in a bandage).[119] Nonetheless, according to Dr. M. Aylward, the synthetic estrogen ethinyl estradiol should be avoided because when there has been any risk, it was connected to the synthetic form.[28] You may wish to discuss with your doctor the possibility of being tested for antithrombin, which identifies women at high risk for thromboembolic complications. The problem is a very rare one, but if you are at high risk, it is useful for you to know that you are.

### Breast Cancer and Benign Breast Disease

Breast cancer is much publicized as a very serious problem for women, but few statistically competent studies have provided data on the occurrence of breast cancer. Conclusions without published hard data state that between 6 and 10 percent of women have clinical breast cancer by the time they reach age 75.[821] But recently one medical group reported investigating, over the course of ten years (1974 to 1983), more than 32,000 consecutive office examinations in a gynecologic practice.[648] Only 25 cancers were found in the 8,757 patients (less than 0.3 percent) during the ten-year study. Statistics for female death rates in the U.S. show a relatively low annual incidence of death due to breast cancer (38,400), as compared to deaths due to cardiovascular disease (485,000). Breast cancer is more an older woman's disease and is most common in the years characteristic of sex hormone decline.

In March 1988, Dr. David Eddy and his colleagues published

the first real set of nonepidemiologic data to defuse the frightening scenario. Publishing in the *Journal of the American Medical Association,* they showed that the chance of a 40-year-old woman getting breast cancer sometime within the next year was extremely low—1.1 per 1,000.[226] Their analysis fits the published studies described above and is in direct contrast to the scientifically undocumented scare statements so commonly seen in the media.

A number of large- and small-scale studies have provided evidence strongly in favor of the value of estrogen with progestin opposition for reducing the risk of breast cancer.* These studies also reveal that estrogen replacement therapy by itself, without benefit of progestin opposition, does not appear to either increase or decrease the risk of breast cancer.

The incidence of breast cancer does seem to vary in women depending on whether they take no hormones at menopause or different combinations of estrogen and progestagens.[284] Table 4 arrays the data of a nine-year prospective study conducted by Dr. Don Gambrell. The study was initiated in order to learn what the breast cancer outcome would be of women in different hormonal groups.[284]

These data seem to suggest that women who take estrogen with progestagen have the lowest incidence of breast cancer (67 per 100,000) and that women who take any one of the HRT regimens seem to be at a reduced risk of breast cancer.[39] But the data are not perfect. There is a possibility of "self-selection," in which women at risk of breast cancer may have been diverted from HRT. We cannot assess that situation in this study.

There are particular groups of women with breast cancer who show an apparent increased risk of cancer through having used estrogens, although this retrospective analysis cannot prove that the estrogens themselves increased the risk of the cancer. Initially it was thought that those who developed benign breast disease (fibrocystic disease) while taking estrogen replacement

---

*Studies include 284, 286, 392, 618, 636, 752, 753, 820, 908.

**Table 4.** *Incidence of Breast Cancer at Wilford Hall USAF Medical Center 1975–1983*

| Therapy group | Patient-years of observation* | Patients with cancer | Incidence (per 100,000) |
|---|---|---|---|
| Estrogen-progestagen users | 16,466 | 11† | 66.8 |
| Unopposed estrogen users | 19,676 | 28† | 142.3 |
| Estrogen vaginal cream users | 4,298 | 5† | 116.3 |
| Progestagen or androgen users | 1,825 | 3† | 164.4 |
| Untreated women | 6,404 | 22 | 343.5 |
| *Total patients* | *48,669* | *69* | *141.8* |

*Patient-years are calculated by adding up the number of years all the patients are followed.
†Includes individuals who were not using hormones at the time cancer was discovered.

therapy would be at an increased risk of developing breast cancer.[392] Subsequent studies showed that the issue was not so simple.

Fibrocystic breast disease is a relatively common condition in which the breast contains lumps of fibrous matter or cysts. One alarming study showed that among women with fibrocystic breast disease, there was about twice the rate of estrogen use among women who had the disease.[422] A closer look at that study by its own authors led them to conclude that the cause might have been a detection bias rather than an effect of estrogen therapy. They explained, quite correctly, that women who begin taking ERT are probably having their breasts examined more often and more thoroughly, and that if they have fibrocystic breast disease, it will be detected more comprehensively than would be the case for the general population. The data showed that in nonusers of ERT, 108 women out of 111,000 in a health practice were revealed to have the disease. This worked out to 1 woman per 1,000 per year among nonusers of estrogen. The rate was higher in users. Out of the 75,000 users of ERT, 34 women were revealed to have fibrocystic breast disease. This amounts to a rate of 1.9 per 1,000 women per year, a higher rate than in the nonusers. So even a doubling in fibrocystic breast disease after estrogen, apparently before progestin was routinely used, yielded a very small impact (1.9 per 1,000) on the incidence of fibrocystic breast disease.

In contrast to this epidemiological investigation, endocrinologists who have been analyzing the relation of benign breast disease to hormones have concluded that disease results from a naturally occurring abnormal hormonal profile (too much estrogen with insufficient progesterone to counterbalance it) that will generally respond to progestin treatment.[563, 920a] In 1986 investigators in France and the U.S. who had both been actively involved in the study of fibrocystic breast disease and its relation to progestins argued for the beneficial role of progestins, particularly the very strongest ones (the nortestosterone derivatives discussed in the next chapter), in reversing fibrocystic breasts to the normal state.[820, 920a] Although these investigators did acknowledge the potential for this treatment to have adverse effects on cardiovascular health, as reviewed in Chapter 9, their conclusion was that appropriately balanced progestins could be used under the care of a knowledgeable endocrinologist to reverse fibrocystic breast disease and still protect the cardiovascular system. If you have fibrocystic breast disease and decide to seek treatment using progestins, you will need to find a knowledgeable physician who is up to date on both the cardiovascular and the breast responses to the hormone.

After hysterectomy, progestin with estrogen is optimal for breast health. Unfortunately there has not yet been enough detail published within the studies to define what the optimal dose is, but the knowledge is growing and your own reactions will probably reveal how your dose should be adjusted. Progestin by itself—that is, without any estrogen to balance it—does not appear to reduce the risk of breast cancer, although it does not increase it either.

Women naturally wonder whether benign breast disease in general predisposes to cancer of the breast, and fortunately some good information has become available.[223] In 1985 Drs. William Dupont and David Page reported, in the *New England Journal of Medicine*, their data on more than 10,000 patients with benign breast lesions; the women were followed for up to twenty-five years to learn which kinds of lesions increased the risk of breast cancer and which kinds did not. The study concluded that most women (70 percent) who undergo breast biopsy for benign disease are not at any increased risk for breast cancer. Specifically it showed that if a woman had a breast biopsy in which the specimen showed "a lack of proliferative disease," these women were not at any increased risk of cancer over those who had no breast disease. In addition, a family history of breast cancer does not increase the risk of breast cancer for those patients who do not have cysts. Unfortunately, the presence of the condition "atypia" (which means irregular, not conforming to type—in other words, proliferative disease), particularly when it is in conjunction with a family history, does place patients at substantial risk of breast cancer. The good news is that proliferative disease was absent in 70 percent of the women with benign breast disease.[223]

One explanation for the requirement for both estrogen and progestin in order to reduce the risk was suggested by Dr. Don Gambrell. One of the effects that estrogen produces on breast tissue is to cause an increase in the development of progestin receptors (tiny substances that attach to progestin and enable hormonal activation). Once the progestin receptors have been developed, progestin hormones can get to work to resist tumor growth.[286]

One other interesting effect has emerged from these studies: When women develop breast cancer, the death rate among those who have been using hormones is half that of the women who had not been using hormones.[287]

### Carbohydrate Metabolism and Diabetes

If your carbohydrate metabolism is functioning properly, any high dose of sugar will be rapidly cleared from your blood. Pancreatic hormones, particularly insulin, are responsible for this capacity to deal with sugar overloads. There has been some

### The Value of Mammograms

There has been some controversy in the biomedical literature as to the value of regular mammograms for women of different ages. It is reasonably well established that once menopause occurs (naturally or surgically induced), routine screening for breast cancer does seem to increase the survival rate (the percentage surviving in a given year) if cancer subsequently develops.[798] Regular screening also benefits women in reducing the death rate throughout the first seven years after detection.[912] One example of this improved prognosis is a study that followed 29,000 women aged 40 to 74. Half of the women were given a booklet teaching them how to do a self-examination of their breasts, and the other half were given no instruction. The results were quite different in the two groups. The women who had the instruction booklet had smaller breast tumors when tumors were detected, and a relative absence of invasive lesions into the lymph nodes.[894] Smaller tumors and less invasiveness are thought to portend well for recovery from breast cancer.

On the other hand, some biomedical experts believe that the simple act of detecting cancer accounts for a longer survival time without enhancing the quality of life. They conclude that while the cancer is discovered sooner and at an earlier stage, this does not actually promote any greater longevity.[821] Women still die of the disease at the same age, but now live with the fear and certain knowledge of their disease. Because the disease is detected earlier, they have the awareness of it but no guarantee of cure. There are those who believe that the constant search for breast tumors actually reduces the quality of life for women, producing a so-called cancer phobia. It is argued intelligently in the scientific literature that the longer survival time may merely reflect the earlier discovery, not an improved rate of cure.[821]

Obviously the fear of breast cancer is profound in many women, and the decision about whether or not to have regular mammograms rests with the woman and her physician. Until 1987 the data were quite clear in showing that the value of regular mammograms in detecting cancer of the breast became significant only after age 50. More recently there has been some suggestion from epidemiologists that women in their forties can profit from having regular mammograms, but the Breast Cancer Detection Project on which these suggestions are based have selected only the very high-risk women for its five annual screenings in the under-50 age groups ("high-risk" meaning an abnormal physical finding or personal or family history of breast cancer). In direct contrast, Dr. David Eddy and colleagues presented an exhaustive analysis of prospective data gathered from the HIP (Health Insurance Plan), a prospective, scientifically valid study of 62,000 women. They showed that there is no value in routine screening mammograms for women under the age of 50.[31, 226] For those at high risk because of family incidence, they can prove no benefit of routine screening but agree that it probably makes sense. I agree with both of these conclusions. Here are some examples of their discoveries for a 40-year-old woman:

| | |
|---|---|
| The chance that a mammogram will detect a hidden breast cancer when the physical examination of her breasts did not: | 3 in 10,000 |
| The chance of getting breast cancer some time in the next ten years: | 13 in 10,000 |
| The chance of dying from a diagnosed breast cancer sometime in the next ten years if she had no mammogram: | 82 in 10,000 |
| The chance of dying from a diagnosed breast cancer sometime in the next ten years if she had ten annual mammograms: | 60 in 10,000 |
| The consequent difference in chance of such death by annual screening with mammogram: | 22 in 10,000 |

While each woman must make her own decision, it helps to have some facts from which to form conclusions.*

*Baker L (1982) Breast cancer detection demonstration project: Five year summary report. *Cancer* 32:194–225

implication that certain oral contraceptive preparations produce bad effects on glucose (sugar) tolerance.[834, 965] Oral contraceptives are sex hormones that are given in very high concentration; they produce blood levels of estrogen and progesterone that exceed normal limits. In contrast, HRT is given in low doses that approximate the levels found among menstruating women. Two studies have been published to show that, in general, HRT regimens produce no danger to carbohydrate metabolism. Eight different regimens have so far been tested. All hormones produce carbohydrate metabolism responses that are within the normal limits.[836, 876]

In 1986 an investigation in Denmark compared diabetic women on sulphonylurea (a Finnish drug treatment) to nondiabetic women and to those with impaired glucose tolerance.[524] All the women were given a natural estrogen (17 B-estradiol) every day in doses that changed from 2 milligrams the first twenty-two days of the month to 1 milligram the last six. The progestin norethisterone acetate (1 milligram) was added for ten of the days each month. No impairment in carbohydrate metabolism was revealed in any of these women during six months of treatment.[524]

### Effects on the Liver

The liver has been studied to address whether HRT is safe, particularly in oral form. Whenever you take estrogens orally, hormones move through your mouth, throat, digestive tract, into and out of the stomach, and on into the intestines. When the hormone reaches the intestines, it is absorbed across the intestinal walls and then enters into the bloodstream. After it crosses the intestinal walls, the first place the estrogen goes in heavy concentration is to the liver. If you take estrogens by some other route, such as a cream, transdermal patch, or injections, the liver receives the estrogen after it has spent some time in the bloodstream and has been diluted by the fluid in the blood. Because oral estrogens reach the liver in much greater concentration than any other kind of estrogen, they have been assumed to potentially hyperstimulate the liver, that is, to cause it to become overactive, secreting excess amounts of the substances it normally produces. It was also assumed that such overproduction would be dangerous.

When hormones are taken orally, the liver does produce increased amounts of protein molecules, known as binding globulins, the function of which is to bind to sex hormones and to cholesterol and to carry these hormones and fats in the bloodstream.[5] However, this increased production appears to be not dangerous; in fact, some of these liver globulins are very beneficial for cardiovascular health. Oral estrogens tend to result in a lower level of cholesterol and a higher level of HDL-cholesterol. Both of these changes increase the cardiovascular health. (These reactions to oral hormones are discussed in chapters 7 and 9.) Moreover, a recent organ study in small mammals revealed that oral ingestion is not the only way of taking hormones that causes "liver effects." Whenever estrogen or another steroid hormone arrives at the liver via the blood circulation, regardless of the amount of time it has spent in the bloodstream, the extraction of hormone from the blood into liver cells is faster and more complete than in other body organs.[846] Therefore, in whatever way hormone enters the blood, it will affect the liver.

The most important point here is that the effects on the liver of oral HRT (provided the estrogen is a natural form) appear safe. No dangers have emerged after two decades of observation.

### Gallbladder Disease

While questions have recently been raised after one epidemiologic study suggested that oral HRT might increase the risk of gallstones, there are no scientifically valid studies comparing women with gallbladder disease who were given hormone therapies with those who were given placebos. In 1974 the epidemiologic Boston Collaborative Drug Surveillance Program created a stir with its suggestion that the risk for gallbladder disease in postmenopausal women who used the natural conjugated equine estrogens was 2.5 times the risk for gallbladder disease in women who did not use the hormone.[68] However, a closer look at the problem reveals a less threatening hormone scenario.

Gallbladder disease is very rare. If indeed it were true that by taking hormones, you increased the risk of a very rare disease from an extremely low level to a still extremely low level, the potential danger might be dwarfed by all the benefits that you achieve when you take HRT. What emerges from one study, however, is that the most significant influence on gallbladder disease appears to be obesity, which has been found to occur in about 75 percent of gallstone patients.[390] In that study, estrogen replacement therapy was found in fewer than 10 percent of the patients. This makes ERT one seventh as common as obesity among gallstone patients. The one repeating scenario that has occurred with the risk for gallstones appears to be the use of synthetic estrogens, specifically ethinyl estradiol. Thus, gallstones do not appear to be a principal risk factor for HRT, unless a woman is obese and takes synthetic estrogen. (See Appendix B for details on gallbladder disease.)

## Alternatives for Women with Contraindications

Some women should not take estrogens because they have an estrogen-dependent disease but can safely take progestagens as an HRT regimen. If you fall into this category, you should understand that there are benefits as well as detriments to such an approach. Taking medroxyprogesterone acetate, one of the commonly prescribed synthetic progestagens (see Chapter 7), does help with hot flashes and with bone metabolism.[83, 614, 775] It does not seem to matter whether the progestagen is taken by injection or pill if the dose is adequate. Unfortunately, side effects of unopposed progestagen are inevitable because the unopposed progestagen will diminish whatever natural estrogen effect your body is receiving from the remaining estrogen output of your adrenals and/or ovaries.[45, 515] High doses of unopposed progestin pose a potential risk to cardiovascular health, depending on which agent is used (see page 165). Also, vaginal atrophy is commonly reported by women who are taking unopposed progestagen.[775]

Women who suffer from dry vagina but have been told they cannot take estrogen might want to look into the vaginal creams containing estriol, one of the forms of estrogen. Research in Europe has shown that when applied at the local genital surfaces,[454, 757] daily doses of 0.5 milligrams of estriol cream will reverse the atrophy, meanwhile providing very little or no stimulatory effect on other body organs. One study showed that within two to three weeks of this dosage in the form of cream or suppositories, tenderness disappeared, painful intercourse was cured, and a normal appearance of the vaginal mucosa was reestablished. At the same time, other parameters of body function, such as results from endometrial biopsies and levels of gonadatropin, showed no change, nor did the estrone or estradiol levels in plasma show any change. You might also massage the vaginal skin (masturbate) regularly but gently. Research has shown that regular massage will help build up the vaginal epithelium in an estrogen-deficient woman. Estriol cream does not appear to be currently manufactured by any American drug company but can be compounded by a pharmacist if your physician special-orders it.

If you suffer from hot flashes but are unable to take estrogens, you might try other agents that do provide some good effects although they have shown themselves to be much less helpful than hormones. Some tests have shown good benefits with clonidine, an antihypertensive drug,[141, 892] although one study showed it to be no better than a placebo.[512] Alternatively, propranolol (a drug used to combat hypertension) was shown to produce some benefit in reducing hot flashes.[145] LH RH analogs (see page 91) have been studied to see whether they might help hot flashes, but they were shown to be not helpful.[799]

After pelvic surgery, many women grow increased facial hair, the result of relatively higher levels of androgens and lower levels of estrogens. If you are taking as much estrogen as you can safely handle and still suffer from this problem, you should seek medical help. A good endocrinologist should be able to evaluate your condition in light of recent discoveries about peripheral androgen conversion, which suggest that the estrogen that is circulating in the blood is converted into androgen at the skin tissue. While several drug therapies are available whose purpose is to alter the endocrine environment that produces the effects, the potential side effects that they entail may make you want to deal with the problem through cosmetic means.

Cosmetic treatments include hair removal through a variety of means, including shaving and using hot wax treatments, which treat the problem only very superficially and temporarily. A new machine appeared on the market in 1987. Priced at about $90, it removes one hair at a time, without burning or scarring the skin, and is as painless as tweezing hair. This machine, sold under the name Finally Free, seems to be an improvement over electrolysis, which requires that a needle be inserted into a straight hair shaft. (Curved hair shafts, which commonly occur, cannot be effectively treated with electrolysis.) This new machine, which has been tested on thousands of women, is effective and painless, and is being very well received. Finally Free works like a tweezers; one grasps a hair in the tweezers, holds it still for seven to thirty seconds, and then plucks out the hair. Widely offered through magazines and mail-order catalogs, it might be a useful approach for you.

Knowledge about HRT has developed enormously, giving medical science a greater capacity to safely and effectively help women live longer and live better. From the earlier use of excessive doses, which led to an increased risk for uterine cancer, to the present level of development, in which sophisticated prescriptions can reduce the risk of even this cancer, we have come a great distance. In large part, the work of thousands of medical researchers—in England, France, Germany, Scandinavia, Italy, Canada, the U.S., and other countries—has provided a better opportunity for hysterectomized women than would have been dreamed possible just ten years ago. Much work remains to be done, and it is important to stay alert to the limitations of current knowledge. Women will need to adjust their HRT regimens as better approaches become available. Even so, we are now at a point when safe and effective HRT prescriptions can be enjoyed. Chapter 7 provides a detailed discussion of hormone types and dosages.

# 7

# *The Hormones Used in HRT*

If you decide to take hormonal replacement therapy after surgery, many questions will have to be answered as you work with medical personnel to establish and adjust your dosage levels and balances. Which hormone or hormones should you take? How often should you take them? How much should be taken? The answers will depend very much on your own hormonal milieu.

Your ideal HRT regimen will be a highly individual design based upon a balancing of factors: your individual needs for cardiovascular and bone protection; cancer risks if you are in a high-risk group; the risk of gallbladder disease; and the way your body reacts to one hormone or another. An optimum regimen should make you feel good and should result in good bones, cardiovascular health, and healthy sexual functioning.

The dose of estrogen, progestagen, or testosterone has a critical impact on the way your body responds. Given in a high dose, a substance may produce unpleasant side effects, while low doses may be ineffective. Another important distinction in HRT regimens is the difference between synthetic hormones and natural hormones. Because most of the negative effects that have been attributed to high doses of HRT have come from synthetic hormones, you should avoid synthetics and instead take a natural form whenever available.

As you and your physician plan an HRT regimen, you will need to consider both your immediate health needs and your long-term health plans. Is your Kupperman score high (see page 124)? Has radioimmunoassay shown your estrogen level to be low? Are your bones dense? Are your blood lipids in good shape? Are you suffering sexually? Are you depressed? As you define your needs and learn what works for you and what doesn't, you can determine which of the three classes of hormones make sense for your circumstance.

There are no clear-cut guidelines yet available to help you and your doctor establish an appropriate starting dose from which you can then work toward adjustment and refinements. Based on my observations at medical meetings and my reading of medical articles, I see a tendency on the part of doctors to seek a few "standard" doses for all patients. Intense competition from the drug companies that manufacture these substances can lead to a disproportionate number of advertisements of one or another of the brands. For these reasons, women need to be aware of the effects of particular hormones as well as the signals their bodies send about their own unique responses. Twice-a-year health checkups to monitor your hormone-responsive systems (bone density, cholesterol levels and blood pressure, sexual muscle function, feeling of well-being) will tell you when you need to increase or decrease the dosages. It is possible that the HRT dose should be lowered as women age, to accommodate lower physiological needs; research studies on this topic are needed.

You will want to watch for side effects, such as breast tenderness, which indicates that you have too much estrogen, or irritability, which may indicate excess synthetic progestin. Sometimes it takes two or three months for your body to adjust to the regimen. Some women do better on one form of hormone than another, and experimentation may be necessary to see what is best for you. It will be important to record your reactions on a calendar and to work with medical personnel who are sensitive to your responses to hormones. Over the years you will want to have an ongoing dialogue as your body's needs change.

Three kinds of hormones (estrogens, progestagens, and androgens, principally testosterone) form the pool from which HRT regimens are built.

- *Estrogen* forms the foundation of HRT regimens because it plays many fundamental roles in maintaining a woman's health and well-being. It causes bone to be dense. It contributes to lower cholesterol levels. It promotes beautiful skin and breasts. It promotes vaginal moisture, and it has many more functions.
- *Progestagens* have many influences that are beneficial when appropriately prescribed, including reduction of the incidence of breast cancer and an apparent improvement of endorphin secretion. If you take estrogen, you should also take progesterone.
- *Testosterone* therapy is relatively unresearched, and while some sophisticated medical centers do offer it, most are awaiting guidance from research publications. If you take testosterone with your estrogen, you won't need progestins.

There are many different kinds of estrogens as well as various forms of progestagens currently on the market. Some have been studied much more extensively than others. The technical information in this chapter will be useful for the woman who is working to establish her ideal HRT prescription with the help of her medical personnel.

Table 5 provides a list of HRT brands and doses currently available in the United States.[283] Some Canadian brands are listed in Table 6.

### WAYS TO TAKE HORMONAL REPLACEMENT THERAPY

Before considering the hormones in detail, let's look at the ways they can be taken.

*Orally.* Taking hormones by mouth is the method that has been most completely studied in the literature.* Both estrogens and progestagens are available as pills to be taken by mouth. The advantages of this route are: it is effective, it is easy, it is clean,

---

*Studies include  231, 241, 242, 289, 311, 408, 409, 553, 669, 770, 918.

**Table 5.** *HRT Brands Sold in the U.S.* *

| ESTROGENS | | | | |
|---|---|---|---|---|
| Name | Estrogen | Mg | Manufacturer | Method of Delivery |
| Premarin | Conjugated estrogens | 0.3 | Ayerst | Oral |
| | | 0.625 | | |
| | | 0.9 | | |
| | | 1.25 | | |
| | | 2.5 | | |
| Estrace | Micronized estradiol | 1.0 | Mead Johnson | Oral |
| | | 2.0 | | |
| Estratab | Esterified estrogens | 0.3 | Reid-Rowell | Oral |
| | | 0.625 | | |
| | | 1.25 | | |
| | | 2.5 | | |
| Ogen | Estropipate | 0.625 | Abbott | Oral |
| | | 1.25 | | |
| | | 2.5 | | |
| | | 5.0 | | |
| Estinyl | Ethinyl estradiol | 0.02 | Schering | Oral |
| | | 0.05 | | |
| | | 0.5 | | |
| Estrovis | Quinestrol | 0.1 | Parke-Davis | Oral |

| Product | Generic | Dose | Manufacturer | Form |
|---|---|---|---|---|
| Premarin Vaginal Cream | Conjugated estrogens | 0.625 mg/gm | Ayerst | Vaginal cream |
| Estrace Vaginal Cream | 17beta-estradiol | 0.1 mg/gm | Mead Johnson | Vaginal cream |
| Ogen Vaginal Cream | Estropipate | 1.5 mg/gm | Abbott | Vaginal cream |
| Ortho Dienestrol Cream | Dienestrol | 0.01% | Ortho | Vaginal cream |
| Estragard Cream | Dienestrol | 0.01% | Reid-Rowell | Vaginal cream |
| Diethylstilbestrol Suppositories | Diethylstilbestrol | 0.1 mg/gm 0.5 mg/gm | Lilly | Vaginal suppository |
| Depo-Estradiol | Estradiol cypionate | 1 mg/ml 5 mg/ml | Upjohn | Injection |
| Delestrogen | Estradiol valerate | 10 mg/ml 20 mg/ml 40 mg/ml | Squibb | Injection |
| Estraval | Estradiol valerate | 10 mg/ml 20 mg/ml | Reid-Rowell | Injection |
| Estrapel† | Estradiol pellet | 25 mg | Bartor, Progynon | Pellet |
| Estraderm | Transdermal estradiol | 0.05 mg/day 0.1 mg/day | Ciba-Geigy | Patch |

## PROGESTINS, TESTOSTERONE (androgens), ESTROGEN/ANDROGEN COMBINATIONS

| Name | Progestogen | Mg | Manufacturer | Method of Delivery |
| --- | --- | --- | --- | --- |
| Provera | Medroxyprogesterone acetate | 10 | Upjohn | Oral |
| Curretab | Medroxyprogesterone acetate | 10 | Reid-Rowell | Oral |
| Amen | Medroxyprogesterone acetate | 10 | Carnick | Oral |
| Aygestin | Norethindrone acetate | 5 | Ayerst | Oral |
| Norlutate | Norethindrone acetate | 5 | Parke-Davis | Oral |
| Norlutin | Norethindrone | 5 | Parke-Davis | Oral |
| Megace | Megesterol acetate | 20 / 40 | Bristol-Myers | Oral |
| Ovrette | Norgestrel | 0.075 | Wyeth | Oral |
| Micronor | Norethindrone | 0.35 | Ortho | Oral |
| Nor-Q.D. | Norethindrone | 0.35 | Dyntex | Oral |
| | Progesterone Vaginal Suppositories | 25 | — | Vaginal suppository |

| Name | Androgen | Mg/ml | Manufacturer | Method of Delivery |
| --- | --- | --- | --- | --- |
| Oreton | Methyl testosterone | 5 mg | Schering | Oral |
| Metandren | Methyl testosterone | 5 mg | Ciba | Oral |
| Halotestin | Fluoxymesterone | 5 mg | Upjohn | Oral |
| Fluoxymesterone | Fluoxymesterone | 5 mg | Reid-Rowell | Oral |
| Depo-testosterone | Testosterone cypionate | 50 mg/ml | Upjohn | Injection |

| Name | Androgen | Mg/ml | Manufacturer | Method of Delivery |
|---|---|---|---|---|
| Delatestryl | Testosterone enanthate | 100 mg/ml | Squibb | Injection |
| Testopel | Testosterone pellets | 75 mg | Bartor | Injection |
| Oreton | Testosterone pellets | 75 mg | Progynon | Injection |

| Name | Combination | Mg | Manufacturer | Method of Delivery |
|---|---|---|---|---|
| Estratest tablets | Esterified estrogens Methyl testosterone | 1.25 mg 2.5 mg | Reid-Rowell | Oral |
| Estratest H.S. tablets | Esterified estrogens Methyl testosterone | 0.625 mg 1.25 mg | Reid-Rowell | Oral |
| Premarin with Methyltestosterone | Conjugated estrogens Methyl testosterone | 1.25 mg 10 mg | Ayerst | Oral |
| Premarin with Methyltestosterone | Conjugated estrogens Methyl testosterone | 0.625 mg 5 mg | Ayerst | Oral |
| Dopo-Tostadiol | Estradiol cypionate Testosterone cypionate | 2 mg 50 mg | Upjohn | Injection |
| Estrapel | Estradiol pellet (given with testosterone pellets) | 25 mg | Bartor Progynon | Pellet |

*Table 5 data courtesy of Dr. R. Don Gambrell
†Temporarily suspended by FDA

*Table 6. HRT Brands Sold in Canada*

## ESTROGENS

| Name | Estrogen | Mg | Manufacturer | Method of Delivery |
|---|---|---|---|---|
| Premarin | Conjugated estrogens | .30 | Ayerst | Oral |
| | | .625 | | |
| | | .90 | | |
| | | 1.25 | | |
| | | 2.50 | | |
| CES Tab | Conjugated estrogens | .625 | ICN Canada | Oral |
| | | 1.25 | | |
| EstroMed | Conjugated estrogens | 1.25 | Medic Lab | Oral |
| Conjugated Estrogens | Conjugated estrogens | .625 | Pharmascience | Oral |
| | | 1.25 | | |
| Oestrogenes Conjuguees | Conjugated estrogens | 1.25 | ProDoc Laboratories | Oral |
| NeoEstrone | Esterified estrogens | .625 | Neolab | Oral |
| | | 1.25 | | |
| Estinyl | Ethinyl estradiol | .02 | Schering Canada | Oral |
| | | .05 | | |
| | | .50 | | |
| Estrace | Estradiol | 1.00 | Bristol Laboratories of Canada | Oral |
| | | 2.00 | | |
| Premarin | Conjugated estrogens | .625 | Ayerst | Vaginal cream |
| Oestrilin | Estrone | 1.00 | Desbergers | Vaginal cream |

## ESTROGENS

| Name | Estrogen | Mg | Manufacturer | Method of Delivery |
|---|---|---|---|---|
| Neo Estrone | Estrone | 1.00 | Neolab | Vaginal cream |
| Oestrilin cones | Estrone | .25 | Desbergers | Vaginal suppository |
| Premarin | Conjugated estrogens | 25.00 | Ayerst | Injection |
| Femogen forte | Estrone | 5.00 | Stickley & Co | Injection |
| Delestrogen | Estradiol valerate | 10.00 | Squibb Canada | Injection |
| Estradiol valerate | Estradiol valerate | 20.00 | K Line Pharms | Injection |
| Femogex | Estradiol valerate | 20.00 | Stickley & Co | Injection |
| Neo-Diol | Estradiol valerate | 20.00 | Neolab | Injection |
| Estraderm | Estradiol | 2.00 | Ciba Pharms Div. of | Patch |
| | | 4.00 | Ciba Geigy | |
| | | 8.00 | | |

## PROGESTINS, TESTOSTERONE, ESTROGEN/ANDROGEN COMBINATIONS

| Name | Progestin | Mg | Manufacturer | Method of delivery |
|---|---|---|---|---|
| Provera | Medroxyprogesterone acetate | 5.00 10.00 | Upjohn Canada | Oral |
| Colprone | Medrogestone | 5.00 | Ayerst | Oral |
| Micronor | Norethindrone | .35 | Ortho Pharmaceutical Canada | Oral |
| Norlutate | Norethindrone acetate | 5.000 | Parke Davis Div. Warner-Lambert | Oral |

**PROGESTINS, TESTOSTERONE, ESTROGEN/ANDROGEN COMBINATIONS**

| Name | Progestin | Mg | Manufacturer | Method of delivery |
|------|-----------|-----|--------------|-------------------|

| Name | Testosterone | Mg | Manufacturer | Method of Delivery |
|------|--------------|-----|--------------|--------------------|
| Metandren | Methyltestosterone† | 10.00<br>25.00 | Ciba Geigy | Oral |
| Metandren | Methyltestosterone† | 10.00<br>25.00 | Ciba Geigy | Buccal (under the tongue) |

| Name | Combination | Mg | Manufacturer | Method of Delivery |
|------|-------------|-----|--------------|--------------------|
| Premarin Methyltestosterone | Methyltestosterone and conjugated estrogens | 5/.625<br>10/1.25 | Ayerst | Oral |
| Ortho 1/35 | Norethindrone and ethynil estradiol | 1/.035 | Ortho Pharmaceutical Canada | Oral |
| Climacteron‡ | Testosterone enanthate benzilic acid and estradiol dienanthate and estradiol benzoate | 150.00<br>7.50<br>1.00 | Frosst Div. Merck Frosst Canada | Monthly injection |

*Information courtesy of the Drug Identification Division in Canada, obtained through Dr. Sabine Swierenga.
†These testosterones are not reported on in the HRT studies reviewed here.
‡This is the injectible used by Dr. Sherwin in her study of treatment for libido loss.

and it seems to protect best against cardiovascular disease by increasing the beneficial lipids in blood and decreasing the deleterious ones (see page 207).

*As a cream.* In the United States and Canada, only estrogen is marketed in cream form. It is generally applied with an applicator at the vagina. In Europe, both estrogen and progesterone creams are available. They are commonly spread over the arms, where they are rapidly absorbed and move into the bloodstream. With the vaginal cream you can achieve beneficial local estrogen effects with a lower dose.[242, 311, 372] For example, if you do not want to have much estrogen circulating in your blood but are experiencing vaginal atrophy and dryness, the application of low doses of estrogen cream directly at the vagina will have effects there without having profound effects on the blood. However, high vaginal doses will enter the blood.

Until natural progesterone becomes routinely available in the United States, it will have to be compounded by a druggist, and this will entail greater cost. Druggists can obtain natural progesterone powder, which is made in a laboratory but is chemically equivalent to the progesterone found in nature. The powder can be blended into a cream base that is applied on the arms for absorption into the bloodstream. In France, natural progesterone and estrogen are routinely manufactured by pharmaceutical companies for this form of hormone delivery. Hopefully, such a route will someday be manufactured by American companies.

Women should be cautioned not to use vaginal creams before heterosexual intercourse. They rub off onto the penis and are absorbed into the man's body, increasing his blood levels of female hormones.[241]

*In a patch.* In 1987 a new form of cream called the *transdermal,* or *patch,* long available in a number of European countries.[119, 242, 487] began to make its way into the United States. The patch comes as an estrogen-filled bandage, about the size of a half dollar, that is applied to the buttocks. The bandage is replaced every one to three days with a new one, and a woman can increase the dose by adding more bandages. The hormone passes through the bandage, enters the skin, and is absorbed into the bloodstream. Some women find this method convenient, but others report that it is annoying, particularly if they are athletically active; swimming can loosen the patch, as can sweating. One other disadvantage of the patch is that it leaves an unsightly mark on the skin that takes several days to fade. The buttocks become covered with fading patch marks.

Several studies of the patch have been published, but we lack a full picture of the benefits and detriments of this route. For example, although the oral form of estrogen and the vaginal synthetic estrogens both have been shown to increase the protective blood lipids that serve to prevent cardiovascular disease, the arm cream forms and the transdermal patch do not usually have this beneficial effect.[119, 241, 487] Why? Apparently the nonvaginal creams gain their entry into the bloodstream, become diluted, and approach the liver—where the blood lipids and binding globulins are produced—only after dilution. Although in the early 1980s it was widely believed that this was an optimal situation, increasing evidence of the benefits of these liver globulins has altered that conclusion. It may be, depending on the particular circumstance, that you want to get increased binding globulins; in other circumstances, you may not want these liver effects. (For further details, see page 140 on binding globulins in the liver, and Chapter 9 on cardiovascular health.)

*In a sublingual tablet.* Certain kinds of estrogen pills are effectively absorbed when placed under the tongue. The pill melts and is absorbed into the mucosa of the cells in the mouth and then reaches the bloodstream.[90] The sublingual route, like the transdermal route, reaches the liver in much lower quantities than the oral dose. Although a number of years ago there was some interest in this route of hormone delivery, there do not seem to be any other studies yet published that evaluate how effective it is.

*Subcutaneous pellets.* These require surgical insertion every month or so. A little pellet of hormones (estrogen, progesterone, or testosterone) is surgically inserted into a fatty region (for example, the lower stomach), just under the skin, where the hormone is slowly absorbed.[519] The advantage is that you do not have to remember to take daily doses. The disadvantage is the inconvenience of requiring medical intervention, as well as the inability to reduce the dose if you feel the need to lower it within the month.

*Injection.* The injected hormone (estrogen, progesterone, or testosterone) is immediately received in the bloodstream where it becomes diluted rapidly and has its effects all over the body. As with the other nonoral routes, the liver receives a diluted dose rather than a highly concentrated dose. With the diluted dose, the liver does not receive as strong a signal to produce the beneficial lipids that promote cardiovascular health.

If you take hormones by one route and find that it is not optimal for you, you can switch to a different route that suits you better.

## THE ESTROGENS

Companies vary in the way they classify the estrogens. One useful way of categorizing estrogens divides them into four classes:[67]
- *The natural estrogens,* which include 17-β estradiol, micronized estradiol, estradiol valerate, estrone, and estriol
- *Conjugated estrogens,* such as Premarin®, which derive from pregnant mare urine
- *Alkyl substituted estrogen steroids,* which include the synthetics such as ethinyl estradiol and mestranol
- *Nonsteroid substances* with estrogen effects, such as DES (diethylstilbestrol)

"Natural" estrogens can be made in laboratories. They are not taken from one person's body for use by another. What distinguishes a natural form from other forms is that in the natural form the molecular configuration is identical to what is found in nature. The synthetic forms were the first to be used. In Great

Britain synthetic use was predominant until the mid-1970s, when a change gradually took place, and the use of natural estrogens has been steadily increasing ever since.[94] This pattern of the gradual acceptance of natural forms is being followed in the United States also.

### Synthetic versus Natural Estrogens

You should avoid synthetic estrogens because they sometimes have adverse effects.[66, 553, 784, 876] For example, in an attempt to adjust dosage to relieve menopausal symptoms, women were tested first with ethinyl estradiol (a synthetic) and subsequently with Premarin® (the natural conjugated equine estrogen). Blood levels of triglycerides increased on the synthetic estrogen, but not on the conjugated equine estrogen.[66] In fact, natural estrogens often reduced triglyceride levels.[67] Although there is probably no danger in an increased blood level of triglyceride when the cholesterol-rich lipids are favorable, the fact that synthetics increase blood triglycerides would caution against them if natural estrogens are available.[174]

Synthetic estrogen replacement produces exaggerated liver and kidney changes. In one study, the synthetic estrogen ethinyl estradiol was applied as a vaginal cream, and it produced profound alterations in liver activity.[784] Although this study was looking at the role of ethinyl estradiol in contraception, the doses in the study were standard for HRT regimens, and the investigators later showed an equivalent effect in HRT regimens. Liver proteins were exaggerated three- to tenfold by conjugated equine estrogen compared to the pure natural estrogens, but synthetic estrogens were even more potent, producing one-thousand-fold greater productions of liver globulins.[553] The study also looked at the way angiotensin responds to the different estrogen preparations (angiotensin increases blood pressure in several ways). The natural estrogens were equally potent. Premarin® (natural) produces 3.5 times greater response in angiotensin, DES (synthetic) produces 13 times greater response, and ethinyl estradiol (synthetic) produces a 232 times more potent response than the natural estrogens.

Glucose tolerance has also been considered in connection with synthetic and natural estrogen therapies. None of the women on Premarin® (conjugated equine estrogen) or the natural estradiol valerate showed abnormal glucose tolerance, but three of the ten women on the synthetic ethinyl estradiol did show abnormal glucose tolerance.[876]

It should be emphasized that even though ethinyl estradiol produced exaggerated liver and kidney responses, studies have failed to show any danger associated with these changes. Still, why use synthetics when natural estrogens are available?

The natural estrogens have the least side effects of any estrogen form and should be considered your first choice when selecting an estrogen regimen. The conjugated equine estrogens appear to be very close to the natural human estrogens.

### Conjugated Equine Estrogens (Premarin®)

Conjugated equine estrogens are considered to be a natural hormone since they are derived from nature (from the urine of horses). However, the conjugated equine estrogens also contain substances, apparently harmless ones, not found in humans. For this reason, they are listed separately.

Conjugated equine estrogens, taken by mouth, have been widely studied and appear to be quite safe on all systems evaluated. The following report shows the kind of scientific investigations being published.

Thirty-six postmenopausal women more than one year past their last menstrual period were studied and compared to twenty premenopausal women who served as controls. The postmenopausal women showed an increased urine calcium loss (a measure of how much calcium is being lost from the body and probably therefore from bone). It decreased when conjugated equine estrogen was given, provided the dose of Premarin® was 0.3 milligrams per day or higher. As the dose got much higher, to

1.25 milligrams per day, there was a significantly greater decrease in the calcium lost.[302] This is good; the less calcium lost, the better. The vaginal cells recovered from atrophy only at the high dose of 1.25 milligrams per day. Thyroid function was not changed after estrogen replacement therapy; the premenopausal control groups were equal to the postmenopausal groups after receiving Premarin®. Liver function did as expected: the three binding globulins that were studied increased. The more hormone taken, the more these liver proteins were manufactured.[302] Renin substrate, also produced in the liver, increased above the premenopausal controls at all doses. In young women, this can cause increased blood pressure and negative blood lipid effects; however, other studies have shown that in menopausal women an increased renin substrate level does not have any negative effects on cardiovascular health.[174]

Natural estrogens do produce one known negative effect. Oral conjugated equine estrogen treatment may reduce the circulating levels of unbound testosterone by about 30 percent[558] because of an increase in the liver protein SHBG (sex hormone binding globulin), which binds up the free testosterone. The testosterone that is produced gets attached to the binding proteins. When testosterone is bound to binding proteins, it is unable to have its usual effect on cells. Only when hormone is traveling free in the blood can it enter cells and do work. This may explain why some posthysterectomy patients who take estrogen replacement therapy have a problem with libido. It may be that the oral estrogen replacement therapy actually reduces the libido by further reducing the levels of free testosterone. Presumably, if conjugated equine estrogen leads to a reduction in free testosterone, other oral estrogen replacement therapy regimens would have the same effect. The specific studies do not appear to have been published as yet, but if you experience a lowering of libido, one remedy is to add low doses of testosterone to your regimen. Another remedy is to switch to the pure natural estrogens, which will not stimulate the liver proteins (SHBG) as much.

### Other Natural Estrogens

Studies of other natural estrogens have shown beneficial and safe results from their use. After ovariectomy, ten women aged 30 to 50 were given a twenty-day treatment of 2 milligrams per day of estradiol valerate, and their blood was measured four different times over the next twenty days. Despite the very high urinary estrogen (taking in more means more is urinated out), there was no significant change in blood cholesterol, triglycerides, or any of the seventeen coagulation (clotting) factors.[770] Another study showed that estradiol valerate pills rapidly increased the blood levels of the estrogens.[231] One study that compared the lipid response to two different kinds of estrogens (oral 17-β estradiol and skin cream 17-β estradiol) showed that both forms, at the doses given, produced a threefold elevation in the average level of estrogen circulating in the blood.[241] This is good news for an estrogen-deficient woman.

Hundreds of similar studies have filled in the picture. Inevitably, when you take estrogen there are effects on a variety of other hormone levels and on the manufacture of proteins in the liver.[234, 709] Generally, the more hormone you take, the greater the effect.[736] Many of these estrogen effects promote health: of bone, cardiovascular system, sexuality, and the feeling of well-being. Each of these aspects is discussed separately in subsequent chapters.

### How Much Estrogen Should Be Taken, and How Often?

Estrogen should probably be taken every day, and women who have undergone pelvic surgery that influences the output of ovarian hormones (that is, ovariectomy or hysterectomy) should take an estrogen regimen that is balanced with progestagens. Before studies revealed the protective role of progestins in balancing estrogen, a few hormone-free days each month were prescribed in order to induce a withdrawal bleed (see page 60) that relieves the potential for excesses of estrogen. Now that research studies have shown that progestin will balance (oppose) estrogen and that progestin has value even when you no longer have a uterus, there is no logical or scientifically validated reason to have hormonal deprivation for several days each month.

Some estrogens are probably optimally taken twice each day—for example, half the dose in the morning and half in the evening. With your doctor's guidance, you will need to experiment before you understand your own body's reaction.

What dose works best for you and at what frequency has to be a very personal response to your individual biology. If your menopausal symptoms are severe, you will probably want to start at a higher dose. If your symptoms are mild, you will probably want to start at a lower dose.

If you are thin you will probably need to take more estrogen than if you are fat. If you are tall—that is, if you have a large body frame to support—you will probably need more estrogen than your smaller friend. Over time you will learn to sense when the dose is right; you will come to understand how the right amount feels, what an overdose feels like, and what too little feels like. Ultimately you will be balancing the protective effects of adequate estrogen (sense of well-being, adequate bone mass, good cardiovascular health) against the negative effects of bloating and nausea. If your symptoms are intolerable, adjust the dosage downward; if they are mild, you might do best to persist for two to three months. If the dose is too low, hot flashes will probably be your signal that your body is not getting enough.

Some women have a problem with fluid retention when they take estrogen. Three remedies are available: take a day or two off hormones each week; take higher doses of progestagen to better balance the estrogen; or lower the dose of estrogen.

When some women take ERT, their breasts become swollen and sore. Several different studies have shown that the tendency to experience this symptom, known as mastalgia, increases in groups of women who take excessively high doses of estrogen[67, 99, 908] and in groups who take high doses of the 19-nortestosterone progestagens.[920] Breast tenderness can be corrected in two ways: by reducing the estrogen or nortestosterone dose, or by opposing the estrogen with the 17α-progestins or natural progesterone.[67, 908]

Women who have had a hysterectomy to correct endometriosis must watch their estrogen intake because estrogen stimulates endometriotic tissue. If any has been left behind and you take estrogen, there is a possibility (apparently quite rare) that you will experience a reblooming of the disease. However, if you oppose the estrogen with progesterone in a dose that does not stimulate the overgrowth, you may be able to manage very comfortably on HRT. In such cases it is important to find a physician who is experienced with endocrine manipulation.

Because estrogen dosing is more an art than a science, respect your own reactions as a valid expression of your unique biology. How long will it take to get the dose right? The answer is as varied as are women. Some are lucky and adjust immediately; others take a longer time.

## THE PROGESTAGENS

Progesterone serves an important role in a well-balanced HRT regimen. Progesterone counterbalances the forces of estrogen in ways that are only just coming to be understood. In concert with estrogen, it promotes secretion of the beta endorphins, substances that enhance the sense of well-being. It also appears to play a significant role in the prevention of female-system cancers.

The three terms *progesterone, progestagen,* and *progestin* are used somewhat interchangeably.

*Progesterone* refers to the natural progesterone made by the body or to the chemical substitute that is identical in molecular form.

*Progestagen* (sometimes spelled progestogen) refers to a synthetic hormone that has effects reflective of the way natural progesterone works in the body.

*Progestin* is a synonym for *progestagen*, and the terms are used interchangeably.

We know less about the progestagens than we do about the estrogens because the use of progestagens is more recent. Progestin opposition is only now being studied for the benefits it brings to a posthysterectomized body. As with estrogens, when the progestins were first used as HRT, synthetic forms were very common. More recently, studies of natural progesterone have been making their way into the biomedical literature (see tables 5 and 6).

Slight changes in the molecular formation have profound influences on the strength and activity of the progestagens.[756] Among the synthetic progestagens, two key classes are commonly prescribed:

*Medroxyprogesterone acetate* (MPA), a progesterone type. Provera® is the most common brand name.

The *19-nortestosterone derivatives* (such as *norethisterone, norgestrel, norethindrone*),[266] which are derivatives of testosterone. Their molecular form is changed into progestins.

The strength of different progestins can be measured by the effects they produce.[227] The progestins serve to maintain pregnancy in an animal, to prevent a premature delivery, and to prepare the endometrium in its buildup of tissue during each nonpregnant cycle. When different progestins have been tested on these three biological systems in order to determine doses, some inconsistencies occur. Compared to other progestins, one form of progestin sometimes has a very strong effect on one system, for example the capacity to maintain pregnancy, while the same progestin may have a weaker effect on another biological system, such as the development of the endometrium.

Another way that progestagens are compared to each other is by evaluating either their *androgenic potency* (the capacity to produce androgen-like biological effects), their *estrogenic po-*

tency, or their *antiestrogenic potency* (capacity to produce effects that mimic what happens when estrogen is diminished, such as dry vagina or aging skin).[72]

Again, there is a lot of overlap between one synthetic form and the other and between the synthetics and natural progesterone.[72] Sometimes a particular progestin is strong in one biological system but weak in another. For example, the 19-nortestosterone derivatives are strongly antiestrogenic and thus can produce vaginal dryness and painful intercourse. Natural progesterone and MPA are not so antiestrogenic on vaginal cells.[72]

Table 9 (page 220) displays the high and low dose levels of the oral progestins based on their cardiovascular health effects.

### Synthetic versus Natural Progestagens

Natural progesterone may be difficult to obtain in the United States in 1988 or 1989, although your druggist should be able to compound it for you. By the early 1990s it should become more easily available. The natural form is available in Europe, in both pill and cream forms.

In the early 1980s scientific papers began to be published evaluating the difference between the effects of the synthetic progestagens and natural progesterone on a variety of body systems.[240, 658, 948] The differences appear to be profound. Among the synthetic progestagens, the 19-nortestosterone type appeared to have the strongest influences on body systems. Some of these were negative, particularly in producing adverse effects on cardiovascular health.[284, 382, 918] The nortestosterone derivatives— among them lynestrol, norethisterone acetate, and levonorgestrel—are the strongest, most potent antiestrogens.[820, 920]

Potent antiestrogens are sometimes desirable in treating fibrocystic breast disease and other estrogen-dependent disease. However, these strong antiestrogens may have adverse effects on cardiovascular health. Natural estrogens tend to promote cardiovascular health, while those agents that are antiestrogenic tend to lower the benefit, sometimes to the point of increasing risk. It all boils down to a relative balance of competing influences: each of the hormones has its value—and when the levels get too high, each of the hormones has its risk. Thus it is not surprising that later studies showed that the negative effects of certain potent progestins come only with the higher doses.*

Natural progesterone is probably better for you than synthetic progestagen unless you are trying to overcome a problem like fibrocystic breast disease (see page 133). One other benefit of natural progesterone, as opposed to a synthetic progestin, was suggested by Drs. Lorraine Dennerstein and Graham Burrows. These Australian investigators have been responsible for educating us about women's emotional responses to progestins. They suggest that natural progesterone has a hypnotic effect, a feeling that is generally perceived as pleasant, while the synthetic progestins may induce a sense of tension and irritability in some women.[203] Unpleasant feelings have been frequently reported in response to synthetic progestins, particularly in the high dose range described in the footnote below.[920] Because definitive research on this subject will probably not appear in the literature before 1992 or later, it is helpful for you to be aware of what hormones you are taking and of how you respond. If one hormone does not work well, a different one may.

In 1980 Dr. Malcolm Whitehead and his colleagues, after studying five postmenopausal women with intact ovaries, concluded: "Naturally occurring progesterone may not [harmfully] alter blood lipids and, as it is stable for two years and cheap, it may be useful for combination with estrogen in the menopausal regimens."[948] Dr. Whitehead's highly respected group works in Great Britain.

Other investigators also have concluded that the natural oral progesterone is preferable to the synthetics.[240]

*High doses include the following: for levonorgestrel, 0.25 mg/day; for norethisterone, 5 mg/day; for norethisterone acetate, 5 mg/day; for norgestrel, 0.075 mg/day; for lynestrol, 5 mg/day.[240, 243, 284, 382, 918, 920] Cyproterone acetate, an antiandrogen that has progestational properties, also is shown to be high in dose when it is given at 5 mg/day; at that level it is responsible for a profound suppression of the estrogen levels.[882]

Several recent research studies that have begun to provide information on both synthetic and natural progestin doses are reviewed on page 168.

What conclusions can we draw about the progestagens? The first is the importance of keeping alert for new studies as they become published. Research on progestagen use in postmenopausal women has only begun to appear in the literature. For this reason, we must realize how sketchy our knowledge is and make the best of what is available. Natural progesterone appears to be the safest way to take this beneficial hormone.

### How Much Progesterone Should Be Taken, and How Often?

How can you know if you are overdosing on this hormone? If you begin to experience antiestrogenic effects, such as dry vagina, it may be that your dose needs to be adjusted downward. If you begin to have negative feelings or irritability, you may want to locate a natural progesterone source.

The more estrogen you have in your system, the more progesterone you will need as a counterbalance. The less estrogen you have, the less progesterone you will need.

The idea that commonly prescribed progestin doses might be too high began to appear in the literature in the early 1980s. The intricate studies by Dr. Whitehead's group led them to suggest that a Provera® dose of 5 milligrams a day might be considered a high dose, judging by the biochemical data. This was half the dose commonly being prescribed at the time (and half the level being routinely recommended for the Progestin Challenge Test; see page 63). They also showed that the 19-nortestosterone doses could be lowered and still achieve the desired effects.[947]

In 1982 Dr. Whitehead's group published a study in the *American Journal of Obstetrics and Gynecology* in which they concluded that they suspected that even lower doses of progestin will be fully adequate; they were currently recommending 1 milligram per day of norethindrone (one fifth the dose reported in other studies described above) and 75 μg of norgestrel (as

### Studies on Synthetic and Natural Progestins

One of the synthetic progestins, *norethisterone,* has been used in menopausal HRT.[2, 242] At a dose of 5 milligrams twice each day for one year, ovariectomized women maintained their bone, in contrast with ovariectomized women on no HRT, who lost bone.[2] However, although the norethisterone was good at maintaining bone, a different group of ovariectomized women in their forties, who took 5 milligrams a day and were compared with a control group, did not do so well on lipids. Their beneficial lipids (HDL-Ch) were reduced in response to the norethisterone, and the dangerous lipids (LDL-Ch) were increased.[243] Thus the same dose that helped bone health hurt cardiovascular health. (Chapter 9 discusses the blood lipids.)

Another synthetic progestagen, *norgestrel,* has also been studied. As an oral contraceptive in doses of 150 μg per day combined with synthetic estrogen, negative effects were revealed in glucose tolerance and in insulin response.[965] Studies of menopausal use of norgestrel showed negative effects on the lipids at doses* of 120 μg per day[240] and 250 μg per day.[658] At doses of 30 micrograms per day, oral *levonorgestrel* was well tolerated when given every day with estrogen cream (1.5 milligrams).[389]

In contrast to the synthetic progestins from the 19-nortestosterone family (norethisterone and norgestrel), the synthetic progestin *medroxyprogesterone acetate* (MPA) has performed better.[303, 657, 873, 949] Both combined with estrogen and used by itself, MPA has been studied to determine its effects on bone health. Provera® (one brand of MPA), in the commonly prescribed dose of 10 milligrams a day for ten days each cycle, did not alter the amount of calcium that was excreted from the urine or any other parameter of bone metabolism. This is reassuring news since estrogen does favorably improve these measures,[394, 601] and Provera® does not alter the benefits of estrogen. The initial doses commonly prescribed for Provera® were 10 milligrams per day for ten to twelve days per cycle; more recent work led Dr. Whitehead and his group to suggest that this dose could be lowered.[949] As Provera® doses are lowered, bone should be fine. Norethindrone and norgestrel doses also, they believed, could be lowered; and when they are lowered, negative effects do not seem to occur.[949] In fact one research group, publishing in 1985, concluded that the adverse effects of these progestagens are dose-dependent for either the 19 or the 17 α form of progestagen.[303, 658] Other experts agree.[284]

More recently, as several reports of the use of natural progesterone have appeared, optimal HRT regimens would seem to favor the natural forms. A study from Sweden showed that the lipid alterations that can be so unwanted (for example, with 250 μg levonorgestrel or with 10 milligrams per day Provera®) did not occur when natural progesterone (100 milligrams twice a day) was taken by mouth.[657] Twice a day doses totaling 300 milligrams per day were also safe.[240] Work from Great Britain has shown that the oral intake of capsules of 100 milligrams of natural progesterone produced progesterone levels in the blood equivalent to a cycling woman's level about seven days before her menstrual period.[948] But higher progesterone doses of 300 milligrams per day for ten to twelve days per cycle may be optimal for many women.[240]

*To convert milligram doses into their equivalent microgram doses, multiply by 1,000; for example, 0.075 mg = 75 μg (micrograms). To convert microgram doses into milligram equivalents, divide by 1,000: 75μg = 0.075 mg.

opposed to either 120 or 250 μg then being prescribed). They recommended that the progestin be taken for thirteen days to achieve the full progestational opposition to estrogen therapy.[950] A later study followed bilaterally ovariectomized women who were prescribed 1.25 milligrams of Premarin® per day, opposed with 5 milligrams of another progestin, medrogestone. Their results showed that the lipids were not adversely affected by this regimen; the investigators considered that these results "may be regarded as entirely favorable."[874]

Biomedical investigators suggest that the natural progesterone dose be divided so that some is taken in the morning and some is taken at night. Progesterone undergoes a rapid metabolic breakdown once it gets into the blood. By replenishing this supply twice a day, one more nearly mimics the natural condition in which ovaries would have been continually secreting the hormone into the bloodstream.

Some of the newer regimens employ continuous estrogen opposed to continuous low-dose progesterone. Others advocate continuous estrogen with thirteen days per month of a somewhat higher dose of progesterone. Either of these two approaches will probably be effective for protecting your overall health. We must await further research studies in order to learn which plan is optimal. For now, you will want to work closely with your physician or health center to adjust the dose to your individual blood lipid levels and to your overall optimal body function.

### TESTOSTERONE

Ovariectomized women commonly report a loss of libido. Many hysterectomized women do, too. In 1973 Dr. C. Lauritzen, in describing the management of postmenopausal patients, commented that estrogen-androgen preparations produce some very predictable effects.* Within a few weeks, women often developed acne and excess hairiness, and showed deepening of the voice and an increased libido.[489] Other investigators have discussed testosterone in women and its relationship to hirsutism (developing a male pattern of excess hairiness). Dr. Ronald Strickler noted that when the total testosterone went above 2 nanograms per millileter in the blood, or the unbound (free) testosterone above 40 picograms per millileter, women tended to show severe hirsutism.[858]

In contrast to these negative effects of extremely high testosterone, more recently Dr. Barbara Sherwin and her colleagues have shown some very beneficial effects of androgen in an HRT regimen after ovariectomy.[805] They found that androgens enhanced the intensity of sexual desire and arousal as well as increasing a woman's experience of sexual fantasies. Their dose of androgen was 200 milligrams of testosterone enanthate given by injection once a month.[804, 805] They reported no negative effects with either a testosterone addition to estrogen or testosterone given alone. (See Chapter 10 for more about libido and hormones.) Dr. Sherwin's group also showed that any of the forms of HRT used in their study (estrogen, estrogen with androgen, or androgen alone) helped overcome the depression that women

*Testosterone is the principal androgen used for HRT; other androgens include dihydrotestosterone, dehydroepiandrosterone sulfate (DHEAS), and androsteredione.

were experiencing. When the hormones were withdrawn, depression returned.[804]

This study provided some very strong evidence for the possible value of low doses of androgen in an HRT regimen for women who have been ovariectomized or who have lost ovarian functioning after hysterectomy. Dr. Don Gambrell also notes a beneficial effect on libido when androgens are added to HRT regimens.[283] Hopefully, other investigators will study this very important hormone.

It makes sense that testosterone replacement could become a useful part of an HRT regimen. Ovaries do produce testosterone. Removing or lessening the production of the ovarian source will diminish the testosterone circulating in the blood. Unfortunately, testosterone therapy is the least studied of the hormonal regimens. If you do decide to take it, you will want to be carefully monitored by your physician to prevent untoward side effects, such as male-pattern hair growth and deepening of the voice. The size of the dose is the critical variable.

## DRUGS THAT AFFECT HORMONAL MILIEU

It is probably true that any time you take a drug, there are alterations in your hormonal environment. The roles of corticosteroids and of diuretics for use by menopausal women with and without HRT are particularly well studied.

The corticosteroids, such as prednisone, are very powerful agents that are given for a variety of diseases, including rheumatoid arthritis. Although there is no doubt that they help the diseases for which they are prescribed, they also produce powerful negative effects on sex hormone–dependent systems.[156, 278] Details of these effects of corticosteroids on metabolic bone health and disease appear in Chapter 8.

Since thiazide diuretics are commonly prescribed for women for a variety of purposes, it is relevant to note some diversity of study results. In four recent studies no serious negative effects on the critical aspects of menopause emerged. Coronary risk factors were not adversely affected by thiazide diuretics.[137] Likewise, bone mineral content and fracture prevalence were not hurt and might even be helped by thiazide diuretics.[763, 886, 931] However, diuretic use was common among men with high cholesterol levels, suggesting that diuretics might contribute to higher cholesterol levels.[310] When these diuretics are combined with estrogen, our best knowledge today suggests they are probably safe.

Because HRT has profound benefits for a woman after hysterectomy, it is well worth your time to become as knowledgeable as possible. Your very sense of well-being depends upon your hormonal environment, and there is so much you can do to optimize your situation.

The remaining chapters will help you to understand the relationships between hormones and the cardiovascular system, bones, sexual functioning in men and women, depression, urinary incontinence, nutrition, and exercise. It will then be possible for you to judge your particular needs within the context of the benefits of different forms of HRT. Your individual need will be a unique combination that delicately balances the competing influences of your life situation.

# 8

## Maintaining Bone Health

Bone health is a particularly critical concern after pelvic surgery, because the surgery can have a significant negative effect on both the density and the strength of your bones. The subject is more complex than current advertisements for calcium supplements would have us believe, and scientists know a good deal about the way that healthy bones are maintained. If women will take the steps recommended in this chapter, they can maximize their potential to have healthy bones throughout their lives.

### OSTEOPOROSIS—THE PREVENTABLE DISEASE

All of the sex hormones—the estrogens, progesterone, and testosterone—play a major beneficial role in maintaining bone mass. Both ovariectomy and hysterectomy, with their pervasive influence in reducing the sex hormones, drastically accelerate bone problems.[163, 180, 395, 810] Even if you had your surgery after age 45 when your estrogen levels were already declining, you still need to be vigilant in protecting your bones.[263]

The highest rates of bone loss occur in the *initial* stages of estrogen decline.* One study showed that within two years after

*Studies include 8, 425, 476, 513, 639, 852.

ovariectomy, women who did not take HRT lost 20 percent of their spinal bone mass[299] (see Figure 13). Other studies have showed that during the first three years after ovariectomy, women who do not take HRT suffer at least twice the amount of bone loss that they will suffer in the next three years.[394, 476] And once bone starts losing its mass, the process continues—a little at a time, year in and year out.

Ideally, a woman should act immediately after surgery to prevent the loss of bone. However, if some time has passed since your hysterectomy and you already have lost bone mass—even if you have already had fractures—there is much that you can do to prevent the further decline of your bone health.

Our bones serve as a kind of bank for calcium and other minerals. Under normal circumstances, in our youth the calcium we take into our diets—as milk, cheese, sardines, eggs, and other foods—gets deposited into the bones. As the bones take in more

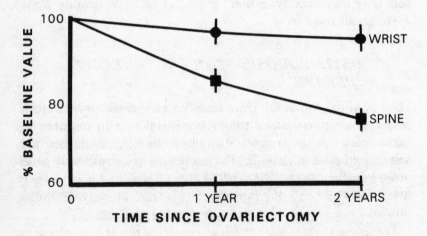

Figure 13. Mineral loss in wrist and spine following ovariectomy

calcium, they grow, both in length and in width. By about age 20, most of us have stopped growing in length. At that point, the bones begin to store the excess calcium, much as a person might store money in a retirement fund. From about 20 until about 35, if our diets are adequate, the bones continue to become structurally thicker and more solid. Sometime after age 35, the flow of currency changes, and our bones begin to lose mass—about 0.5 to 1.5 percent a year.[330, 733]

When the average life span was shorter, this loss rarely reached significant proportions. Most women died before bone loss affected their health. But now, with life spans routinely passing age 60, the loss of bone can make a real difference in the quality of life. In the late twentieth century, we are confronted with a worldwide medical problem in the form of osteoporosis, the disease of porous, brittle bones. About half of all white women over the age of 60 have bones that show osteoporosis.[291] By the time a woman dies, if she has not used estrogen or other hormonal replacement therapy, she will have lost about half her spinal bone mass and about one third of her arm bone mass.[733]

The term *osteoporosis* creates some confusion because there is no precise definition (or threshold amount) of bone loss after which healthy bone is considered osteoporotic. In general, the term is used to reflect a condition of porous bone sufficient to render its victim at high risk for nontraumatic bone fracture. The less mass your bones have, the weaker your bones are. When bones become very porotic, the least little activity, such as bending over to lift a chicken out of the oven or enjoying a gentle hug, can cause them to break.[582] The bone loss problem needs to be understood for what it is: a slow and progressive loss of bone mass. By the time it shows, in reduced height or bone breakage, the disease has already reached an advanced stage.

The loss of bone mass is something akin to the drying out of a piece of fruit; for example, after an apple dries out, it crumbles because it is so fragile. Fractures are common in "dried out" bone. Each year in the United States, more than 1 million people (mostly women) are afflicted.[174] The fractures occur as follows:

| Fractures of the spinal vertebrae | 538,000 cases |
| Fractures of the hip | 227,000 cases |
| Colles' fractures (wrist fractures) | 172,000 cases |
| Fractures of other limbs | 283,000 cases |

Similar data have been collected all over the world.[174]

There are genetic and gender differences in bone makeup. The bone is systematically thicker in black and thinner in Mexican-American, Japanese, and Chinese men and women.[291] Men usually have thicker bones and muscles than women. Throughout life, men are less subject to the devastation of osteoporotic immobility, in large part because their sex hormone, testosterone, exerts a more powerful influence than the female sex hormones estrogen and progesterone in building thicker bones and thicker muscles. As men age and their testosterone level declines, they also lose bone, but except for Oriental men, rarely is the bone loss sufficient to cause osteoporotic fractures;[174] in a very real sense, the male "bank of bones" has so much more on deposit that the subsequent withdrawals do not damage them. Men who develop diseases that diminish their ability to produce testosterone, however, may suffer from reduced bone formation or reduced bone mass.[269, 326, 366] Testosterone therapy can help them.

Certain regions of the body are more vulnerable than others because of their underlying structure. The spinal bones (vertebrae) and the wrist bones often reveal the first signs of osteoporosis. Figure 14 shows the startling rapidity of bone loss experienced by a woman with a bent back, or "dowager's hump." What has happened is that the woman's vertebrae have broken and fused together, shortening the length of her back and distorting her posture. Sometimes vertebral osteoporosis is painful, but often it is not. Wrist fractures, common among women in the early stages of estrogen decline, are often painful during the healing process, which can take several months.

Hip fracture is associated with diminished hip density, just as spinal fracture is associated with diminished spinal density[584]

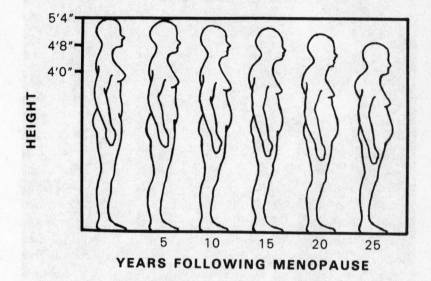

HEIGHT

YEARS FOLLOWING MENOPAUSE

Figure 14. Postural changes associated with spinal osteoporosis if no hormonal therapy is used.

(see page 180 and Figure 15). Fractures of the hip account for 80 percent of the estimated $10 billion annual cost of osteoporosis in the United States,[564] as well as causing the confinement to wheelchairs, the immobility, and the loss of freedom that so many women suffer in their later years. Moreover, hip fracture kills.

Half of the victims of hip fracture do not return to independent living after the fracture. And sadly, the survival after hip fracture has not improved in twenty years. Six years after hip fracture, more than half the patients die of heart attack, pneumonia, or other acute illnesses.[388] Perhaps the most important contributing factor in these deaths is the immobility necessary while the bone is setting. Immobility reduces a person's maximum oxygen consumption (the maximum amount of oxygen the lungs

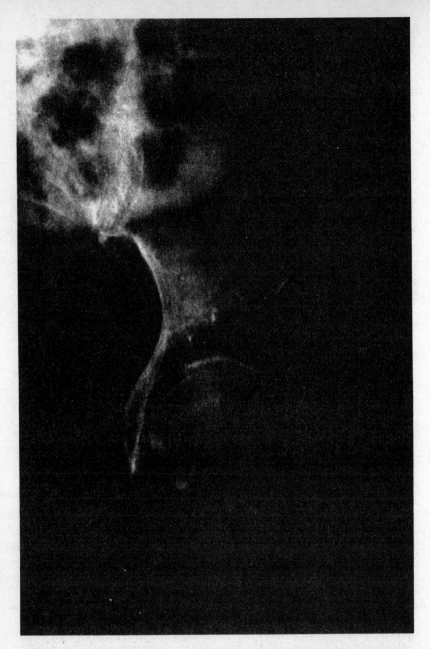

Figure 15. The hip socket showing the femur (top of thigh bone) where it inserts into the pelvic connection at the pubis bone. (The left is from a postmenopausal woman who broke her hip on the non pictured side. The right is from a healthy postmenopausal woman.) Courtesy of Dr. Frederick Kaplan, chief of metabolic bone disease at the Hospital of the University of Pennsylvania.

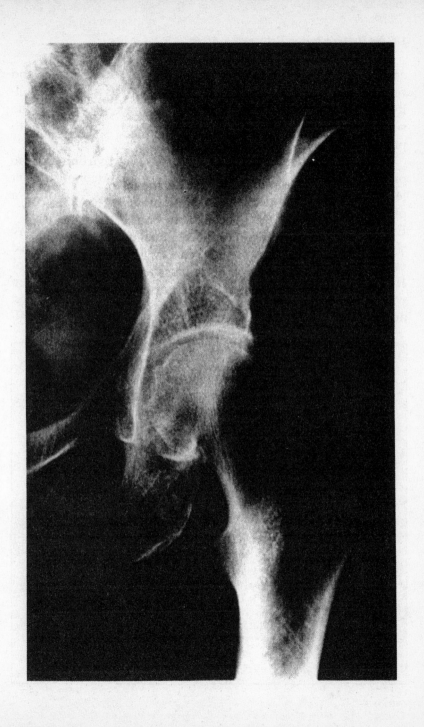

can deliver to the blood per minute) to half the normal level, and reduced oxygen consumption seriously threatens the body's ability to fight life-threatening disease. The bleak statistics on the survival rate after hip fracture demand that we pay attention to preventing it.

A variety of diseases that alter the hormonal environment also produce predictable declines in bone mass.[76] Alcoholism that leads to cirrhosis of the liver reduces bone mass,[384] as does a pituitary tumor resulting in reduced gonadatropic hormones.[575] Endometriosis has adverse bone effects; afflicted women have significantly lower vertebral bone mass and are usually denied estrogens because these aggravate the disease, yet this denial of HRT results in further bone loss[668] (see page 86). For women with endometriosis, progestins will help the bones, but estrogen and progestin together are probably ideal, provided that the bal-

---

### Hip Fractures

Two different kinds of hip fractures commonly occur: the *femoral neck fracture* (also called the transcervical fracture) and the *intertrochanteric fracture*. The femoral neck fracture occurs at the point where the femur (thigh) bone attaches to the pelvic bones. Common in women between ages 60 and 75, it is not particularly painful, perhaps because that part of the bone is encapsulated in a protective cushion. With femoral neck fractures, about forty-eight hours pass before healing gets well under way. Depending on the degree of displacement of bone, the orthopedic surgeon may insert pins to connect the broken pieces, allowing the patient to move around during the healing process.

The second kind of hip fracture, the intertrochanteric, occurs toward the top of the long thigh bone, and commonly occurs in men and women between the ages of 70 and 85. Perhaps because there is no capsule surrounding this part of the bone, this fracture leads to more blood spilling, swelling, and pain. Although it is more painful, the fracture generally heals by itself, thanks to the tremendous blood supply. Sometimes the bone is bolted back together by the surgeon using a "femoral compression screw." Generally the healing requires six to twelve weeks of immobilization.

These two kinds of hip fractures together occur 227,000 times a year in the United States.

ance between the two hormones is monitored to prevent or reverse any regrowth of endometriotic tissue.[701]

## THE BASICS OF BONE METABOLISM

Bone is active tissue that is very much alive. Although we may think of it as a solid, hard structure, in fact bone is composed of a complex, well-ordered matrix of tissue that has nerves and blood vessels running through it. A cascade of influential molecules controls when bone tissue breaks itself down and when it builds itself up. Two major types of bone cells, the *osteoclast cells* and the *osteoblast cells,* work in synergy with each other.

The osteoclasts are small cells whose major function is to chew bone into tiny particles. The osteoblasts are small cells whose major function is to take those tiny particles and build them into new bone. One might think of this as a sort of ongoing recycling process. Hormones and vitamins control the direction of the action. The hormone *calcitonin,* produced in the thyroid gland, seems to be involved in turning on the osteoblasts to do their job of building bone. Another hormone, *parathyroid hormone* (PTH), which is produced in the parathyroid gland, appears to have a critical role in turning on the osteoclasts, which calcitonin turns off. In normal healthy bone, these two bone hormones play complementary roles in controlling bone cell metabolism.

The sex hormones—estrogen, progesterone, and testosterone—appear to stimulate calcitonin secretion. Because of its effect on estrogen levels, ovariectomy triggers a decline in calcitonin secretion,[301, 852] and since the uterus influences the ovaries, hysterectomy probably also inhibits calcitonin. Although no study has yet tested for a reduced level of calcitonin after hysterectomy, such reductions most probably do occur. After about three months of therapy, estrogen raises the calcitonin level,[224] which both increases the bone-building activity[848, 850] and slows down the osteoclastic chewing.

At every age, women have about twice the level of PTH that

men have. As women get older, their PTH levels increase.[958] Increased PTH levels are also found in women with certain diseases of the kidney,[767] and such women are inclined to have osteoporosis. The net effect of these increases is that bone building will not be able to keep up with bone breakdown, and the loss of bone will make bones vulnerable to fracture.

## PROTECTING YOUR BONE MASS

Beginning immediately after hysterectomy, you can act to prevent osteoporosis. Even if you suspect that you have already lost bone and even if you have suffered a fracture, you will benefit from taking action.

Four major positive influences work together to help protect the strength of your bones, and you can exert control over each. There are also two risks to avoid. These six considerations are discussed in the sections that follow:

• You need to maintain a positive calcium balance.
• You need to ensure adequate amounts of vitamin D.
• You need to have adequate levels of sex hormones, which control the bone hormones calcitonin and PTH.
• You need to engage in adequate exercise.
• You need to avoid smoking.
• You need to be aware that certain drugs and diseases increase bone loss.

### Maintaining a Positive Calcium Balance

Calcium plays a critical role in bone health and strength. Every day calcium leaves the body through the urine, feces, and sweat. If you don't take in enough calcium to compensate for the amount that is leaving, you will have a negative calcium balance. The level of calcium in the bloodstream will remain relatively constant, but the bones will give up calcium and become proportionately less dense.[236, 741] Calcium balance is affected by a number of different elements, particularly the sex hormones and your diet.

Calcium balance was studied in 170 nuns beginning at around age 35 and at subsequent five-year intervals to age 55.[361, 362, 363] In hospital tests, every food item consumed was measured for calcium content, and the calcium balance was computed by subtracting the calcium content of each woman's excretions from the content of her dietary intake. Several important findings emerged:

Most of the women consumed about 661 milligrams of calcium a day.

Their bodies absorbed about 32 percent of their calcium intake; the rest was excreted.

On average, even before their menopause, the women were in negative calcium balance, losing from 40 to 50 milligrams per day.

The more calcium a woman ingested, the more likely she was to be in positive balance.[362]

Perimenopausal women required about 990 milligrams a day, on average, in order to be in positive calcium balance.

Once they became estrogen-depleted, through either natural or artificial menopause, the women's calcium requirement increased to about 1,500 milligrams per day.[361]

What can we conclude from these data? When women are estrogen-deficient, they need more calcium than when they have adequate levels of estrogen. But each woman is different, with an individual need for calcium. Although average values can be obtained, there is a wide variation from one woman to the next. This study used a very special group of presumably celibate women without HRT. Since regular sexual activity increases the estrogen levels,[167, 171, 177] the calcium need is probably lower in sexually active women who still have their ovaries.

*Calcium therapies alone do not prevent or reverse osteoporosis.* Without adequate estrogen, other sex hormones, or calcitonin, no dose of calcium is able to prevent the degeneration of bones.[236, 305, 741, 849, 928] Even intravenous calcium infusions to postmenopausal women with osteoporosis aren't able to help to decrease bone loss or improve calcium balance;[491, 622] in men, they do help.[928]

Yet, although calcium alone is not sufficient to combat bone loss, it is one of the essential components. After a hysterectomy, it is probably wise to consume about 1,200 to 1,500 milligrams a day if you suspect that you are estrogen-deficient[132]. If your estrogen levels are judged to be adequate (either by means of a blood test or by the absence of menopausal symptoms), 750 milligrams per day will probably be adequate. Three 8-ounce glasses of skim milk per day provide close to 1,000 milligrams and only 240 calories. Many other foods are also rich in calcium; Table 7 shows food sources of calcium.

A well-balanced diet can maximize your calcium balance. Learn which foods provide substantial amounts of calcium. Once you know this, you will be able to calculate the average daily calcium intake that is natural for you. If you are not consuming enough, you can then adjust your diet (see page 283).

Calcium supplements are available in drugstores, but two factors should caution you against their indiscriminate use: dissolving rate and absorptive capacity, both of which vary depending on the form of the tablet.

On January 27, 1988, the *New York Times* published an article that provided data developed by Dr. Ralph Shangraw as he tested currently available calcium pills to see how easily they dissolved in a solution designed to approximate what happens in the stomach. Table 8, redrawn from that article, shows how variable the different products are. Some seem to be a clear waste of money because of their failure to adequately dissolve.

The form of the tablet, whether a carbonate form (such as calcium carbonate) or an acid form (such as calcium citrate), may affect the ability of your body to absorb the calcium. No study equivalent to that of Table 8 has yet been published to show the absorptive capacity of different tablets. If you decide to take calcium carbonate, it would be wise to enhance its absorp-

***Table 7.*** *Calcium Values of Common Food Sources\**

| Food | Portion | Calories | Calcium (milligrams) |
|---|---|---|---|
| ***Breads & Cereals*** | | | |
| Cream of Wheat Instant | 1 cup, cooked | 130 | 185 |
| Pabulum cereal | | | |
|   Barley or rice | 3/4 cup, cooked | 108 | 188 |
|   Oatmeal or mixed | 3/4 cup, cooked | 110 | 188 |
| Thomas Protein Bread | 1 slice | 45 | 78 |
| ***Dairy Products*** | | | |
| Cheese | | | |
|   American | 1 oz | 107 | 195 |
|   Cheddar | 1 oz | 112 | 211 |
|   Cottage, creamed | 1 cup | 239 | 211 |
|   Edam | 1 oz | 87 | 225 |
|   Swiss | 1 oz | 104 | 259 |
| Ice cream (chocolate) | 1/6 quart | 174 | 131 |
| Ice milk (vanilla) | 1/6 quart | 136 | 189 |
| Milk | | | |
|   Buttermilk, from skim | 1 cup | 88 | 296 |
|   Skim | 1 cup | 89 | 303 |
|   Whole, 3.5% fat | 1 cup | 159 | 288 |
| Vanilla pudding | 1/2 cup | 139 | 146 |
| Yogurt from skim with nonfat milk solids | 1 cup | 127 | 452 |
| Goat milk | 1 cup | 163 | 315 |
| ***Eggs*** | | | |
| Scrambled, milk & fat | 1 medium | 112 | 52 |
| ***Fish & Shellfish*** | | | |
| Flounder | 3 oz | 61 | 55 |
| Mackerel, canned | 3 1/2 oz | 192 | 194 |
| Oysters, raw | 5–8 medium | 66 | 94 |
| Sardines, canned | 8 medium | 311 | 354 |

**Table 7.** *(Continued)*

| Food | Portion | Calories | Calcium (milligrams) |
|---|---|---|---|
| Scallops, cooked | 3 1/2 oz | 112 | 115 |
| Shrimp, raw | 3 1/2 oz | 91 | 63 |
| *Fruits & Seeds* | | | |
| Figs, dried | 5 medium | 274 | 126 |
| Orange | 1 medium | 73 | 62 |
| Sunflower seeds | 3 1/2 oz | 560 | 120 |
| *Syrups & Sweets* | | | |
| Blackstrap molasses | 1 tbsp | 43 | 116 |
| Maple sugar | 4 pieces (2×1×1/2 in) | 348 | 180 |
| Chocolate candy | 1 bar (2 oz) | 296 | 52 |
| *Vegetables* | | | |
| Artichoke | edible portion (base & soft end of leaves) | 44 | 51 |
| Beans | | | |
| Lima, green, cooked | 6 tbsp | 111 | 47 |
| Snap, green, cooked | 1 cup | 31 | 62 |
| Wax, yellow, cooked | 1 cup | 22 | 50 |
| Beet greens, cooked | 1/2 cup | 18 | 99 |
| Broccoli | | | |
| Raw | 1 stalk (5" long) | 32 | 103 |
| Cooked | 2/3 cup | 26 | 88 |
| Cabbage, Savoy, raw | 2 cups shredded | 24 | 67 |
| Chard, cooked | 3/5 cup | 18 | 73 |
| Chicory | 30–40 inner leaves | 20 | 86 |
| Collards, cooked | 1/2 cup | 29 | 152 |
| Endive | 20 long leaves | 20 | 81 |
| Escarole | 4 large leaves | 20 | 81 |
| Fennel, raw | 3 1/2 oz | 28 | 100 |
| Leeks | 3–4 (5" long) | 52 | 52 |

| Food | Portion | Calories | Calcium (milligrams) |
|------|---------|----------|----------------------|
| Lettuce, romaine | 3 1/2 oz | 18 | 68 |
| Mustard greens, cooked | 1/2 cup | 23 | 138 |
| Parsley, raw | 3 1/2 oz | 44 | 203 |
| Parsnips, raw | 1/2 large | 76 | 50 |
| Rutabagas, cooked | 1/2 cup | 35 | 59 |
| Sweetpotatoes, baked | 1 large | 254 | 72 |
| Watercress, raw | 3 1/2 oz | 19 | 151 |

*From: Cutler, García, and Edwards, *Menopause: A Guide for Women and the Men Who Love Them.*

tion by taking it with a meal.[722] You can take calcium citrate at any time during the day. For both forms, be sure to drink at least 12 ounces of water every time you take a 1,000 milligram tablet. This amount of water will dilute the calcium and help prevent the very slight risk of high doses causing kidney stones.[630] Large doses of calcium supplements should be unnecessary because of the wide range of calcium-rich foods. The supplements are expensive and wasteful, and they may result in your getting too much calcium, which in rare cases can cause kidney stones.

### *Getting Adequate Vitamin D*

In its active form, vitamin D promotes the absorption of calcium from the intestines into the bloodstream. Our natural source of vitamin D is ultraviolet radiation from sunlight. When sunlight hits the surface of our skin, a very interesting chemical reaction takes place. Some of the cholesterol near the surface of the skin is transformed into molecules, sometimes called "previtamin D," which move away from the surface of the skin into the bloodstream, changing into an intermediate form of vitamin D[189] and traveling in the bloodstream until they reach the liver. Enzymes in the liver further convert the molecules, which then

***Table 8.*** *Calcium Supplements Are Not All Equal*

| Brand Name (listed alphabetically)* | Ranking | Milligrams of Calcium (when available) | Dissolution Rate (percent in 30 minutes)§ | Vitamin D |
|---|---|---|---|---|
| AARP Pharmacy Service Oyster Calcium | 33 | 250 | 8 | Yes |
| American Stores Oyster Shell | 37 | 500 | 6.2 | No |
| Ames Calcium | 46 | 600 | 2.9 | Yes |
| Ames Natural Super Oyster Shell | 47 | 500 | 2.8 | No |
| Approved Pharmaceutical Calcium Oyster Shell | 45 | 250 | 3 | Yes |
| Caldor Oyster Shell Calcium | 34 | †NA | 7.5 | Yes |
| Cambridge Vitamin Calcium Oyster Shell | 48 | 600 | 2.5 | No |
| Fields of Nature Oyster Shell | 9 | 500 | 90 | No |
| Foods Plus Natural Calcium | 18 | 600 | 66 | No |
| Foods Plus Oyster Shell | 20 | 250 | 54 | Yes |
| Foods Plus Oyster Shell Calcium | 31 | †NA | 9.1 | Yes |
| Freeda Vitamin Calcium | 25 | 650 | 20 | No |
| General Nutrition Centers Natural Sales-Sea-cal | 44 | 500 | 3.7 | No |
| General Nutrition Centers Potent Calcium (Lot 3G6797EM) | 41 | 600 | 5 | No |
| General Nutrition Centers Potent Calcium (Lot F15952CO) | 22 | 600 | 42 | No |
| General Nutrition Centers Calcium | 51 | 600 | 2 | Yes |
| Giant Foods Natural | 1 | 600 | *107 | No |
| Giant Food Oyster Shell (Lot 22225) | 24 | 250 | 20 | No |
| Giant Natural Calcium | 11 | 600 | 87 | Yes |
| Giant Calcium Oyster Shell | 12 | 250 | 86 | Yes |
| Hudson Calcium Concentrate | 10 | 600 | 89 | No |
| K-Mart High Potency Calcium | 13 | 600 | 79 | No |
| K-Mart Natural Oyster Shell | 26 | 250 | 18 | Yes |
| K-Mart Extra Strength Oyster Shell | 42 | 500 | 4.3 | No |
| K-Mart Calcium | 43 | 600 | 4 | No |

| Brand Name (listed alphabetically)* | Ranking | Milligrams of Calcium (when available) | Dissolution Rate (percent in 30 minutes)§ | Vitamin D |
|---|---|---|---|---|
| Lederle Laboratories Caltrate | 14 | 600 | 77 | Yes |
| Long's Drug Calcium Oyster Shell | 27 | 250 | 18 | Yes |
| Marion Laboratories Os-cal | 2 | 500 | *104 | Yes |
| Medicine Shoppe International Calcium | 21 | 600 | 43 | No |
| Medicine Shoppe International Oyster Shell Calcium | 29 | †NA | 15 | Yes |
| Medicine Shoppe International Calcium Oyster Shell | 49 | 250 | 2.3 | Yes |
| Medicine Shoppe International, Inc. Calcium Oyster Shell | 50 | 500 | 2.2 | Yes |
| Miles Laboratories Inc. Biocal | 40 | 500 | 5.3 | No |
| Nature Made Nutritional Products Oyster Shell Calcium | 6 | †NA | 99 | Yes |
| Norcliff-Thayer Tums | 3 | 200 | *102 | No |
| Norcliff-Thayer Calcimax | 8 | †NA | 91 | No |
| L. Perrigo Nature's GLO High Potency Calcium Formula | 17 | 600 | 67 | Yes |
| Revco Calcium | 16 | 600 | 76 | No |
| Revco Calcium Oyster Shell | 36 | 250 | 6.6 | Yes |
| Rite-Aid Calcium Oyster Shell | 15 | 250 | 77 | No |
| Rite Aid Hi-Cal | 23 | 500 | 24 | No |
| Rite Aid Corporation Calcium Carbonate | 35 | †NA | 7 | No |
| Rite Aid Corporation Calcium Plus | 30 | 600 | 13 | Yes |
| Roxane Labs Calcium Carbonate | 5 | 1250 | 100 | No |
| Rugby Laboratories Oyster Shell | 52 | 500 | 1.8 | No |
| Safeway Calcium | 32 | 325 | 9 | No |
| Safeway Natural Oyster Shell | 39 | 250 | 5.4 | Yes |
| Safeway Hical | 4 | 250 | *102 | Yes |
| Sun Pride Nutrition Oyster Shell | 28 | 500 | 15 | No |

**Table 8.** *(Continued)*

| Brand Name (listed alphabetically)* | Ranking | Milligrams of Calcium (when available) | Dissolution Rate (percent in 30 minutes)§ | Vitamin D |
|---|---|---|---|---|
| Vitaline Corp Oyster Shell | 38 | 250 | 6 | No |
| Warner-Lambert Company Suplical | 7 | 600 | 98 | No |
| Your Life Oyster Shell (Lot K62541) | 19 | 500 | 56 | No |

*Dissolution Rate*
The research, conducted by Dr. Ralph Shangraw, chairman of the department of pharmaceutics at the University of Maryland School of Pharmacy, was done between March 1987 and January 1988. Dr. Shangraw said that some of the companies, whose products did not meet standards set by United States Pharmacopeia, a nonprofit group that sets drug standards, have reformulated their products since the information was made public. According to the standard, 75 percent of the calcium should dissolve in 30 minutes. Dr. Shangraw offers a simple way for the consumer to test the dissolution rate of her own batch of calcium tablets. Place one tablet in a glass of vinegar at room temperature. Stir vigorously every few minutes for 30 minutes. If the tablet has not disintegrated into fine particles by this time, it probably won't dissolve adequately in the human digestive system.
*The lot number is included if a different batch of the same product was tested separately and also appears on the chart showing disintegration rates only.
§Number 1 has the highest dissolution rate, Number 52 the lowest. The higher the percentage rate, the more likely the body can absorb the calcium. Where the percentage adds up to more than 100 percent, the actual milligrams of calcium were more than what is stated on the label.
†Not available.

travel in the bloodstream until they get to the kidneys, where another enzyme converts them into the final active form of vitamin D, known generically as calcitriol. People with liver and kidney diseases commonly suffer from bone problems. One reason is likely to be the involvement of these two organs in converting vitamin D into the active form.

Under normal circumstances, natural exposure to sunlight provides us with enough vitamin D. In the United States and Canada, milk is supplemented with the active form of vitamin D, but in Great Britain it is not. Cheese does not usually contain supplements of vitamin D in the United States, Canada, and Great Britain. Studies in Great Britain have shown that in the winter months, the blood levels of the active form of vitamin D severely decline among the general population and that in the sunny spring and summer there is an increase.[174]

Taking too much vitamin D by supplement can be very dangerous, causing calcium to leach out of bone into the blood and increasing the risk of osteoporosis as the kidneys rapidly dispose of it via the urine. Our daily need for vitamin D, which appears to be about 400 IU, is easily supplied with fifteen minutes a day in the sun or, in the United States and Canada, with milk.

### The Need for Adequate Sex Hormones

In a healthy woman, it is only when her estrogen and progesterone levels begin to show the declines characteristic of the menopausal transition that bones begin to lose their mass. Although research studies have not yet been done to evaluate exactly how each of the components of bone health respond to gain and loss of estrogen, the pervasive influence of the sex hormones is very well established.

If you are estrogen-deficient, you should consider taking HRT. Estrogen replacement therapy with or without progesterone slows or halts further loss of bone whenever it is begun, provided the dose is adequate.* Progestin and androgen therapies also have produced positive results.[305, 622]

Three principal forms of estrogen are naturally produced by the ovary: *estrone, estradiol,* and *estriol.* Estradiol is generally thought to be the strongest, most biologically active estrogen. However, in four studies that compared blood levels of estrogens to bone mass, estrone was shown to be most closely associated with bone mass.[423, 424, 546, 548] Fortunately, your body converts a significant portion of the estradiol into estrone.

In the middle to late 1970s, four investigators reported that

---

*Studies include 2, 7, 24, 70, 132, 134, 135, 280, 393, 394, 476, 477, 509, 550, 574, 576, 603, 619, 723, 739, 801, 851.

estrogen therapy helped in the long-term prevention of post-menopausal osteoporosis. The investigators followed women prospectively (before and then continuing through treatment) with control groups for comparison; in some studies, the estrogen was accompanied by calcium. All four showed the same thing: the higher the dose of estrogen, the more effective the therapy was in maintaining bone mass or preventing bone loss.[236, 393, 509, 723] At low doses of ERT, bone was lost but not nearly as severely as among placebo users. Low doses (0.3 milli-

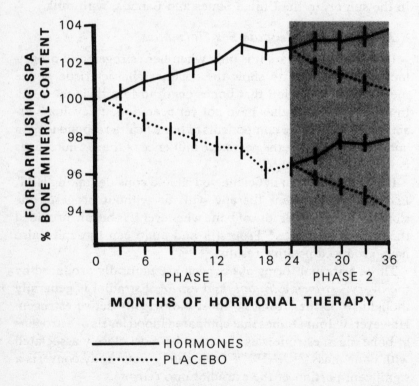

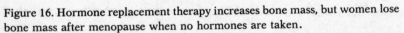

Figure 16. Hormone replacement therapy increases bone mass, but women lose bone mass after menopause when no hormones are taken.

grams per day conjugated equine) combined with very high calcium (1,500 milligrams per day) were also protective.[236] Whenever the estradiol form is used, whether synthetic or natural, the bone is protected. In contrast, estriol, the weakest estrogen, failed to produce bone benefits.[511]

In the early to middle 1980s, further studies established a relationship between estrogen and the maintenance of bone health, not only in inhibiting the excess breakdown of bone but also in stimulating the formation of bone[394, 801] (see Figure 16). Dr. Claus Christiansen and his colleagues showed that hormone users actually increased their bone mineral content. In his study, women took estrogen combined with progestin, and their wrist bone measurements were compared with those of a control group who took a placebo. After two years, some of the women received the opposite treatment, some placebo users getting hormone and some hormone users getting placebo. Whenever hormones were given, bone mass began to increase. At any point that hormones were withheld, bone mass declined.[134] The hormones used were a European mixture of estradiol and estriol with a progestin (norethisterone acetate) in opposition. The women took estrogen every day and progestin ten days out of each month, and received 500 milligrams of calcium per day. An androgen used in Europe (nandrolone decanoate, a 50-milligram injection every three weeks) also increases bone mass in osteoporotic women with vertebral fractures.[305, 622]

The effect of progestin alone has been studied. Norethisterone acetate (a strong progestin) increases bone mass.[734] It appears to increase the intestinal absorption of calcium[885] yet not affect the urinary excretion of calcium.[601] Happily, progestin reduces the breakdown of bone by osteoclast cells.[508]

While progestins and androgens alone (without simultaneous estrogen) do protect bones, the side effects they produce, such as vaginal dryness, make them less desirable choices for a posthysterectomized woman. If you can't take estrogen, then other options, such as calcitonin therapy, may be sensible (see page 198).

## The Importance of Exercise

Regular exercise helps prevent bone fractures for several reasons. Osteoporotic women fall down more, and nerve and muscle weaknesses may contribute to the breaking of bones in women whose mass is already low.[425] Exercise stimulates both blood circulation and muscle tone; it makes the nerves and the muscles strong and healthy. If you engage in a regular, disciplined exercise program several days a week—such as swimming, taking a two- to three-mile walk, or other equivalent exercise—you are likely to experience profound benefits to your bone health. Although the mechanism by which exercise enhances bone strength is not well understood, the fact that exercise helps bones is clear from several research studies. For example, athletes have higher bone mineral content than controls (office workers) when the athletic activity is cross-country running. The biggest difference in stronger bones is found in the parts of bone that are most susceptible to fracture.[181]

Although inappropriate exercise—that is, exercise that is excessive or done improperly—should be avoided because it can do more harm than good,[817] there are certain activities that are very helpful for maturing women (see Chapter 15). Generalized fitness promotes higher spinal and hip bone density in older women.[694] One study evaluated women in the age group 50 to 73 who had had a forearm fracture. The women were divided into two groups. One group was prescribed exercise; in the other, the women were left to their own activity patterns. After eight months, both groups had their spinal bones read (a second time) by dual photon absorptiometry (described on page 196). The exercise program was very effective in increasing the density in the spinal vertebrae.[473]

Another investigation compared athletic women to nonathletic women in two age groups: 40 to 55 years old and 50 to 75 years old. "Athletic" signified that the women exercised for an hour at least three times a week, for eight months per year, for a minimum of three years. Athletic women were shown to have better bone density than those who were not athletic.[411]

Regular exercise promotes and maintains healthy bones. Chapter 15 describes how to set up a safe exercise plan not only for your bones but for your overall health.

### The Dangers of Smoking

Smoking has terrible effects on bone health. Among women with bone fractures, the overwhelming majority is always made up of women who smoke. When women take HRT, nonsmokers show blood levels of estrogen that increase in proportion to the therapy dose; smokers do not show these benefits. Somehow, a smoker does not seem to metabolize the estrogen therapy in a similar fashion to a nonsmoker. Smoking also reduces a woman's maximum oxygen consumption; as a consequence, a smoker will not experience the increase in bone mass that is a benefit of regular exercise. If you want good bones, you must not smoke. To stop smoking is tough; to become immobilized after a hip fracture is tougher. (See Chapter 14.)

### Drugs Known to Cause Bone Loss

Thiazide diuretics, which are commonly prescribed to women for hypertension, have been shown to be potentially helpful in maintaining bone mass when combined with estrogen.[763, 886] Although too few studies are currently available to draw firm conclusions, if you are taking thiazide diuretics with estrogen, there is no evidence that they will be harmful and there is some preliminary evidence that they may be helpful. However, be warned. One diuretic, furosemide (not a thiazide diuretic), causes a loss of calcium through the urine. If you need a diuretic, ask about its impact on calcium loss, and read the package insert yourself to be sure.

A large literature has emerged that shows that the glucocorticoids, or corticosteroids (such as cortisone and prednisone), which are prescribed for the treatment of rheumatoid arthritis and other diseases, are bad for bone metabolism.* It appears that they are responsible for at least seven dangerous side effects:

*Studies include 6, 49, 101, 127, 130, 196, 271, 278, 343, 416, 461, 546, 616, 661, 867.

they elevate the parathyroid hormone, increase bone resorption, inhibit calcium absorption, increase the urinary loss of calcium, lower the body's level of estrogen, reduce bone mass in the forearm, and impair osteoblastic bone-building activity.

What can you do? Avoid harmful drugs. If you cannot avoid them, be aware that HRT may be helpful. Unfortunately, very little literature is yet available to guide in the treatment of osteoporosis in corticosteroid-treated patients.[174] If your doctor believes that you need these drugs, ask for a counterbalancing force—that is, HRT—to preserve your bones. And insist on regular evaluation of your bone mass to be certain that your HRT is adequately dosed.

## HOW TO TELL IF YOUR BONES ARE HEALTHY

If you want to know whether you are currently at risk for osteoporosis, you should probably have your bones tested. The spine is the region of most critical early interest. Dual photon absorptiometry (DPA) repeated every six months should provide

---

### Bone-Testing Terminology

*Densitometer* machines are so named because they measure density. The word *absorptiometer* refers to the same machine but describes the method used (the measurement of absorption of particles of radioactive material). Some machines (single photon) beam a single radioactively labeled photon (particle of light); others (dual photon) beam two different kinds of radioactively labeled photons. The measurements that arise are then abbreviated as SPA (single photon absorptiometry, or densitometry) and DPA (dual photon absorptiometry, or densitometry).

*Quantitative computerized tomography* (QCT) X-ray provides a picture of what a cross-section of the body would look like. Because it provides a visual image, even though it does not actually measure density it is useful for detecting fractures in bone.

SPA is used mainly to evaluate the radius bone of the forearm. DPA and QCT X-ray are used to evaluate the spinal and hip bones.

you with accurate information about changes in spinal bone mass. The spinal and hip bones can be evaluated using DPA or the QCT X-ray (see page 196). The radius bone of the forearm can also be evaluated, using single photon absorptiometry (SPA).

While there is agreement in the literature that SPA gives an accurate reflection of bone density in most regions of the body, controversy exists about its value in screening for spinal density via the measurement recorded at the arm.[48]

If the objective is to get an immediate, accurate baseline report to use as a basis for comparison with subsequent reports, you will probably want to have your spinal or hip bones evaluated. Likewise, repeated measures, every six months, of both the end and middle part of your forearm will reveal whether your body is maintaining, gaining, or losing bone and at what rate.[564] These readings should continue until you show a stabilized level for three consecutive tests. After that, every twelve to eighteen months should be sufficient. If you are healthy and can manage to have regular, repeated measurements of SPA, you will probably have sufficient information from this cheapest and fastest assessment to guide your hormonal, nutritional, and exercise planning.[564]

All of these methods are painless. If you have your arm evaluated using SPA, the procedure should take about fifteen minutes. Your arm will be placed in an armrest while a scanner silently moves above the arm. If you have your spinal or hip bones read by DPA or by QCT, the procedure will be a bit less convenient, requiring that you lie down on a table and maintain a still posture for twenty to thirty minutes while a scanner moves above your body.

These noninvasive measures involve the beaming of radioactive material at the bone in question as a computer system calculates bone density. The radiation exposure with QCT is relatively high (500 to 1,000 mRems). Even though with the newest and best equipment the QCT dose reduces to 100 to 300 mRems, that is still a high exposure. (A standard chest X-ray provides 70 to 100 mRems.) DPA provides less than 10 mRems, while the single photon densitometer scanning the forearm is even lower, 3 to 5 mRems.[630]

SPA is more accurate than DPA, which is more accurate than QCT X-ray unless the DPA beam is reading a compression site. (If you have suffered a compression fracture, after which two spinal bones then fused together, your DPA report may provide one or two readings [out of five or six] that are falsely high, in response to the high density created at the compression site. Such a reading does not represent strong, thick bone.) The main value of the QCT X-ray is in its ability to show where fractures have occurred. In general, QCT X-ray is relatively uninformative about density until more than 50 percent of the bone mass is lost.

As research continues to develop our understanding of appropriate ways to use single photon absorptiometry as a screen for spinal density, SPA is likely to become a common first line of evaluation for bone mass for many women.*

Bone can be analyzed in other ways. Histochemical techniques, in which laboratory experts examine pieces of bone that are removed from the body, can provide important information about bone disease. Such analysis is generally done on portions of hip bone when there is already a serious condition that needs to be further evaluated. Other forms of biochemical methods to either detect osteoporosis or predict the predisposition to it are currently in experimental stages and not yet biomedically useful.

## WHAT IF YOUR BONES ARE LOSING MASS?

You may be reading this book after already having developed osteoporosis. Or you may be a candidate for the disease because estrogen therapy is not an option for you and because you do not want the negative sexual and cardiovascular effects associated with unopposed progestin therapy. Women already

---

*The first study published in 1988 provides preliminary evidence to show how SPA can be used to screen for spinal bone loss.[163]

suffering from osteoporosis or at high risk for the disease should consider the full arsenal of treatments their doctors have available understanding the strengths and dangers of each.

### Hormonal and Calcitonin Therapy

If, after doing all you can with healthful habits of diet, regular exercise, and nonsmoking, you find that you are losing bone, then HRT should be the first choice for medical treatment. If you take estrogen replacement therapy and your hormonal milieu is normal, the estrogen will cause your calcitonin level to increase automatically. As has already been discussed, some women hesitate to consider estrogen therapy because they fear that estrogen will cause cancer. This fear is no longer warranted. When estrogen is appropriately opposed with progestin, the risk of cancer is lower than when women take no hormones. This knowledge should be reassuring in light of the benefits that estrogen offers with respect to bone metabolism.

If you can't take estrogen, because of a disease or condition that is sensitive to it, then calcitonin hormone therapy should be seriously considered. The hormone calcitonin, normally manufactured in the thyroid gland[855] and sometimes produced in the parathyroid gland,[850] appears to be involved in turning on the osteoblast cells, which build bone. Except when women are pregnant, men have higher levels of calcitonin than women.[366, 530, 850] Under normal circumstances, calcitonin levels rise whenever you consume calcium,[197] as part of nature's way of dealing with increased dietary calcium, which is to store it as increased bone mass. A series of recent studies provides new data on the potential value of calcitonin in the treatment of osteoporosis. Calcitonin is only a second choice to the sex hormones because, although it will preserve your bones, it will not help with the other posthysterectomy problems. (See page 200.)

Currently, calcitonin is available only in injection form, a nuisance because the injections must be given daily. Some physicians have begun to adjust from daily to weekly dosages, but no published study has yet allowed for a careful evaluation of ap-

### Calcitonin Therapy and Bone Health

Fortunately, bone health may be maintained through calcitonin therapy.[131] Although women with normal bone showed a rapid increase in the blood calcitonin levels when calcium was infused intravenously, osteoporotic women did not.[869] The conclusion: osteoporotic women have a calcitonin deficiency.

Studies of the use of long-term calcitonin therapy in postmenopausal osteoporosis have noted some beneficial effects.[329] Calcitonin helps the kidneys to convert pre-vitamin D into the active form.[850] Bone biopsies, in which pieces of hip bone were removed and studied under microscopic conditions, showed that women who received calcitonin had the benefits of a significant decrease in areas of bone that are breaking down and no change in the formation rate.[329] This combination of effects would increase bone mass.

In 1987 several more studies were presented to the convening scientists at the International Menopause Society Meeting. These studies showed further benefits of calcitonin therapy in women who cannot take estrogen.[301, 488, 852] Calcitonin stops the reduction of bone loss at the spine, it decreases the urinary loss of calcium, and it helps to serve as an analgesia (painkiller) for bone pain. (Adequate dietary calcium is just as necessary with calcitonin therapy as with HRT.)

The future looks bright for the potential of calcitonin to move from the experimental state in a few highly sophisticated medical centers into actual use in mainstream health care centers.[848, 851]

proaches. Research is under way to provide an intranasal spray, and so far the results look promising. Experiments in four different centers in the United States are showing that the spray is well tolerated and is likely to be a useful route for taking this hormone. Unfortunately, an intranasal spray is not likely to be available in the United States before 1991 or 1992.

### Vitamin D Treatment

Vitamin D deficiencies often appear among elderly people,[282] especially those who avoid the sun and have inappropriate dietary levels of the vitamin.[44] D deficiencies are particularly pronounced among people who have a high risk of osteoporosis.[82] When osteoporotic women consume either normal or low-calcium diets, the vitamin D level plummets.[639]

Although vitamin D levels are low among elderly people with osteoporosis, vitamin D therapy has not shown itself to be an effective solution.[622] Approaching osteoporosis with vitamin D therapy is difficult. If the active form of vitamin D is increased too much, it causes a further breakdown of bone.[640] In one study, one group of women was given 1 μg of active vitamin D with 2.5 grams of calcium carbonate per day, and a control group was given a placebo coupled to calcium.[387] The effects of vitamin D were both good and bad. The good effect was an increased rate of fracture healing among osteoporotic people. But unpleasant drug reactions were severe for a significant number of participants,[387] and there was no measurable increase in bone density (in the wrist area) after six months. Thus, although the idea of vitamin D therapy appears to have some validity because it can promote healing, it can simultaneously lead to bone loss and is rarely effective anyway.

For most women, vitamin D therapy will not be useful. If you are elderly, you should try to get your vitamin D through fortified dairy products and/or regular sunshine. Only after you have tried these sources might it be appropriate to consider vitamin D therapy, and then only under the care of your physician.

### Fluoride Treatment

Sodium fluoride treatments have been reported to have some beneficial effects on bone health. Unfortunately, more than 40 percent of the treated groups reported severe side effects, which included recurrent vomiting, bleeding ulcers, anemia, and painful ankles.[183, 740] (Side effects halted within a few weeks after stopping the treatment.) One study evaluated thirty-six patients with osteoporosis and treated them with a combination of calcium, sodium fluoride, and vitamin D. Another study evaluated the possible benefit of sodium fluoride to postmenopausal osteoporotic women.[183] Although there was a clear increase in bone mass after three years of treatment, the bone mass appeared to be gained only at certain sites and not others. More recently, a comparison of bone mass in middle-aged women who regularly drank well water showed that communities with high fluoride in the well water suffered twice the fracture rate.[831] Additional research is under way. Meanwhile, the effects and side effects of fluoride treatment require longer and more thorough study before it can be considered useful.[132] Although a slow-release form of fluoride made available in 1987 seems less toxic, by 1988, after ten years of research, sodium fluoride remains an experimental drug for the treatment of postmenopausal osteoporosis. The scientific results look poor.

After hysterectomy, you need to pay special attention to the health of your bones. You should be certain to include adequate calcium in your diet, preferably from a wide variety of calcium-rich foods. If it is necessary to take calcium supplements to meet your needs, then divide the dose up during the day to maximize your body's ability to absorb the calcium. Be certain to develop a regular exercise program that builds your muscle tone and strengthens your bone mass. Your intake of vitamin D should be sufficient but not excessive; fifteen minutes a day in the sun will suffice. As far as your bone health is concerned, any of the sex hormones are effective, but you will need to be aware of the hormones that are particularly dangerous to cardiovascular health and those that are particularly beneficial. Since HRT can now be prescribed in ways that enhance your overall longevity, it makes sense to seriously consider its use for maintaining your bone health. If you are unable to take HRT, you should search out medical centers that have experience with calcitonin therapy.

As recently as ten years ago, osteoporosis was an expected fact of life for 60 to 70 percent of the aging female population. Today, with sophistication and planning it is no longer a necessary reality. You can enjoy the benefits of good bones as you age. Even if you have already lost bone mass, with proper measures you can largely halt the further degeneration of your bones.

# 9

# *Protecting Your Cardiovascular Health*

Your most serious concern after hysterectomy should probably be cardiovascular disease, which claims the lives of more than 485,000 women each year in the United States. All of the reproductive-system çancers combined (breast, uterus, cervix, and ovaries) add up to less than one-eighth this number: 60,000 a year.

Most of us take good health for granted until disease forces a different focus. After menopause, cardiovascular health becomes a looming problem for large numbers of women.[190] Because hysterectomy produces an earlier menopause, it significantly increases a woman's chance of developing cardiovascular disease. Fortunately we know about many of the risk factors, and you can take protective action.

## *THE HEALTHY CARDIOVASCULAR SYSTEM*

Under healthy circumstances, the cardiovascular system provides an extraordinary range of critical life functions. *Cardio* refers to the heart, and *vascular* to the vessels—the arteries, arterioles, capillaries, venules, and veins that form the "pipes" through which blood flows all over the body. The heart is a hollow, four-chambered muscle that receives and disperses blood through a well-organized series of muscle contractions. When blood is in the chambers and the heart contracts, the liquid is forced out into the vessels. The blood is a richly complex liquid that derives its color from a particular group of cells (the red blood cells) that travel within the fluid. But the red blood cells form only a small part of the dynamic. A great many other molecules travel within the blood. Some are extremely tiny, such as the sex hormones. Others can be quite large, such as globules of cholesterol.

When your body is healthy, blood circulation serves a number of critical functions. First, the blood transports substances from one part of the body to the other. Second, changes in blood flow regulate your body temperature. Third, blood serves to deliver oxygen and other fuels to your cells and to take away waste from your cells. These are vital physiologic functions that maintain your life, and if any part of the system becomes nonfunctional, your health must suffer. If the heart muscle cannot contract properly, your health is at risk. If the blood vessels are clogged with cholesterol or if they are torn and damaged, blood cannot circulate freely, and your health is at risk.

Cardiovascular disease is the number one killer of women and men in the United States. Although men are vulnerable earlier in life, with the onset of menopause and hysterectomy women soon catch up and overtake them.

## CORONARY HEART DISEASE

The development of coronary heart disease, like osteoporosis, is the end result of a degenerative process that includes angina (pain), coronary insufficiency, and heart attack.[111] In atherosclerosis, the blood vessels of the heart become clogged with fats at the site of tears in the vessels and then thicken, preventing the smooth flow of blood and leading to coronary heart disease.[744]*

For some years biomedical researchers have been aware of the relationships among increased fats in the blood (hyper-

---

*The term *arteriosclerosis* describes this condition within the walls of arteries; *atherosclerosis* is specific to arteries of the heart muscle.

lipidemia), increased blood pressure (hypertension), obesity, diabetes, atherosclerosis, stress, cigarette smoking, and physical inactivity—all of which lead to coronary heart disease.[891] Hysterectomy increases the incidence of many of these factors and therefore mandates our attention here.[835] Figure 17 depicts the relationship of these elements.

Although coronary heart disease is progressive, you can influence many of the factors that can contribute to it. Especially after hysterectomy, you should take control of the several elements that protect cardiovascular health.

### *Hormonal Deprivation*

Estrogen deprivation induced by pelvic surgery increases the risk of heart attack. As early as 1959, published studies revealed an increased incidence of coronary heart disease (diseased heart muscle) in women who had had their ovaries removed prior to menopause.[744] There was also an increased incidence of athero-

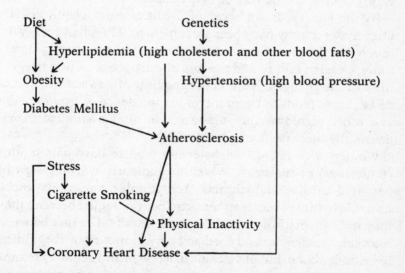

Figure 17. The relationship of risk factors for coronary heart disease

sclerotic disease (clogging of the coronary arteries) in ovariecto-mized women. Even the less invasive surgery of hysterectomy (while retaining the ovaries) was discovered to increase the risk of several forms of cardiovascular disease, including atheroscle-rotic disease, heart attack, and angina pectoris (pain in the chest).[744]

Although in women cholesterol normally increases with age, surgery that incapacitates the ovaries accelerates the problem.[337] Younger women show the most severe increases.[713] Ovariecto-mized women have 20 percent higher levels of LDL-Ch, the dan-gerous type of cholesterol, as compared to intact women of the same age.[9, 116, 316, 534, 710, 713, 751]

By 1981 at least six different studies had been published to show that hysterectomy with or without ovariectomy profoundly in-creases the risk of cardiovascular disease.[9, 190, 534, 744, 751] For example, 122,000 women with surgically induced early meno-pause were studied to determine their risk for heart attack. In this group, estrogen replacement therapy after ovariectomy signifi-cantly decreased the risk of heart attack.[32]

By the late 1980s, an array of cardiovascular health deficits after hysterectomy have been documented. The situation is very much like the one that exists for women's bones after hysterec-tomy. Ovarian failure and the loss of estrogen secretion triggers most of the changes. With increasing time after a natural meno-pause, there tends to be an increased incidence of hypertension and other cardiovascular diseases, but after a surgical meno-pause, the increase is much worse.[915]

Women with estrogen deficiencies tend to have palpitations (flutterings) of the heart, which are an early warning sign of potential cardiac arrhythmias. Arrhythmias, variations in the normal rhythm of the heartbeat, can be frightening because they may indicate malfunction of the heart muscle. The link between estrogen deficiencies and cardiac arrhythmias is only beginning to be understood, but physicians in a few health centers are now experimentally using estrogen to treat arrhythmias, with some success. Although this research is still in the experimental stage,

HRT regimens recommended for a posthysterectomized woman will treat this problem, too.

### Lipids and Your Health

The terminology surrounding the lipids (fats) is sometimes confusing, and because the terms are widely used in blood test reports it is helpful to understand them. *Lipid* is a general term encompassing many different fats. A *lipoprotein* is a molecule formed from the combination (attachment) of a lipid to a protein. A *triglyceride* is a complex molecule composed of three fatty acids attached to other substances. *Cholesterol* is a pearly fatlike substance found throughout the body (in the brain, fats, oils, liver, kidneys, and so on). Most of the body's cholesterol is manufactured in the liver, rather than—as is commonly supposed—derived from dietary cholesterol. Although cholesterol is chemically a fatlike substance, it is not a lipoprotein. When cholesterol attaches to (or combines with, or is carried by) a lipoprotein molecule, the name of the resulting large molecule is lipoprotein-cholesterol, or *lipoprotein-Ch.* Molecules of lipoprotein-Ch are generally referred to in one of three categories, named for their density (the relative amount of protein): the *high-density lipoprotein cholesterol* molecule, abbreviated HDL-Ch; the *low-density lipoprotein cholesterol* molecule, abbreviated LDL-Ch; and the *very-low-density lipoprotein cholesterol* molecule, abbreviated VLDL-Ch.

Cholesterol is an important substance because it is a principal component in the membranes that surround all the cells of the body.[146] It also serves as the material from which the steroid hormones (estrogen, progesterone, and testosterone) are manufactured. Cholesterol travels in the blood in free form as well as attached to lipoproteins and other blood proteins such as albumin. The term *total cholesterol* (or total plasma cholesterol) reflects the sum of all of the cholesterol that is traveling in the blood.

We need some cholesterol. The question is, when is "some" too much? In men, the lower the cholesterol level, the lower the risk of death; the higher the cholesterol, the increasingly higher the risk of death.[842] And the same principle apparently holds true for women.[545, 743] A cholesterol level that is less than 180 milligrams per deciliter (mg/dl) protects your cardiovascular health.[522]

The levels of the three principal classes of lipoprotein-cholesterol are generally measured when your blood is taken and sent to a lab for analysis. Your levels can be used to predict your risk of cardiovascular disease.

*LDL-Ch*, the low-density lipoprotein cholesterol, is the principal molecule that carries cholesterol in blood, usually accounting for 70 percent of the total cholesterol in the blood.[522] LDL-Ch has a tendency to increase with age.[926]

*VLDL-Ch*, the very-low-density lipoprotein, is a triglyceride-rich lipoprotein secreted by the liver. These very big molecules can make your blood look turbid (cloudy) when drawn into a test tube.

*HDL-Ch*, the high-density lipoprotein cholesterol, the smallest and the most dense, appears to play a role in transporting the cholesterol from the peripheral tissues to the liver to be excreted from the body.[522]* You might think of HDL-Ch as a vacuum cleaner, removing excess cholesterol and preventing clogging of the blood vessels.

Although a number of studies have shown that as the LDL-Ch level increases, the risk of heart attack increases in women, the LDL-Ch level is generally in proportion to the total plasma cholesterol level. When one is high, the other is high. And when one comes down, so does the other.[315, 337, 883] Some studies focus on the LDL-Ch, others on the total plasma cholesterol. Either way you look at it, high levels are dangerous, and surgical menopause increases the levels of both.

In contrast, as your HDL-Ch level increases, your risk of coronary heart disease decreases.[110]

---

*The HDL-Ch molecule has been shown to form a class of substances, and some studies attempt to show that certain subgroups of HDL-Ch are more protective than others.

## Triglycerides

Although high blood triglycerides have been shown to be a risk factor for subsequent heart attack in young men, the same has not been shown to be true for women. In fact, investigators in the Framingham Study have clearly shown that for women triglyceride levels are irrelevant when the HDL-Ch level is known.[315] The importance of triglyceride levels to your cardiovascular health seems less critical than that of total plasma cholesterol, LDL-Ch, or HDL-Ch.

## Hypertension

Hypertension (high blood pressure) is dangerous because it increases your risk for cardiovascular disease, as well as for stroke.[687]

In blood pressure readings, the larger number is the *systolic* measurement, and the smaller number the *diastolic*. The systole describes the maximum amount of pressure that is achieved against the walls of the arteries as the heart pumps blood throughout the vessels. The diastole reflects the elasticity or bounce-back that the stretched vessels are able to maintain. It is rather like a balloon: the maximum amount of air you might blow into it reflects its systolic pressure, while the lowest pressure after you let go of the spout would reflect the diastole. The analogy can only go so far; in a perfectly elastic balloon, the diastolic pressure might actually go as low as zero if the balloon completely flattened out when you let go of the spout; in the arteries, the bounce-back of the vessel walls is less elastic and the lowest recorded measurement might go as low as 50 or 60 millimeters of mercury (mm Hg). The two measures together describe how healthy your vessels and pushing force are. If the systole (pushing force of blood as it passes through your arteries) is too high, you run the risk of tearing blood vessels, just as you risk bursting a balloon if you blow too hard. If the diastole (pressure measured during the elastic rebound) is too high, the arteries have lost elasticity and, in becoming rigid, no longer can promote healthy blood circulation. Good cardiovascular health demands elastic blood vessels because the vessels have the critical job of transporting the blood to nourish all the cells of the body.

In one study, high blood pressure was defined as a systolic pressure greater than 145 mm Hg or a diastolic pressure greater than 95 mm Hg. Using this definition, less than 7 percent of premenopausal women showed hypertension; by menopause, the incidence had quadrupled.[915] At younger ages, a high diastolic blood pressure is probably more predictive of cardiovascular disease, but the situation reverses with aging; after about age 70, it is systolic hypertension that is most prevalent.[754]

The interrelationship between atherosclerosis, hypertension, and heart attack should begin to make sense. As arteries become sclerotic (clogged), blood pressure tends to increase in order to compensate for the difficulty of blood in passing through the clogged vessels. This pressure causes tears in the blood vessels. Where vessels are damaged, high pressure that shoves at the lumps of cholesterol can push them against weakened tissue and cause further tears. Torn vessels build scar tissue, and this scarring further narrows the passage. Lumps of cholesterol get caught in the tears, adding further to the clogging of the vessels. The greater the clogging (and consequent narrowing) of the vessels, the harder the heart must work to pump blood through; the blood pressure tends to increase; and ultimately the heart muscle itself is unable to receive sufficient blood circulating within its own clogged vessels. Lacking adequate blood, oxygen is denied to the needy heart muscle and parts of the muscle then die from lack of the vital oxygen. As the heart loses partial function, it no longer can pump blood adequately to the rest of the body. The term *heart attack* denotes this condition. The term *stroke* represents a similar sudden attack—a loss of vital function and cell death in a particular region of the brain, with subsequent effects in other areas of the body.

### Other Factors

Several diseases have been associated with a low HDL-Ch level and a high risk of coronary heart disease. They include diabetes mellitus, kidney disease, and chronic cholestasis (a liver disease). Also, a number of coronary risk factors are generally found among people with low HDL-Ch levels; these include obesity, physical inactivity, cigarette smoking, and a family history of coronary heart disease.[599]

## WHAT YOU CAN DO TO PROMOTE CARDIOVASCULAR HEALTH

A vigorous approach to your own health care requires that you have a regular evaluation of your cardiovascular system. Internal medicine specialists are probably an ideal resource for this evaluation. Other physicians, such as general practitioners and cardiologists, also have training in the cardiovascular system. Some gynecologists are sophisticated about cardiovascular health promotion, but many are not. Ask!

There are five actions that you can take to protect your cardiovascular health. Working together, they will enhance the strength of your cardiovascular system and the length of your healthy life.

- Through good nutritional habits, you need to maintain a proper lipid and cholesterol balance in your diet, and to be aware of the impact of both vitamin C and salt.
- You need to engage in aerobic exercise.
- You need to avoid smoking.
- You need to regulate your blood pressure, if necessary with a prescription from your doctor.
- You need adequate levels of sex hormones and should consider taking HRT to protect your cardiovascular health.

After a hysterectomy, you should have regular medical exams, ideally twice a year. There are several cardiovascular risk factors to be on the alert for. You will want to be certain that your plasma lipids do not put you at a high risk of cardiovascular disease; the way to do this is to have the levels tested, by evaluation of a sample of your blood. Blood pressure measurements will determine if you have hypertension. A baseline electrocardiogram (EKG) to provide information for your health history makes sense. Even though your health insurance may not pay for these diagnostic and preventive measures, it is a cost that you should see as necessary and wise for maintaining your cardiovascular health.

### Proper Diet

A large body of recent research data has shown that certain fats in your diet increase plasma cholesterol and LDL-Ch levels, while other fats decrease these levels. The HDL-Ch can also be manipulated through the diet. The cholesterol content of the foods in your diet appears to be much less important than either the type of fat or the proportion of the different fats that make up your diet. Certain foods, including fresh apples, bran muffins, and cooked oatmeal, serve to clear cholesterol from the blood. If you can include these in your regular diet, your cardiovascular health will benefit. (Chapter 13 provides the details of both the lipid levels and the foods that manipulate them.)

The question of reducing salt intake has stirred a good bit of controversy. Although self-help magazines commonly advise women (and men) to reduce their salt intake, in 1986 a review in the *Archives of Internal Medicine* on sodium (salt) and hypertension suggested an approach tailored to an individual's situation. In some people, hypertension can be caused by abnormal salt metabolism; for them, restricting the salt intake can effectively lower the blood pressure. Particularly susceptible groups include those with a family history of hypertension, the elderly, blacks, and those with low renin–hypertension disease. Moderate salt restriction will significantly reduce blood pressure in a large percentage of these people. But not everybody needs to restrict their salt, and a severe restriction of salt is not necessarily helpful. If you are in one of these susceptible groups, then reducing your level to a moderate amount may help you. Otherwise, salt change is probably irrelevant.[398]

A deficiency of vitamin C (ascorbic acid) promotes the ability of fats to be deposited in blood vessels. This clumping of fat triggers atherosclerosis even when cholesterol levels are normal.[794] Adequate ascorbic acid is also needed to maintain the structural material of the blood vessels. When the ascorbic acid is depleted, the structure weakens (as is the case for bone) and the vessels become more vulnerable to the tears that lead to cardiovascular diseases. Thus, coronary atherosclerosis can result in part from a deficient consumption of ascorbic acid.[794]

Your need for vitamin C varies and depends on stress, disease, smoking habits, the requirements of wound healing, and dietary habits. After a hysterectomy, you should be certain to consume adequate vitamin C. If you are a nonsmoker, 500 to 1,000 milligrams per day is probably at the low end of what you need. If you smoke, your requirements double. Your bowel tolerance level will guide you (see page 306).

Total calorie intake also influences cardiovascular health. In one twelve-year study in Sweden, women who ate too little (as shown by their being in the lowest quintile of calories consumed) experienced four times the heart attack rate of those in the higher calorie groups.[482] On the other hand, excessive weight exacerbates and sometimes even causes hypertension. (Chapter 14 may help if you are overweight.)

### Exercise and Relaxation

Aerobic (air-burning) exercises—those that cause you to breathe deeply and heavily—serve your cardiovascular system in several ways. They increase your oxygen consumption, bringing more oxygen into your bloodstream to nourish cells throughout your body—including your heart muscle, which when it receives plenty of oxygen functions with less chance of harm coming to it. They help the blood to remove waste (carbon dioxide and other metabolic waste) more efficiently. They reduce the dangerous lipids in blood and increase the protective ones. They lower blood pressure and prevent heart disease.[660, 813]

Promoting muscle relaxation through exercise also helps to lower blood pressure. You can take advantage of this physiological mechanism by setting up your own pattern of regular exercise. If you take a swim or a long walk every day, your muscles will enter a state of relaxation automatically. Muscle relaxation affects all the muscles of the body, including the muscular blood vessels. In addition, as we relax and lower our adrenalin-related nerve transmissions, the electrical signals that control the generation of pressure in the heart muscle change into the kind that promote lower blood pressure.

To maximize your cardiovascular health, you need at least three hours of athletic activity per week. However, you don't need to go through the pain and stress of very strenuous exercise classes. You can engage in a pattern of regular, pleasant physical activity, such as swimming, walking, or dancing. (See Chapter 15 for advice on planning an exercise regimen.)

During the past ten years, a number of biofeedback experiments have attempted to learn whether people can be trained to lower their blood pressure levels through behavioral means. The answer is yes—under certain conditions. In one study, patients went off their hypertension medication for six weeks. Progressive muscle relaxation techniques were then introduced, and the patients were asked to do these at home twice a day for twenty minutes. The people who responded to this kind of training were those who originally had higher norepinephrine levels in their blood. Norepinephrine, also known as noradrenalin, is similar to adrenalin; it appears that it can be lowered when one learns how to relax in a disciplined way.[150]

Stress can be understood as the body's physical reaction to the threat of danger. When unbalanced by compensatory relaxation, it is very dangerous to the cardiovascular system. In the face of stress, the particular chemicals that promote the body's ability to fight or to run (for example, adrenalin) get turned on and are secreted in very high quantities, accelerating the heart rate and

blood pressure. In large part, our mental and emotional perceptions control our reactions to external events. One woman may
be emotionally overwhelmed by a situation that would not even
"ruffle the feathers" of another, and the one who reacts excessively puts an additional burden on her physiological system.

To control stress one needs to exert effort in a variety of ways.
Some people are able to achieve a change of philosophy or attitude, thereby gaining access to a heightened capacity to cope
with life's difficulties. For some people, a religious orientation
helps the soul to find rest. The practice of regular, quiet medita-
tion can help to lower the blood pressure, as can biofeedback
training. Supportive therapy—whether through a group, a psychotherapist, or courses of study—can help one to reorient attitudes. How one learns new ways of looking at oneself is less
important than the actual capacity for changing. Sometimes it is
helpful to change one's physical environment and retreat from
stress-induced situations.

Regular physical exercise promotes the physiological systems
that permit stress to be handled more easily; it also changes the
way we perceive, as our brain chemistry is flooded with the beta
endorphins that produce feelings of well-being. And then there
is love, the greatest stress reducer of all when it is well received.
If you are not receiving love, then find someone to give love to,
perhaps through community or social service volunteering. Giving another person a sense that you accept them as they are
serves a double purpose: it is a blessing to the receiver and to the
giver. This kind of giving always helps focus priorities differently, and in the process stress is lessened.

### Avoiding Smoking

When we inhale smoke, our bodies take in carbon monoxide,
a deadly gas that attaches tightly to the red blood cells, making
them unable either to retrieve carbon dioxide waste or to receive
oxygen. In consequence, the cells throughout the body become
vulnerable and begin to die of asphyxiation and disease. Because
smoke asphyxiates all the cells of the body, smoking forces the

physical machine, especially the heart, to work against a debilitating force. Chapter 14 reviews what you can do if you are a smoker and want to quit. It will be very, very difficult, but the rewards are life itself and the vigor that is a part of a healthy life.

### Regulating Your Blood Pressure

A low blood pressure lowers the risk that dangerous lipids can damage your cardiovascular health.[438] When the blood pressure is high, the pushing force of the blood against clumps of cholesterol causes tears in the vessel walls, producing more damage than when pressure is lower. If you have high blood pressure, you should take action to bring it down.[688]

If your blood pressure remains high after you have taken positive steps in terms of diet, exercise, stress, and smoking, you may need a medical prescription for reducing blood pressure. There are a number of medications currently available, and your doctor will help you choose one that is appropriate. But it would be better to create such good physical and mental health habits that you do not need them. Drugs correct the symptom, but they do not address the cause.

### Hormonal Replacement Therapy

Properly selected types and dosages of hormonal replacement therapy will help cardiovascular health. If you want HRT to affect your cardiovascular system, the estrogen should be oral.[241, 710] Creams and patches generally do not help the cardiovascular system (see chapters 6 and 7). The progestin does not have to be oral, but that route may be your only option in any case.

While most hormones decrease the risk of cardiovascular diseases, some increase the risk. It is important to avoid high concentrations of either the synthetic estrogens or the 19-nortestosterone progestagens unless you particularly need them in addressing another problem (for example, see "Breast Cancer and Benign Breast Disease," page 133). The synthetic estrogens (ethinyl estradiol, DES, mestranol, and sometimes estradiol valerate) have each been shown to have some adverse effects.

Fortunately, many HRT regimens, principally the natural estrogens and progesterones, either reduce the risk of cardiovascular disease or show no negative effect on it.*

## The Estrogens

The early forms of HRT, especially after hysterectomy, used only estrogens. For this reason a number of studies were done on only ERT, and these are discussed first.

Because hypertension tends to increase in menopause, it was logical to consider that the condition might result from estrogen deficiency. As early as 1958, investigators had evaluated the use of a high dose of natural ERT (up to 2.5 milligrams of Premarin® per day) for women who already had coronary atherosclerosis. ERT reduced the cholesterol levels.[545, 743, 955] Normally cholesterol rises with age,[9] and ovariectomized women are even worse off with age.[380] Cholesterol levels do not increase when such women take ERT[337, 713, 927] and are usually reduced within several months. The lower levels remain as long as the studies have tested them, so far up to three years.[465, 921]†

Likewise, in most cases hypertension is not increased and may even be decreased for most women who use natural estrogen therapy. However, exceptions do occur.[643, 901] There does seem to be a group of women who are at risk for increasing their blood pressure when they take ERT (stopping it produces a recovery from the phenomenon within several months).[154, 901, 919] But this is rare, occurring in only 4 percent of ovariectomized ERT users.[901] If you do take estrogen therapy after hysterectomy, it will be important for you to keep track of your blood pressure to see whether you are in this rare group for whom estrogen

---

*Studies include 32, 476, 618, 688, 716, 750, 843.

†The lowering of the total plasma cholesterol occurred on ethinyl estradiol (0.01 mg per day);[745] mestranol (20 to 40 µg per day);[9] estriol succinate (2 mg per day);[710] and conjugated equine estrogens (ranging from 0.625 to 1.25 mg per day).[745] Estrogen therapies also reduced the LDL-Ch level.[337, 883] And estradiol treatment of postmenopausal women with high total plasma cholesterol levels decreased their cholesterol.[883]

therapies produce an increase in pressure. It is not necessarily appropriate to stop estrogen therapy even if your blood pressure does increase, according to at least one investigator, who said: "In our opinion, whenever hypertension appears under estrogen treatment, estrogen medication should not be stopped at once. Salt intake, however, should be reduced to a maximum of 3 gr a day. Should this prove to be insufficient, antihypertension drugs should be added to hormonal replacement therapy."[919] You might want to discuss such an approach with your health care team. Since hormones have such great value, if there is a way to continue taking them, you may well want to do so. (It should be mentioned that the literature, while overwhelmingly favorable to the effects of ERT on cardiovascular health, has produced one confusing exception, which appears to show that ERT increases the risk of heart attack.*)

The data now published on studies of many thousands of women appear to be generally consistent in showing that if you have had a hysterectomy and/or an ovariectomy, you are at risk for having a cardiovascular disease. The same set of data most strongly suggests that ERT will not only cause you no increased risk, provided the estrogen is a natural form, but will actually reduce a number of the risk factors for cardiovascular disease. Therefore, I agree with the conclusions of Dr. Meir Stampfer and his colleagues, as published in the *New England Journal of Medicine:* "The data support the hypothesis that the postmenopausal use of estrogen reduces the risk of severe coronary heart disease."[843]

---

*Different publications surrounding the Framingham Study (an epidemiologic study), as it continues to follow an aging population, have produced some data that appear to be somewhat internally contradictory. In 1985, in a report of a study of 1,200 postmenopausal women, ERT was shown to lower both the total plasma cholesterol and the LDL-Ch levels while increasing the HDL-Ch.[955] These results were consistent in showing that ERT was associated with reduced risks. However, in this study the authors concluded that ERT increased the risk of cardiovascular disease. A publication by the same authors in 1976 came to opposite conclusions,[750] and in 1978 they concluded that ERT increased the risk of nonfatal heart attacks.[420] I believe the problem of contradictory conclusions (that estrogens lower the risk factors for heart attack but increases the risk of heart attack) comes from limitations of the study design. For further details of the biomedical analyses of this work, the reader is referred to reference 174.

Although estrogen appears to be helpful for your cardiovascular health profile, a really complete HRT regimen should include estrogen with progestin.

## Estrogen with Progestin Opposition

Several forms of progestagens have been studied for their effects on the lipids in the blood. Most have been studied in opposition to an ERT regimen, although occasional studies of the effects of progestagen alone have appeared. Table 9 shows the different progestins that have been studied, grouped into three categories.

High doses of these hormones, whether alone or in opposition to various doses of different estrogens, sometimes produce adverse effects, increasing the total plasma cholesterol and the LDL-Ch and lowering the beneficial HDL-Ch. However, low doses of any of these agents appear to have none of these adverse effects on the plasma lipids. It should be noted that medroxy-progesterone acetate (MPA), commonly sold as Provera®, only rarely produces unwanted lipid changes in the high dose range, whereas the high doses of 19-nortestosterone frequently show these adverse effects. When the MPA dose of 10 milligrams is divided, half in the morning and half in the evening, the negative effects on cardiovascular health are stronger; there was an 18 percent reduction in the protective HDL-Ch levels.[658] Why should dividing the same dose in half and taking it every twelve hours have a generally stronger effect than taking the full dose every twenty-four hours? Apparently when you take it all at once some of it never gets to work; perhaps it does not get absorbed fully, or perhaps the system gets so overloaded it can deal with only about half the amount.

In contrast, even the highest doses of natural progesterone, when given in doses of 100 milligrams twice a day and opposed to 2 milligrams a day of estradiol valerate, were shown to have no negative effects on the plasma lipids (neither cholesterol nor LDL-Ch rose, and the HDL-Ch did not decline).[657, 658]

It has become increasingly clear that the androgenic progestagens (norethisterone acetate, norgestrel, and others) are decid-

**Table 9.** *Oral Progestins*

| Hormone Used (usually 10 to 13 days per month) | High Doses | Low Doses | References to Studies |
|---|---|---|---|
| *19-nortestosterones* | | | |
| -medrogestone | 5 mg | | 874 |
| -norethisterone acetate | 5–10 mg | 1 mg | 71, 383, 811, 968 |
| -d Norgestrel | 1.8 mg | | 811 |
| -levonorgestrel | 120–250 μg | 30 μg | 240, 383, 658 |
| *17α progestagens* | | | |
| MPA (medroxy-progesterone-acetate) Provera® | 10 mg or 5mg twice/day | 2.5 mg twice/day | 383, 658, 811 |
| *pure natural progesterone* | | 100mg twice/day | 657, 658 |

edly stronger than the 17-α progestagen MPA. With the trend toward the use of natural preparations (which began with the estrogens and which is becoming more common internationally with progestagens), it seems reasonable to suggest the following:

• Until natural progesterones are available in the United States and Canada, MPA will probably be your best option unless you already have a disease for which a stronger progestagen is to be prescribed (for example, cystic glandular hyperplasia) or unless you have a libidinal deficit that impels you toward the 19-nortestosterones. High doses of MPA appear to be better tolerated and are less likely to increase your cholesterol levels.

• If you take lower doses of MPA, 2.5 milligrams twice a day will probably be optimal for protecting against adverse lipid effects. Likewise, low doses of the 19-nortestosterones may be quite satisfactory, particularly for libidinal stimulation, although research has not yet addressed this potential.

- The duration of progestagen use should probably be between ten and thirteen days per month, although some investigators have suggested that very low progesterone, opposed to estrogen, be given every day. Studies are needed to determine the best approach.

The issue of how many days of the month a progestagen should be taken (every day versus half the month) has not yet been resolved, and we must stay alert to the results of future studies. Testosterone therapy, useful for libido and muscle strength after surgical depletion of ovarian hormones, has not yet been studied for dose/response on cardiovascular measures. Such studies are badly needed.

## Oral Contraceptives

Although the development of our knowledge has shown that appropriately dosed oral HRT regimens are healthy for the cardiovascular system, the same has not been universally true of oral contraceptives. Because of the awareness that oral contraceptives have had negative effects on cardiovascular health, it may be useful to briefly review that literature to assure you that HRT is different from oral contraceptives. Oral contraceptives use synthetic estrogens and progestins; HRT should use naturals wherever possible. Oral contraceptives produce artificially high sex hormone levels in the blood; HRT produces levels below those of normally cycling women.

Oral contraceptives sometimes produce dangerous lipid changes, including increases in both total plasma cholesterol and LDL-Ch, as well as decreases in the useful HDL-Ch.[465, 921, 926] The culprit in the contraceptive appears to be the synthetic hormones, particularly their progestin component. When the progestin (norethindrone acetate) dose of oral contraceptives increased, the incidence of stroke increased proportionately, albeit the incidence was still low.[572] But HRT users need not be concerned. Norethindrone acetate, a form of progestagen that derives from the 19-nortestosterone form, is not recommended for HRT regimens in the high doses (2 to 4 milligrams per day) that were commonly used in oral contraceptives.

It has been long noted that thromboembolic phenomena (clots) have been associated (rarely) with oral contraceptive use in young women but not in women on HRT.[642] In fact, one study showed that the stronger oral contraceptive doses led to increases in a specific blood globulin, "clotting factor VII," that leads to an increased risk of thrombosis.[573] This risk appears to exist for some users of oral contraceptive estrogens; it does not appear to be a concern for users of HRT.

Blood pressure, both systolic and diastolic, increases among almost all women who take oral contraceptives and then decreases within three months after stopping the hormones.[938] In contrast, for 98 percent of HRT users, blood pressure does not increase on HRT regimens.

In spite of the risk factors that oral contraceptives can be shown to induce for some women, no significant difference in overall death rates has emerged between oral contraceptive users and nonusers when matched for age.[228] In fact, the incidence of heart attack would be significantly reduced if known special risk groups did not take oral contraceptives. The groups that should probably avoid the use of oral contraceptives include women past the age of 35, particularly if they smoke; hypertensives; diabetics; women with hypercholesterolemia (high levels of blood cholesterol); and those with a family history of coronary heart disease.[179]

Fortunately, postmenopausal women taking natural estrogen, alone or with small amounts of progestagen, have not exhibited the increased risk of coronary heart disease shown by oral contraceptive users over the age of 35.[693] For most women, the use of HRT after a hysterectomy is beneficial to cardiovascular health. And even among women with coronary heart disease, natural HRT regimens appear useful and safe for protecting blood lipids and blood pressure.[687]

## COAGULATION FACTORS IN BLOOD

The ability of your blood to clot, or coagulate, is an essential health requirement. However, excess clotting can be dangerous. Studies have been conducted to evaluate whether HRT interferes with the clotting process, and the results are essentially consistent in finding safety. One exception, published in 1976, reported on an increased tendency to clot among a group of menopausal women who were given conjugated equine estrogens in doses of 1.25 milligrams per day;[844] it was particularly the young women who seemed to be at risk. None of the other investigations have agreed with that result. For example, the Boston Collaborative Drug Surveillance Program has concluded that ERT does not affect thromboembolic events (those caused by clotting).[68] Others have provided data in agreement that HRT is safe.[28, 644, 770]

Dr. John Studd and his colleagues, after investigating six different estrogen preparations, some of which were opposed by norethisterone or testosterone, concluded, "This study does not reveal any change towards hypercoaguability [increased clotting] in any of the parameters with the treatment regimens studied." In 1986 investigators reporting in the *New England Journal of Medicine* also concluded that there were no clotting factor changes on any dose of any preparation when they compared oral estrogen in the conjugated equine form to transdermal estrogen.[119] Nonetheless, according to the conclusions of Dr. M. Aylward,[28] the synthetic estrogen ethinyl estradiol should be avoided because, when there has been any risk, it was due to the synthetic form. You may wish to discuss with your health care center advisor the use of antithrombin screening tests, which allow the identification of women at high risk for thromboembolic phenomenon. The problem is a very rare one, but if you are at high risk, it is useful for you to know it.

Cardiovascular disease is the biggest killer of posthysterectomized women. In order to avoid the long, degenerative process that results in coronary disease, you can take several positive actions.

You should have your blood pressure and your blood lipids checked to learn whether or not you are at an increased risk of cardiovascular disease. Your nutritional choices should include substances that will maintain a low total plasma level of cholesterol (less than 180 mg/dl) and high levels of the beneficial HDL-Ch. (See Table 12, page 289, which shows the relationship between a relatively high HDL and a relatively low total plasma cholesterol.) If you smoke cigarettes, you should seriously consider stopping or significantly lowering your intake of these contaminants. Avoid routine passive exposure to other people's smoke; it, too, is bad for you. A program of regular exercise will help to keep your blood pressure low and your lipids in healthy order. If you are obese, you should diet to lose weight.

HRT has very beneficial effects on the cardiovascular health profile. An ERT regimen, coupled with appropriate progestagen, should help to improve the various preventive factors. A healthy cardiovascular system pays a rich dividend in promoting your ability to live and to be well.

# 10 🌿

# *Sexual Life After Hysterectomy*

🌿 Because of its delicate, private nature, sexual life is perhaps the most difficult subject for both women and their health advisors to address. Does a hysterectomy alter your sexuality? It certainly should, if you consider that parts of your sexual anatomy have been removed. Does hysterectomy necessarily diminish the quality of your sexual life? The answer to this question is much more complex and will depend on you, the availability of a partner, the attitude of your partner, and the sophistication of your physician.

Here is how one woman in her mid-forties described her reaction:

> Before my hysterectomy/ovariectomy ten years ago, at the age of 35, I used to have a wonderful sexuality. I had no hang-ups about the surgery, in fact welcomed it, as birth control had caused me a lot of grief. Since the surgery, I have experienced a dramatic impairment of several specific components of sexual response. These are: mental desire (I never have any sexual feelings or needs now), the ability to be aroused through touch, and the lubrication response (I have to use a lubricant).
>
> I expect that someday this sad side effect of hysterectomy may be worked out and treatable. For now, research (and I suspect interest among physicians) is lacking. I feel cheated of the best years of my sexuality.

She is right on several points. Most physicians do not have training that enables them to help you enhance your sexual life after pelvic surgery.[440] There are no certification requirements to ensure that physicians maintain awareness of developments in the field of sexual health.

Meanwhile, the work of biologists and biopsychologists has moved forward to provide important perspectives on sexual function. For a woman who has had a hysterectomy, state-of-the-art medical care is important because science is only now providing solutions to the sexual problems that hysterectomy can cause. The woman with concerns about her sexual life after hysterectomy will need to learn the facts and then to ask prospective physicians about the methods they employ to help with her specific problem. Knowledge empowers a woman to discern whether she is in an appropriate medical office when she has a medical problem related to her sexual life.

## *HORMONES AND SEXUALITY*

The study of the interactions between reproductive-system hormones (the estrogens and androgens) and various aspects of sexuality has a history that is rich and complex. Sexual behavior between couples and their chemical signaling to each other have been well investigated. We know that hormonal changes cause sexual behavior changes, and that changes in sexual behavior can alter the hormones.*

Yet, while some areas of human sexual behavior are conducive to scientific study, others are not because of the intensely personal and variable nature of the experience.[391, 690] And because of normal age-related changes in sexuality, it is easy to overlook the changes that are induced by surgery. Women who do not have hysterectomies commonly experience sexual problems as they age, but problems are even more common among women who have undergone pelvic surgery.

*Studies include 147, 459, 591, 592, 593, 594, 595, 692.

## SEXUAL RESPONSE CHANGES WITH AGE AND HORMONAL DECLINE

Ideally, lovemaking should be the central focus of sexuality, and lovemaking should get better with the wisdom that comes with maturity. If you are blessed with a compassionate partner, you are very fortunate. Even so, it helps if you understand the underlying sexual system and if that system is working at its healthiest level. Four components make up the cornerstones of the female sexual system:

• *Libido*—the mentally and psychologically based drive to engage in sexual activity

• *Arousability*—the physical and emotional capacity to be aroused

• *Genital tissue response*—the ability to produce sexual wetness and the other related physical components of sexual arousal

• *The capacity for orgasm*—the ability to experience the full range of reflexes associated with a complete sexual encounter

As we age, there are inevitable changes in each of these dimensions. The frequency of sexual activity may diminish, but the capacity for sensual joy need not. Sometimes less quantity becomes more pleasure in terms of the quality and the tone of the experience. Let's look at the age-related changes in each aspect of sexual life.

### Libido

As women grow older, most experience some loss of libido (interest in sexual activity).[29] Not everyone does, but by about age 54, whether or not they have had pelvic surgery, 75 percent of women no longer have the same level of interest in sex that they once had.[346] In fact, a decline in libido is what most commonly brings women to sexual health clinics.[29, 331, 478] The loss of libido is generally more sudden than gradual—rather like walking through a door and finding oneself in a completely different room. It seems to happen at the point when the sex hormone levels have completed their transition to the markedly lower postmenopausal levels.[164, 567] Until then, for heterosexual women with an available partner, there appears to be no loss in the dimensions of sexual desire, sexual response, or satisfaction with sexual life.[164]* Once the hormones reach the low postmenopausal level, there is even a significant decline in the numbers of sexual thoughts and fantasies. About half of postmenopausal women who are not taking hormonal replacement therapy also show signs of genital atrophy, the problem occurring most commonly in sexually inactive women.[341]

At about the same time, there is usually a decline in coital frequency within stable and loving relationships, from an average of about two times a week to less than once per week. Why does frequency decline? Usually, although the libido may be lower, the capacity to respond to a sexual advance is not diminished; often the woman is willing but her partner is not, and the couple settles into a routine that matches the lowest level of desire for coitus.[690, 769] Data show that only when women have younger (male) partners does the frequency tend not to decline as the woman grows older.[769] Although estrogen therapy will improve lubrication and perhaps orgasm, there is a general agreement that it will not help with the loss of libido that is very common after pelvic surgery.[206, 207]

### Sexual Arousal

Under normal circumstances, sexual arousal is accompanied by a delicious sensation as blood rushes from other areas of the body into the groin. As local blood flow increases, the vaginal tissues *transude,* or sweat, a wetness that comes from blood fluids being pushed through the tissues. Menopause changes some of the elements of this pelvic vasocongestion.

Dr. William Masters and Ms. Virginia Johnson, in their classic

---

*No data on menopausal or hysterectomy-induced influences on lesbian sexual activity have yet been published in scientific or medical journals.

work *Human Sexual Inadequacy,* published in 1970, quantified the physical changes in response to aging:[557]

- It takes longer to become wet. Instead of the young woman's fifteen- to thirty-second response time for sexual stimulation to produce vaginal lubrication, with age it may take five minutes or more of "nondemanding sex play" for any degree of lubrication to occur.
- This is similar to the man's delayed onset of erection. It takes him longer to become erect as he ages.
- The vaginal walls become thin and deteriorate, turning pink instead of purple as the estrogen levels diminish.
- HRT reverses many of the effects of aging on physical sexual response.

Recently some thoughtful and thorough experiments have been published to show that the vaginal blood flow increases when ERT is given.[791] The Kegel exercises also increase the vaginal blood flow (see page 239). As the vaginal blood flow increases, the lubrication response improves.

### Genital Tissue Response

A man's and a woman's sexual arousal reactions are physically similar.[391] In both cases, blood rushes to the genitals. For the man, the blood fills the capillaries of the penis, thereby producing an erection. For the woman, blood rushes to the genitals, swelling the labia and vagina and increasing the fluid pressure against the capillary walls; the increased pressure leads to sexual wetness. (Scientists who study sexual response use established techniques in private laboratory settings in order to evaluate genital changes during particular circumstances, such as during estrogen depletion or replacement.[818])

With the aging that results from estrogen deprivation, the vagina shortens by about 40 percent of its younger length. Simultaneously, the vaginal tissue thins. In addition, during the excitement phase of sexual arousal, when the vaginal barrel typically expands (much like a balloon and similar to your throat just before the climax of a yawn), the capacity to expand is reduced with age. Although the clitoral size enlarges throughout life,[399] the clitoral response to sexual excitement tends to decline with age.[556]

If you don't have an available sexual partner, masturbation will either prevent genital atrophy or, at the least, minimize it.[493] Studies have shown that masturbation is very common. Generally 25 percent of women in their seventies acknowledge the behavior.[441] Masturbation, although it does not affect the hormonal environment, is similar to partner-induced sexual activity in that it increases the flow of blood into the genital region. It also keeps the cellular structure healthy.

ERT, when given in sufficient quantity, corrects the lubricative dysfunction that is common among hormonally deprived women.* The cellular structure of vaginal tissue that becomes atrophic (deteriorated) and produces vaginitis (inflammation of the vagina leading to pain) does respond to ERT, but it seems to take a rather high dose to achieve this effect. One study showed that only doses of 1.25 milligrams a day or higher of conjugated equine estrogen were sufficient to improve atrophic vaginitis in women who had already developed the condition.[302] Estrogen cream applied directly at the vagina appears to produce a good result with a lower dose.[317] (Vaginal estrogen should not be applied before sexual intercourse because it will rub onto the penis and be absorbed by the man.)

A sexually active couple should realize that until lubrication is achieved, intercourse should be postponed. Otherwise, the pressure of an erect and dry penis against a dry vagina can easily cause vaginal abrasions (cuts and tears) that will make subsequent sexual activity even more painful. Although lubricants can be purchased that will overcome this friction, it might be more thoughtful for the male partner to await natural lubrication as a signal of the woman's needs.

*Studies include 206, 207, 302, 430, 557, 791.

### Capacity for Orgasm

The actual physical response of a genital orgasm can be likened to the physical response in the throat during a yawn. In both, there is an increasing tightening of the muscle structure, followed by a spasm in which the tightness is released. The orgasmic response in women is a reflex that, once set in motion, is usually capable of going on to completion, just as a yawn generally begins and is followed by completion.

Another familiar reflex is the "knee-jerk" response. Reflexes generally require some stimulation through the nerves going to the spinal cord; this stimulation is followed by nerve impulses firing back on the muscles near the place where the stimulation originated, triggering them to contract. In many ways, the orgasmic reflex follows this pattern. Although orgasm carries emotional and spiritual aspects, the mechanical process is pretty similar. Debate has been waged for years concerning exactly where the stimulus should be applied in order to trigger orgasm. It now appears that there are several different routes: one at the clitoris; one inside the vagina, particularly at the G Spot location (discussed later in the chapter); and one, in estrogen-rich women, at the cervix. Repeated tapping or rhythmic massage at any of these three regions can produce a subsequent vaginal and/or uterine orgasm.[174, 679] But here too, aging changes things.

Unlike a yawn, which produces a single spasm, orgasmic spasms often come in multiples. In the estrogen-rich woman, orgasmic contractions will generally occur five to ten times; in the estrogen-depleted woman, orgasmic contractions are fewer, occurring three to five times. As estrogen levels decline, the intensity of sexual response also diminishes.[556] But if there are 50 percent fewer vaginal contractions during orgasm, this does not necessarily produce a reduction in the experience of pleasure. The music produced by a string quartet is no less harmonious or delightful than that made by a full symphony.

## POSTHYSTERECTOMY SEX DIFFICULTIES

After a woman has a hysterectomy, she may experience two forms of sexual difficulties: those that are immediate and generally recoverable; and those that are long-term and, if left alone, may never recover.

Immediately after surgery you must allow yourself time to heal. Even assuming that you have an excellent surgeon, the abdomen may feel easily bruised, and it can take three to four months before coital pressure is enjoyed rather than just tolerated. This is probably due to a temporary shrinkage of the vagina, which produces a shorter and narrower vault.[15] In one study, the kinds of difficulties that were encountered in more than half of the women included difficulties with the penis entering the vagina, dryness in the vagina, painful intercourse, reduced libido, and coital bleeding.[153] Yet for women in stable heterosexual relationships, within two months after hysterectomy more than half are sexually active; within four months, 90 percent are.[153]

Adhesions (internal scar tissue) are also a common result of surgery and occur in about half the women who undergo pelvic surgery.[213] They can be painful, and sometimes further surgery is necessary in order to remove them.

Radiation therapy may lengthen healing time. One study showed that one year after cancer surgery, differences emerged among patients who had undergone radiation therapy compared with those who had not. The irradiated patients experienced significant decreases in sexual enjoyment, ability to attain orgasm, libido, frequency of intercourse, sexual opportunity, and sexual dreams.[787] Because it prevents cell division, radiation interferes with healing; therefore a longer period of pain is to be expected. In addition, the irradiated groups had greater stress and anxiety, which contribute to a slower healing time.

In the longer term, there has been a well-documented decline in the physiologic dimensions of sexual function after hysterectomy.

## *Libidinal Deficits*

After your surgery, you may experience a loss of sexual appetite that does not recover. Decline in libido after hysterectomy has been carefully studied. Close to half of all women experiencing a hysterectomy, with or without an ovariectomy, report the deficit.* It may take some time before the loss of libido is revealed. Perhaps because the slow recovery period can confuse lassitude with loss of libido, studies of sexual response shortly after the surgery are less likely to show deficits than studies that follow women for up to two years after their hysterectomy.

ERT does not improve the problem after hysterectomy. Double-blind, placebo-controlled studies have established that whatever the factors are that control the libidinal aspects, they are not estrogen-dependent,[206] and if you want to experience a higher libido, you will have to consider androgen therapies.

Testosterone, predominantly a male sex hormone, probably plays an important role in female sexuality. Ovariectomized women lose an important source of testosterone. So do hysterectomized women who retain ovaries that then become sluggish.

Androgens, particularly androstenedione and testosterone, have been shown to be related to libido in women. Medical experts, drawing on observations of patients, have commented that although libido may increase or decrease with aging, it does appear to be related to a woman's blood levels of androgens.[323, 441, 764] Three prospective studies have been published evaluating the influences of testosterone on sex drive in women.

The first study, published in 1977, involved British women complaining of a loss of libido after hysterectomy. They were provided with hormonal implants of estradiol mixed with testosterone.[859] A significant improvement in libido occurred in 80 percent. (The study had excluded women who reported marital difficulties in order to focus on women who said they had good marriages but were distressed about libidinal deficits.)

In 1982 a study in Philadelphia explored the relationship be-

*Studies include 206, 351, 459, 896, 897, 900.

tween the blood levels of testosterone and ongoing sexual behavior in women.[680] Two groups of healthy married women, thirty years apart in age, were evaluated. The study showed no relationship between estrogen level and sexual appetite, but higher levels of sexual desire were associated with higher circulating levels of testosterone.

More recently, investigators in Montreal have published a double-blind study of fifty-three women who had hysterectomy.[805] The women were assigned to four different treatment groups, one receiving estrogen, one androgen (testosterone), one a combined estrogen/androgen therapy, and one a placebo. Testosterone (but not estrogen) therapy enhanced the intensity of both sexual desire and arousal, as well as increasing the number of sexual fantasies in hysterectomized/ovariectomized women. The androgen affected only libido, not the physical response (such as sexual wetness) or other interpersonal aspects of sexual behavior.

The studies seem to agree that there is a relationship between sexual desire and androgen levels. It should be noted that ERT has a chemical effect of reducing the amount of circulating free testosterone in the blood.[558] Therefore, if you take estrogen your testosterone level may drop. For this reason, some scientists suppose that testosterone would be beneficial as an adjunct to ERT, instead of progesterone. Certain health centers routinely offer estrogen with testosterone, but most do not yet have familiarity with this method. Moreover, although the data of all of the possible side effects of taking testosterone have not yet been published, there is a demonstrated risk associated with taking testosterone therapy. If a woman wants to try testosterone, she will need to empower herself with the knowledge found in this book and then she will need to seek out sympathetic medical people.

When the concentrations of testosterone exceed the usual female levels, there is a tendency for a woman to develop a male pattern of hairiness, a deeper voice, and other male attributes. Because there are only two studies in the literature in which testosterone therapy has been administered to women,[805, 859] not enough information has been compiled to assess dosage, duration of therapy, and the side effects that occur from testosterone therapy. For these reasons, testosterone should be used with caution. A natural form should be taken, and blood levels of testosterone and lipids should be monitored every six months or so to be sure that your cholesterol level does not get too high. Meanwhile you will know if you are taking too much because of the side effects (a reversible increase in hairiness or deepening of the voice).

### Vaginal Problems

Vaginal problems, including painful intercourse *(dyspareunia)*, can have several different causes. To solve the problem, you need first to define its cause. It can result from the presence of uterine tumors, from a change from celibacy, from estrogen deficiency, or from fear.[479]

### Uterine Tumors

Sometimes intercourse becomes painful before hysterectomy, such as when fibroid tumors are crowding against nerves; in such cases, the surgery often relieves the pain. In one study of women before hysterectomy, many were experiencing painful intercourse. Of those who had a complete hysterectomy with removal of uterus and cervix, half reported improvement. For those who had preoperative dyspareunia and a supravaginal hysterectomy (one that retained the cervix), even better response was noted: six months after the surgery, 13 percent had dyspareunia; by the twelve-month point, only 6 percent were still experiencing it.[458]

Although the dyspareunia was relieved by either operation, and more so by the supravaginal procedure that retained the cervix, the authors did not evaluate why retaining the cervix would yield a lower rate of coital pain. One reason may be that when the cervix is removed, the vaginal canal is shortened, and a shorter vagina may be unduly stressed by coital thrusting.

When the cervix is retained, the preoperative length of the vagina is better retained. In addition, the cervical mucus (see Figure 8, page 31) may be still available to lubricate the tissues.

## Renewal of Sexual Activity

After a period of celibacy, you should be careful and gentle in resuming genital stimulation. Tissues become thinner when they are unused. They thicken when rubbed, but if there is too much rubbing, or if such stimulation is resumed too soon, genital massage can cut and tear the delicate skin. Your partner needs to understand why patience is necessary. After a few weeks of gentle genital stimulation, the vigor of the tissue will return.

## Estrogen Deficiency

The structure of the vaginal lining is in many ways similar to the structure of the mouth lining. Oral problems (dryness, bad taste, burning sensations, and viscosity of the saliva) were common among postmenopausal women who were estrogen-deficient.[691] Those with complaints may have a thin, atrophic (deteriorating) epithelium (a layer of specialized cells that line the mouth and the vagina). One study showed that cream of placebo, estrogen, or estrogen with progestin, massaged into the gingiva (mouth tissue) three times a day, restores the mucosa. Apparently it is the massage of the ephithelium layer that causes the cellular lining to toughen and grow. Massage also increases the flow of saliva.[691] Similar results have been shown for vaginal massage, through either intercourse, sexual play, or self-stimulation.[493, 556] In fact, while it is well known that deficient levels of estrogen inevitably produce vaginal thinning, absence of adequate lubrication, and subsequent abrasions during intercourse, those women who maintain regular vaginal stimulation often avoid these abrasions and escape dyspareunia in spite of estrogen deficiencies.

Dyspareunia after hysterectomy can result from estrogen deficiency. When there is inadequate estrogen, there is likely to be vaginal dryness. If so, intercourse can be painful and cause abrasions. If the dose is high enough, dyspareunia usually gets better after ERT, as greater vaginal lubrication occurs during intercourse.[206] A progressive improvement was shown each six months up to the eighteen months of one study in which ERT was given.[790] When estrogen levels get low after a hysterectomy, women commonly experience intense itching of the genital skin.[209] ERT will correct this.

Because dyspareunia generally appears before there is any cellular evidence of vaginal deterioration,[790] it may not be obvious to a physician who tests the vaginal cells using the vaginal maturation index (VMI), a test designed to evaluate vaginal deterioration. The VMI is determined by taking a smear of vaginal mucus and cells, placing it on a slide, and looking at it under the microscope. The microscope reveals the condition of the cells and will show when the cellular condition is deteriorating. However, two careful studies intending to find that the VMI and the estrogen levels in a woman's blood would be correlated reported that they were not related.[504, 855] The VMI will not give reliable information about your estrogen level. It may provide useful information about vaginal deterioration, but your own sexual discomfort will tell you sooner—and without the expense of a test.

A variety of acid substances thrive in the vaginal moisture. These include acetic acid, aliphatic acids, and lactic acids. An acid environment is healthy because it protects against the growth of bacterial infections. Your vaginal lactic acid increases as your estrogen level increases.[47] A hysterectomy, which generally leads to deficient levels of estrogen, can be expected to alter the acid environment of the vagina, making one more vulnerable to vaginal infection. ERT helps.

## Fear

Being afraid can cause vaginal problems. If you are apprehensive about the sexual encounter and your muscle strength is adequate, you can tense up and consequently find intercourse painful. It may be possible, if you understand the cause and have a considerate and gentle partner, to overcome the fear with patience and with love. You may need help from a sexual therapist or from a psychotherapist. You will have to select the approach that fits your circumstance.

Estrogen emerges as a necessary hormone for maintaining adequate sexual function in women whose estrogen has declined below minimum levels. Progestin therapies will not benefit the sexually responsive tissue and may even cause vaginal atrophy, but they are important in forming a complete HRT regimen. For this reason, if progestin is taken along with estrogen, it needs to be carefully balanced so that it does not produce too much estrogen opposition. Since each body is different and metabolizes substances differently, it would be wise to be alert to how your body responds if you are taking both hormones. The role of testosterone therapy in an HRT regimen does appear to be helpful for the sexual life of a woman, although potentially dangerous for other body systems. Hopefully, in the next few years studies will expand our understanding of which doses are able to provide benefits without danger. For now, testosterone therapy should be considered only if there will be careful monitoring of its effects and a readiness to rapidly respond by changing dosages as necessary.

### Difficulties in Achieving Orgasm

After surgery, your internal anatomy will be changed. These changes, as well as the hormonal changes that follow, will probably combine to alter your orgasmic experience. The joy that comes from an intimate sharing of lovemaking should take priority emotionally over the mechanical responses. Even so, there are things that you can do to improve your physical reactions.

In 1981, publishing in the *Journal of Sex Research,* Drs. John Perry and Beverly Whipple published a now-classic study in which they proved that there are two forms of sexual stimulation, carried on two different nerve networks. Either can produce orgasm.[679] In a way, one could think of this as the solution to the old question of whether there are two different kinds of orgasm, clitoral and vaginal, and whether one is "better" than the other. In fact, that old argument really misses the point because both orgasms described by Perry and Whipple involve vaginal stimulation. What distinguishes them is that one can be triggered by clitoral or vaginal stimulation, which fires the *pudendal nerve,* while the other can be triggered by either vaginal or cervical stimulation, which fires the *pelvic nerve.*

This finding was proved with Valium. When women took Valium, it interfered with the firing of the nerve in the clitoral/ vaginal area, but not with the firing of the pelvic nerve.[679] These data, collected in women who had not lost their uterus, helped to show that there is a uterine orgasm and that two different sensory nerves influence orgasmic responses in different regions of the genitals. After hysterectomy, the pelvic nerve, which connects to the rear two-thirds of the vagina, to the bladder, and to the uterus from the spinal cord, may be damaged. But all should not be lost; usually the pudendal nerve is still fine. You will be able to improve your orgasmic pleasure by strengthening the muscular part of the reflex and by teaching your partner how to massage your G Spot.

## The PC Muscles

The pubococcygeal (PC) muscles form a very important muscle band that courses through the genital region, encompassing the bladder, the vagina, and the anal region (see Figure 18). They connect to the pubic bone at one end and the coccyx at the other, and wrap around the three openings of urethra, vagina, and anus much like the figure eights of an ice skater. Strong muscles promote and enhance the quality of orgasm. The greater your PC muscle strength, the easier it is to achieve orgasm through clitoral and/or vaginal stimulation.[320, 679, 939] (Chapter 12 provides a detailed discussion of the pioneering work of Dr. Arnold Kegel and the exercises he developed to strengthen the PC muscle system.)

Sexual position also may be relevant. If one's legs are spread

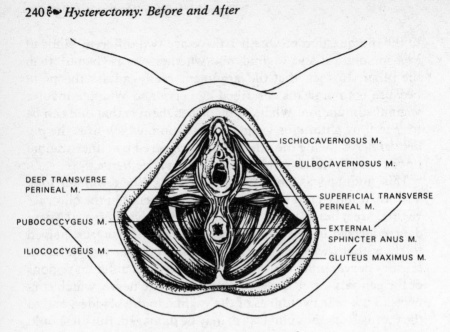

Figure 18. Pubococcygeus muscles

with one's feet above the body, as when lying on a gynecological examination table with the feet in stirrups, one may be unable to contract the muscles adequately. Although this may be something women surmise from their personal experience, no studies have addressed whether sexual position variations alter the quality or strength of orgasm; but since position affects muscle strength, one can expect that sexual position could be demonstrated to affect orgasmic response, too. No studies have addressed the degree to which different forms of pelvic surgery disrupt either the PC muscles or the nerves that control their contraction. The likelihood is high that some surgical procedures do interfere with PC muscle function and that this function can be regained or enhanced after hysterectomy with biofeedback treatment.

At the start of biofeedback therapy, the physiologist or physician identifies the PC muscle for the patient by inserting a finger into the patient's vagina, asking her to contract the muscle

around the finger, and letting her know when she has successfully achieved a muscle contraction. The next step is to insert
into the vagina the tamponlike end of a measuring device called
a perineometer, in order to objectively measure the strength of
the contractions. (The perineometer measures the strength of
the muscles of the *perineum,* the region between the pubic bone
and the coccyx bone.)

The modern perineometer has a graph attachment that allows
a woman to see recordings on a computer screen as she contracts
her muscles, so that she can learn how strong or weak the muscles are. (The regular contracting of the PC muscles is referred
to as Kegel exercises.) This biofeedback approach has been
shown to be the fastest and most effective way to develop the
strength of these muscles. You need to have an immediate feedback measure in order to know how well you are doing. In 1986,
publishing in the *American Journal of Obstetrics and Gynecology,*
Dr. Kathryn Burgio and her colleagues demonstrated that
women who did not have the biofeedback apparatus when they
were attempting to train their muscles did less well than women
who did.[88] (Chapter 12 contains details of that study as well as
relevant information on retraining urinary stress incontinence
problems.)

Recently, an electromyographic (electronic graph of *myo,* or
muscle, contraction) perineometer has been developed that automatically averages and digitizes the measurements, thus
greatly improving the accuracy of the instrumentation.[678] A
major advantage of the electromyographic perineometer over
the original air-pressure perineometer invented by Kegel is that
the new version also measures pelvic muscle tension, which can
often be a problem, just as muscle tension is a problem in other
parts of the body, and which is correctable with exercise. This
new machine is currently available in certain biofeedback centers in the U.S., and a portable electronic perineometer that can
be purchased and used at home will be available in late 1988 or
1989. With this new equipment, investigators were able to demonstrate, as shown in Table 10, a relationship between the mus-

cle strength achieved during a ten-second contraction (in which the woman holds the muscle taut) and the level of sexual functioning.[678] The higher the muscle strength during the contraction, the greater the chance of experiencing orgasm during sexual intercourse.

Some women express embarrassment because they release a sudden emission of fluid at orgasm and fear that this is urine. Usually it isn't. For some women, particularly those with high PC muscle strength, there often may be an ejaculate, which is expelled through the urethra, just as the male ejaculate is.[939] And as in the case of the male, the female ejaculate is not composed chemically of urine but of a different substance that is very low in urea (the basic substance of urine) and high in acid phosphatase.[939] Thus, the fluid that is expelled through the female urethra during orgasm is not urine but a true ejaculate. On the other hand, women who have "stress" incontinence (see Chapter 12) may very well leak small or even large amounts of urine during orgasm. Female ejaculate and urine, besides being produced in different organs, smell and taste quite different. The ejaculate is almost always described as "sweet"; urine seldom so.

What causes the PC muscles to be strong or weak? Your own pattern of behavior. A study published in the *Lancet* in 1985

**Table 10.** *PC Muscle Strength and Sexual Functioning*

| Pubococcygeal Muscle Strength (in microvolts) | Predicted Level of Sexual Functioning (stimulation required to achieve orgasm) |
| --- | --- |
| 2 to 4 microvolts | No form effective (nonorgasmic woman). |
| 6 to 8 microvolts | Orgasm requires direct clitoral stimulation. |
| 10 to 12 microvolts | Clitoral or vaginal penetration can produce orgasm. |
| 15 or more microvolts | Multiorgasmic; any form of genital stimulation yields orgasm. |

showed that the various procedures that accompany childbirth—episiotomy (a surgical cut in the vagina that is resewn once the baby is born), vaginal birth without episiotomy, and cesarean section (which bypasses the vagina)—were not significant factors in whether a woman had PC muscle strength twelve to fourteen months after childbirth. In most cases the stretching or cutting of the muscle bundle had fully healed within a year. What did vary was whether a woman got regular exercise, such as running, jogging, swimming, or dancing. Women who engaged regularly in vigorous exercise showed significantly greater PC muscle strength, in spite of having done no conscious Kegel exercises.[314] There are no equivalent studies published to guide our understanding of the posthysterectomized woman, but there is reason to expect that equivalent exercise should be helpful.

## The G Spot

During studies of PC muscle functioning, Perry and Whipple discovered—actually rediscovered—the Grafenberg Spot as a particularly fine site of vaginal sexual response. They demonstrated and published the results of a study that showed that about an inch and a half inside the abdominal side of the vagina, there exists an area of tissue that becomes engorged with blood and swells (similar to the swelling in a man's penile erection). This area forms a mound about the size of a quarter or half dollar when a woman is sexually aroused and properly stimulated by gentle repeated stroking of that spot. Dr. Perry named this the Grafenberg (G) Spot after its original discoverer,[679] and other investigators subsequently confirmed his findings.[939, 943] Normally, the G Spot is routinely massaged during coital thrusting. If the penis has a ridged head (from circumcision), the ridge will "tease" the G Spot each time it withdraws. If no ridge is present, the stimulation will be somewhat less intense. The muscular contraction of the PC muscle is a reflex response to G Spot stimulation.

The particular rhythm of the thrusts is important. If the rhythm of sexual intercourse follows a regular, repeated harmonic pattern (as contrasted with a stop-and-start pattern), then the nerves will be "recruited" with ever-increasing stimulator effect. Scientists who study nerves (neuronal physiologists) have learned that it is the inherent rhythmic harmony of nerve firing that allows the nervous system, like a harp, to produce a resonance. One of the wonderful aspects of a long-term sexual relationship is the opportunity it offers for lovers to develop a virtuoso skill in playing their sexual harps. When a man develops a sophisticated sensitivity in stimulating the G Spot through a harmonious rhythm of coital thrusting, he will be rewarded with a spasmodic series of seven to ten orgasmic contractions of the PC muscle around his penis; these in turn can stimulate his own orgasm. (This knowledge of sexual resonance through harmonious coital thrusting is not new. It appears in early Taoistic writings of two to three thousand years ago.)

Recently Drs. Beverly Whipple and Barry Komisaruk have provided evidence that direct physical stimulation of the G Spot also serves to decrease pain.[943] In that study, the regular repeated massage of the G Spot did not diminish sensitivity to touch; it only diminished sensitivity to pain. These results suggest that the stimulation fires nerves that have a simultaneous effect of increasing the resistance to pain. It is likely that these nerve impulses trigger the release of the endogenous opiates, although no research reports have yet analyzed the question directly.

The PC muscles appear to be profoundly important for sexual physiology. There are no published studies that evaluate whether different forms of hysterectomy interfere with PC muscle strength, but the likelihood is high that some surgical procedures do interfere either with the muscles or with the nerves impinging on the muscles. If you find that your orgasmic capacity has declined after hysterectomy, the first logical action would be to attempt to strengthen your PC muscles. Considering the recent studies showing that training without biofeedback information produces much less desirable results than that undertaken with biofeedback,[88] it would be wise to try to locate a biofeedback center or physiologist who could work with you to get you started. Alternatively, you might buy a portable electronic perineometer. (For information on the portable at-home electronic perineometer, write to Leslie Talcott, M.S., R.N., The Perineometer Research Institute, 242 Old Eagle School Road, Strafford, PA 19087.)

## MALE SEXUALITY

Men undergo changes parallel to the ones women experience. These include declines in androgen levels, in libido, and in both the speed and the frequency with which an erection is achieved. If your sexual life is showing a decline, one part of the reason may be your partner's changing sexuality. If you are sensitive to these age-related changes in men, you can better enjoy the many sensual opportunities that do come with maturity.

Men, like women, show a clearly defined pattern of physiological aging within their reproductive and sexual systems. In fact, there is a remarkable parallel between the two genders, with one critical difference. Because men lack a regular monthly cycle, strictly speaking they undergo no menopause; instead they experience an ongoing and steady change. Their gonads (sexual organs), sexual behaviors, and hormones change with age.

### The Gonads and Genitals

Like the ovaries, the male gonads (the testes) shrink with age. In consequence, sperm production also declines in the advanced years.[621] Although the individual cells that manufacture sperm maintain their vigor in producing healthy sperm even into old age, as men get older they produce fewer of them. Vascular (blood vessel) degeneration in the gonadal region also occurs with age.[428, 627] The physical structure of the testes, when examined under a microscope, shows an aging pattern very similar to the structural change in the ovaries (described in Chapter 2). In both cases, the structure of the tissues that formerly produced both genes and hormones takes up less of the space. Meanwhile the mass of other tissues, which make neither hormones nor sperm, expands.[429] Therefore, as the gonads age, the tissue for producing sperm and hormone diminishes.[187, 475, 620, 665, 760] There are corresponding changes in the penis, the prostate (a gland that contributes substances that liquify the ejaculate), and the seminal vesicles (the tubes that produce and house the sperm), and after age 80 the ability of sperm to move and swim becomes very impaired.[620, 783] Nonetheless, unlike women, most men retain the ability to contribute their genes into at least their late seventies.

Penile erection, which is a physiological reflex response, can be triggered in either of two sensory (nervous system) pathways: either through mental processes (imagination, viewing an erotic film or woman) or through physical touching and stroking of the penis, which stimulates sensory nerve endings. The particular muscles that are reflexively triggered near the penis are on the blood vessels, which close and open to direct the flow of blood. When blood flows rapidly into the penis, erection results. And when the erections occur during the dreaming stage of sleep, the testosterone level rises.[772]

For most men, the number of orgasms and the number of morning erections decline with age. The change from the forties to the sixties is quite noteworthy—about a 50 percent decline in the number of orgasms and morning erections. By the time a man reaches his seventies, his amount of sexual behavior is about one-sixth what it was in his forties.[64, 188]

### The Male Hormones and Male Sexual Behavior

As men age, for most there is a clear decline in their sexual function. This decline is noted in the hormone levels, the frequency of desire for intercourse, the capacity for erections, and the frequency of intercourse.

Most boys show very large increases in their testosterone levels beginning at adolescence. Men in their twenties, thirties, and forties demonstrate a wide range of individual testosterone levels that differ from one man to the next. Some are very high, others less so, but almost all men circulate at least forty times more testosterone than women. After the age of 50, the high levels are rarely seen, and most men begin to show a decline in testosterone level.[33] There are exceptions. Some men with vigorous health and regular exercise show no decline of testosterone with age,[352] but most men do show declining levels of the hormone with the advancing of years.[913, 914] This effect is shown whether the man lives in a home for the aged, in the general population, or in a monastery.[913] It occurs regardless of diet; no differences were found in any of the age-related hormonal changes between men on vegetarian, macrobiotic, and high-fat diets.

With the advancing of the years, men show hormonal changes that are very similar to those of women. The sex steroids decline, and the pituitary gonadotropins (luteinizing hormone and follicle-stimulating hormone) increase.[33, 352]* Just as in women, scientists do not yet understand the effects that these increasing levels of LH and FSH have on male mental and physical functions.

The frequency with which most men seek sexual intercourse tends to decline as they age.[188, 441, 462] There have been some documented relationships between men's testosterone levels and their sexual behavior. In general, when men become celibate, their sex hormone levels drop.[406] When they become more sexually active, their testosterone levels increase.[680] This parallels the studies that show that women who have regular weekly sex with men tend to have higher levels of estrogen, and that women who receive testosterone tend to have an increased interest in engaging in sexual behavior. (See "Sexual Behavior Affects Hormones," page 41.)

While in most men there are some subtle but predictable relationships between hormones and sexual behavior,[187, 465] in men with impotence the relationships appear to be different.

*The gonadotropins act in men in a fashion similar to the way they do in women: they stimulate the production of gonadal hormones and the genetic cells, or sperm.

### *Impotence*

Impotence, the inability to attain or maintain an erection (also called erectile failure or erectile dysfunction), is defined in different ways by different investigators.[502, 786] The problem is widespread, estimated to occur in 35 to 40 percent of all men past age 40.[822, 857] The problem of impotence is not necessarily related to a lack of sexual desire.[822] If a man in your life has a problem in achieving an erection or maintaining it as long as you want, there are now many solutions that were previously unavailable. And according to one large study at the Veterans Administration, about 90 percent of the time the problem seems to have a physiologic cause and a physiologic cure.[822]

At what age does a man tend to suffer from this problem? Figure 19 gives some idea of the age distribution. The years between 50 and 59 are the most vulnerable ages for developing impotence, but older and younger men also seek help.[607, 822]

Although we might be tempted to, we cannot conclude that testosterone treatment will help all men who want to increase their sexual performance. In those rare cases in which an abnormally low natural testosterone level (less than 2 mg/ml) exists, androgen therapy does seem to help overcome impotence in men, but it also produces some negative effects.[87] Testosterone therapy has been shown to inhibit the development of sperm and may cause a rise in both the free plasma cholesterol and triglyceride levels.[87] Both of these lipid changes increase the risk of coronary heart disease.

In order to achieve help in overcoming impotence, you need to seek the expertise of specialists in this field. Unfortunately, many physicians are not specialists and may not be aware of how to locate a specialist. Armed with the information in this chapter, you should be able to use a telephone to find urologists, endocrinologists, and psychotherapists who are experts in sexual medicine, who specialize in erectile problems, and who are familiar with this research. Ask them about their methods and

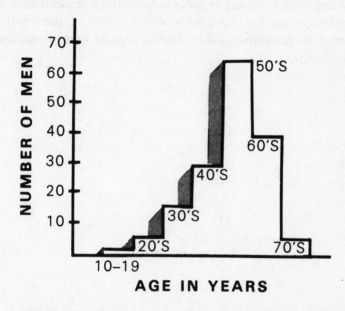

Figure 19. Impotence is most common in men in their fifties.

about their success in treatment. Currently fewer than half the men with erectile problems are willing to seek help. It is hoped that, with the encouragement of their partners, more will take advantage of the help that is available.

A sexual relationship is not available for every woman as she ages, and women who have undergone a hysterectomy seem to be particularly at risk of losing a fulfilling sexual relationship. In part, this may be attributed to the declining capacity of men as they age. In addition, women live longer than men, and with each passing year fewer men are available. Until single women turn to younger men as sexual partners, there will simply not be enough men to go around, and many women will find themselves celibate. Celibacy is not necessarily an undesirable state of existence, but for those who seek a sexual relationship, the information provided in this chapter should help to maximize the possibility.

# 11 ❦

# *Overcoming Depression*

❦ It is natural for hysterectomy to have an impact on your emotional life. If your presurgical condition included pain, excessive bleeding, and a general malaise, resolving that problem probably will have increased your sense of well-being. Often, however, the surgery promotes depression.

If you have undergone a hysterectomy, with or without an ovariectomy, and are suffering from a diminished sense of well-being, you are certainly not alone. You are part of a very large group of women who suffer silently, out of embarrassment or a sense of futility. Take heart. There is much that you can do to overcome these sad or pessimistic feelings and to change your life into an exhilarating one.

Depression is a disease in the deepest sense of the word—a distinct lack of ease with life. Its victims suffer from persistent dreary feelings and a pervasive sense of gloom. Psychiatrists identify depression by evaluating the intensity, duration, and frequency of a composite of behaviors, including depressed mood; an increased amount of time spent sleeping; and decreases in motor activity, cognitive efficiency, appetite, sociability, speech rate, and level of optimism.

But even without the benefit of medical expertise, you know when you are depressed. You know when you do not seem to have the energy or the interest to get moving with your life, to undertake new projects, and to carry out old ones. You know when smiles do not come easily and when you are experiencing a general sense of melancholy. You know when it takes real effort to get out of bed in the morning because of an overwhelming lack of energy.

We are affected by all of life's experiences, and a cyclic variation between emotional highs and lows is part of being human. What matters is the degree of depression, the range of the swing from high to low. It is possible for even a lay person to distinguish depression that is normal and transient from a depression that is more serious and should be treated. In serious depression, although highs may still occur, the lows go much lower than among normal, nondepressed people, robbing one of any sense of joy in living. And they linger. One woman had this to say:

> I think the most significant change in my life since the surgeries [complete hysterectomy and bilateral ovariectomy] is the feeling of hopelessness. I feel like a good part of my life is all over and done with. . . . I used to have such a bubbly, outgoing personality. Now I just get through one day at a time. Is there any help available to me?

Depression is a pervasive female experience even without hysterectomy—probably caused, in part, by the cyclic variation in beta endorphins, as well as their severe decline when the sex hormone cycle is disrupted. Beginning in the menopausal transition years and continuing on, roughly from the age of 47 to 54, women tend to experience the greatest amounts of depression in their lives. As many as 40 percent of nonhysterectomized women undergo a depression during that stage of life.[174] Fortunately, for most women the depression characteristic of those years diminishes in time.

Likewise, the depression related to hysterectomy tends to diminish. Women ultimately do adjust. But it is possible to take action to accelerate the recovery process. Effective action begins with acknowledging the problem.

## *HYSTERECTOMY AND DEPRESSION*

How often does a hysterectomy show a relationship to severe depression? The data are incomplete, but for women under 40 years old, some good information has been published. Within three years of a hysterectomy, more than half the women in one study developed depression.[730] In a follow-up study, investigators concluded that 70 percent of hysterectomized patients suffered a severe depression within three years of their surgery—more than double the rate of age-matched controls who became depressed in the same span of time.[731] Clearly the problem is pervasive.

Unfortunately, many well-meaning physicians are not aware of the true and documented relationship between hysterectomy and depression. Why? Because the physicians who do the surgery or who recommend the surgery tend not to follow the cases of these women two or three years after their surgery, and the depression usually begins after the last postsurgical checkup. Surgeons generally "sign off" on a patient after six months or one year, and depression generally emerges at the two- to three-year point.[39, 444, 578, 609]

Although it is reasonable for a woman to experience depression if surgery has interfered with her desire for pregnancy, the fact is that many women who have no wish for further pregnancy also suffer depression after hysterectomy. Something is happening that cannot be explained by the loss of the ability to gestate babies.

As early as 1968, the biomedical literature revealed that hysterectomy seemed to be associated with more postoperative depression than other forms of surgery.[39] Several studies were published throughout the 1970s and into the early 1980s, all showing similar phenomena. The number of women affected went beyond what one would expect in these age groups, and the number affected was more substantial than the number affected after other surgeries.*

*Studies include 18, 34, 444, 578, 609, 730, 731.

The health of the uterus turns out to be one factor in predicting who will suffer a postoperative depression. It appears that hysterectomized women who had no pathology in their uterus are the ones who are particularly at risk for a depression after their uterus is removed.[39, 730] Why? Perhaps the hysterectomy did not solve anything. Bleeding is a symptom, and simply stopping the bleeding by hysterectomy may not change the underlying psychophysiology that led to the problem. And while the problems that prompted the search for medical help remain, there is now another set of physical, biochemical, and emotional adjustments adding to the total burden.

Although hysterectomy has been shown to increase the incidence of postoperative depression within three years of the surgery, particularly for women who had no uterine pathology, the reverse also has been documented. Women who had uterine pathology, such as fibroid tumors or very heavy bleeding, show an improvement in physical vigor within one to two years after surgery.[147] Thus the issue is not simple. If hysterectomy has improved your physical health, you may feel better in spite of the organ loss. If nothing was wrong with the uterine tissue, then the failure to solve a problem, coupled with the loss of an organ and its associated nerve and hormonal networks, can be expected to cause a problem.

But beyond the issue of the relative state of well-being before and after surgery, why does hysterectomy appear to increase the risk of depression? What are the chemical and nervous-system changes that a hysterectomy might produce that could lead to a depression? And how can one overcome the problem? Let's first focus on some brain biochemistry as we explore safe ways to overcome depression.

## BRAIN BIOCHEMISTRY AND HORMONAL REPLACEMENT THERAPY

The cause of depression in hysterectomized women appears to be largely biochemical. Studies of the neuroendocrine (nerve and hormone) system have provided a body of data that may help to explain the depression problems that follow the surgery and consequent sex hormone deficiencies.

Neuroendocrinologists investigate the nervous and hormonal systems and how they interact with each other. Typically, nerves can "fire," serving as something like a spark that "ignites" the endocrine glands to release hormones. In turn, hormones seem to alter the firing pattern of the nervous system. It is a circular system in which changes in one factor (that is, either the nerves or the hormones) inevitably produce changes in the other factor. Surgery cuts nerves, and it removes endocrine (hormone-producing) organs. Pelvic surgery would be expected to alter your neuroendocrine system. How could it not?

Studies show that HRT can relieve depression that coincides with sex hormone deficiencies.[244, 779] Estrogen combined with progesterone appears to serve as a kind of "concertmaster," controlling the interactions that promote a healthy functioning of the nervous system. HRT helps to correct inappropriate levels of several substances that have been shown to relate to sad and negative feelings, increasing substances that coincide with a sense of well-being and lowering those associated with depression.

### Tryptophan

Tryptophan, an amino acid produced in the brain, appears to be a critically important wellness substance, and tryptophan deficiency seems to cause depression. Among perimenopausal women, estrogen in the blood and tryptophan in the blood appear to interact. As estrogen levels rise, tryptophan levels rise; as estrogen levels fall, tryptophan levels fall.[878] It has been known for at least ten years that depressed patients often improve when they are treated with tryptophan or another substance called a monoamine oxidase (MAO) inhibitor.[92] HRT is often similarly effective: by increasing the tryptophan and inhibiting the MAO, it relieves depression.[463, 464]

For women who have not had a hysterectomy, the highest risk

of becoming depressed occurs during the roller-coaster estrogen declines that occur from about ages 47 to 54. In this age group, tryptophan is significantly lower than in any other age group.[959] As depressed people recover from their depression and feel better, their blood level of tryptophan increases. If you are taking lithium for depression, research shows that estrogen also helps to increase the level of tryptophan in comparison to lithium without estrogen.[959]

If your HRT estrogen dose is relatively high, you would probably be wise to include a daily dose of 100 milligrams of vitamin $B_6$ to protect against a possible $B_6$ deficiency, which can result in reduced secretion of tryptophan.[325]*

Other hormones also interfere with tryptophan metabolism. It has long been known that the hormones cortisone and ACTH, which are sometimes given to treat other diseases, often cause severe depression, and it has been suggested that alterations in tryptophan metabolism are the cause.

### The Beta Endorphins

Other wellness substances, the beta endorphins, have recently come to public light through reports in the scientific literature. Like tryptophan, they are dependent on the harmonic pattern of sex hormones. The beta endorphin system is a likely source of the depression that is common to women after hysterectomy.

Recently scientists began asking why human beings are receptive to a plant narcotic like opium. In order for a body to be receptive to a substance, it must have receptors, molecules that can receive that substance and produce action as a result. The scientists hypothesized that if the human brain had receptors for substances like opium, then the human body must manufacture something opium-like. Research studies that proved the exis-

---

*Certain forms of oral contraceptives (which contain levels of estrogens and progestagens that are much higher than those in HRT regimens) have been shown to produce a vitamin $B_6$ deficiency.[5] While we do not yet know whether typical menopausal doses of HRT will cause tryptophan deficiencies, the sensible approach is not to stop taking estrogen, but to add vitamin $B_6$ at about 100 mg per day.[325]

tence of opiate receptors in the brain led to the search for endogenous (internally produced) opiates and to discoveries that the body manufactures opium-like substances (endogenous morphines) referred to as the *endorphins*. These substances are just beginning to be studied, but the relationship between endogenous opiate levels, well-being, and the sex hormones is now scientifically accepted. (See page 39.)

While postmenopausal women have much lower levels of beta endorphins than young cycling women, in terms of endorphin levels and depression it probably does not matter what your steady-state amount of endorphins is. The cyclic depression that women feel before menstruation is probably the effect of the withdrawal from a high level to a lower level, rather than a reflection of some exact amount. It is the change, the pulling back of a hormone, that can cause a problem. Once a woman gets used to a lower level, provided the lower level stays steady, there is probably less trauma than that produced by the withdrawal from a high to a medium level.

In humans, ovariectomy produces a significant reduction in the beta endorphin levels within six months after surgery[300] (see Figure 20). Hysterectomy also probably reduces the endorphins, particularly in the 50 percent of women whose ovaries stop cycling. Perhaps the two- to three-year delay in the onset of post-hysterectomy depression reflects the typical two- to three-year span before retained ovaries usually become sluggish. If you have had only a hysterectomy and your ovaries are intact, your body's production of beta endorphins depends on whether or not your ovaries are functioning optimally.

Ovariectomy can be expected to lead to a dramatic reduction in the endogenous opiate levels of women, unless both estrogen and progestin or testosterone therapy is taken. Estrogen alone is probably not as helpful in restoring your sense of well-being as estrogen in combination with progesterone. Progestins alone have been shown to increase endogenous opiate activity in postmenopausal women,[107] but more studies are needed before we can learn the optimum HRT dose range to maximize the endor-

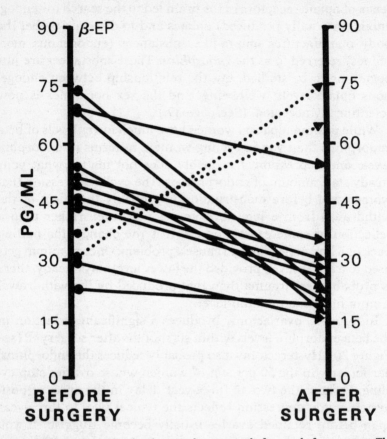

Figure 20. Beta endorphin levels in twelve women before and after surgery. The dotted line reflects the occurrence of a hot flash.

phins. Still, HRT that fails to include progestin may not adequately protect against the loss of beta endorphin production in the brain.

No studies have yet evaluated testosterone replacement, and research dollars are needed. The likelihood is great that, if the doses are appropriately low, testosterone will help because it increases vigor, both through its relationship to the endorphin system and through the building of muscular and cardiovascular strength.

## WHAT CAN BE DONE TO OVERCOME DEPRESSION?

If you are suffering from sad and pessimistic feelings, you should seek relief. The actual decision to take action can in itself begin to counteract depression. Talking with your medical advisors and establishing beneficial patterns of behavior will give you a sense of taking charge of your problem and gaining some control over it. You will do best to approach depression on several fronts:

- *Hormonally,* by having your estrogen level tested to see whether it is low, and by taking the appropriate HRT regimen
- *Physically,* by establishing a habit of regular exercise
- *Nutritionally,* by following a proper diet
- *Through work with and service to other people*
- *Emotionally,* through women's support groups
- *Through psychotherapy,* which may be helpful if carefully selected

### Hormonal Replacement Therapy

Estrogen replacement therapy with progestin or testosterone opposition is the most helpful treatment for depression in women who are sex-hormone-deficient. If you start taking HRT, you will probably notice the beneficial effect on your mood within four to ten weeks, provided the dosage is correct. Some lucky women respond more quickly. One "fast responder" had this to say:

Thank [you] for giving me the moral support necessary to confront my doctor. I was able to get many of the answers I so desperately needed, and he immediately started me on .625 mg of Premarin (on 21 days, off 7 days), as well as 10 mg of Provera (taken the last 5 days of the 21-day cycle). Within 48 hours, I became a new person.

He also arranged for me to take a series of blood tests to check my bodily functions (adrenal gland, thyroid gland, etc.), and we discovered that my thyroid is very underactive, and I am now taking medication to correct that dysfunction. I am delighted to report to you that my hot flashes have all but disappeared, I am sleeping at night now. . . . I have more energy than I've had in many, many months. I am also taking a prenatal vitamin . . . as well as calcium. And I haven't had one headache since I began taking the hormones. Needless to say, it's been a long time since I've felt this good.

One very elegant research study conducted in the mid-1970s in Scandinavia analyzed the value of estrogen for well-being and mental performance in estrogen-deficient postmenopausal women.[244] All the women were told that they were getting estrogen treatment, with one of two doses of progestin opposition, but some were given a placebo instead. All were assessed at the outset and then at one-, three-, and six-month intervals. The women who took the hormones began to have increasing levels of estrogen circulating in their blood, and within about six months the circulating estrogen had reached maximum levels. Estrogen users became more extroverted; placebo users did not. Estrogen users became less neurotic, according to a standard personality test, whereas placebo users became more neurotic. In general, the sense of well-being improved among the women who took estrogen, and it did not improve among the others.

In 1987 a different investigator reported a similar set of results in a group of women 55 to 65 years old.[514] Estrogens improved the mood and sense of well-being much more effectively than placebo. Other investigators have also confirmed the "mental tonic effect" of estrogens when given to women after ovariectomy.[70, 898] HRT also improves the quality of sleep and reduces anxiety.[879] If you are very depressed, you may need other types of help in addition to HRT. If your depression is milder, HRT will probably be sufficient to enhance your sense of well-being.[779]

If you are taking HRT and still feeling depressed, you may need an adjustment in your dosage. You may do better with a higher intake of estrogen, or perhaps you should take it every day of the month. You may have better results if you lower the synthetic progestin dose, switch to a natural progesterone, or increase the duration of low-dose progestin to thirteen days or more each month. You may want to add a *low*-dose natural testosterone. Many women find that their depression lifts once their hormones and nutrition are adjusted, but each body metabolizes hormones differently. The dose that works for you will not necessarily match somebody else's routine prescription. Be prepared to experiment until you find your dose. And be aware that you will need to locate compassionate medical personnel who will respect the validity of the reactions you describe as you search for an optimal HRT regimen.

Be cautious about the kind of HRT regimen you accept. Synthetic progestins (see Table 5) sometimes produce negative feelings, whereas natural progesterone does not seem to have this effect. If you feel unhappy, irritable, or depressed on an HRT regimen of estrogen and synthetic progestin, ask your physician to arrange for you to switch to (the more expensive) natural progesterone. (See page 165.)

### Exercise

Regular exercise has been repeatedly shown to improve women's sense of well-being and joy of life. Drs. Gloria Bachman, Sandra Leiblum, and colleagues have specifically showed that rigorous exercise training produced clear improvements in the well-being of postmenopausal women.[29] It seems likely that one of the mechanisms that account for this improved well-being is the increased level of beta endorphins that results from exercise that is done in a repeated and disciplined way. When a person first starts to do exercises, there is an immediate rise in the blood levels of beta endorphin and a larger rise in the blood levels of the molecule (beta lipotrophin) from which the beta endorphins are made.[106] Training—that is, the systematic and disciplined scheduling of exercise to increase one's aerobic capacity—enhances this effect.[106]

If you have feelings of depression, you certainly should begin a program of regular exercise. Simply taking a daily walk, one that keeps you in constant motion for about an hour, will have profoundly beneficial effects. Swimming is another nonstressful exercise that helps, without risking bone breakage or muscle tears. You will notice elevations in mood within two or three days of starting. Chapter 15 describes how to design an exercise program tailored to your needs and your lifestyle.

### Nutrition

The kinds of foods you eat affect the way you feel. Recent work conducted at the Monell Chemical Senses Center in Philadelphia has focused attention on the roles of different nutritive and non-nutritive substances in promoting general health, appetite, and well-being. Although the research is currently at too early a stage for specific conclusions to be drawn, it is becoming clear how powerfully our eating habits affect our lives. High quantities of sugar will probably cause extreme mood swings. "Diet foods" and high doses of artificial sweeteners in sodas may increase your appetite for sugar. If you eliminate high-sugar items and cut down on artificially sweetened foods, you will probably feel better. A healthy diet is a requirement for well-being. (Chapter 13 provides a detailed discussion of nutrition.)

### Work and Service

In addition to safeguards for your physical health, you need caring and personal attention, in the form of supportive and loving human contact.[147, 879] People need other people in a regular and ongoing way in order to feel okay, and as a source of positive reinforcement and loving-kindness.

Loneliness produces depression. If you are seriously depressed, people may avoid being with you in order to avoid becoming depressed themselves. To escape that vicious cycle, it is appropriate to turn to professional help. If you are not seriously depressed but are feeling quite down, the efforts you make to get out into the world and interact with people will surely help.

Happiness is a by-product of living well, and the feeling that your life is useful to others is an important element in your sense of well-being. We may well ask how life can be meaningful unless we find a way to be of use to others. Although the idea is a difficult one to prove through rigorous double-blind research, it is so intrinsically sensible that it hardly requires scientific investigation. However, one study of more than 8,000 women, entitled "Women in Work: An Investigation of the Association Between Health and Employment Status in Middle-Aged Women," did find data to support the premise that women who work are healthier than those who do not.[417]

For those who work for a living and those who do not, volunteer service is an excellent way to be of use to people and causes outside your immediate circle. You can begin through charity groups, houses of worship, local libraries and schools, political groups, and public service agencies. All have a great need for volunteer help.

### *Support Groups*

If you are feeling down, lonely, and lackluster, consider forming a support group with other women who you suspect are feeling the same way. If one or two of your friends are interested, you could arrange a meeting to which you each invite one or two others. You might want to meet on a weekly basis for a couple of hours, discussing your feelings and what you can do about them. Support groups often provide great resources of strength that promote the well-being of the members. The suggestions that women make to each other can often be very effective, and sharing feelings with people who are undergoing similar experiences is frequently very helpful. The power within a group of women is rich and you can tap into it.

Women's support groups (especially menopausal support) may already be available in your community. Check your Yellow Pages or write to HERS, the Hysterectomy Educational Resource Service, 422 Bryn Mawr Avenue, Bala Cynwyd, PA 19004.

## Psychotherapy

There is a bewildering array of psychological approaches to helping people feel better. If you are going to seek help through psychotherapy, you need a plan for approaching the professional therapeutic community.

If you are fortunate enough to have a health center that can both prescribe HRT and provide counselors on staff, that may be your best option. Otherwise, you will need to put together your own health care team: HRT physician (gynecologist, endocrinologist, or internist) and someone capable of evaluating and treating the psychological component of your depression. So many of the studies discussed in this chapter have been published after 1980, and some after 1986, that unless a therapist keeps up with this literature he or she may be unaware of the biochemical situations that may be causing your depressed feelings.

First, consider what sort of therapist you might best find a fit with: psychiatrist, counselor, psychologist, social worker? The academic degree is probably less important than the therapist's awareness about posthysterectomy depression. Second, compile a list of recommended professionals from friends and doctors. *Ask for help and you will find it.* Gather information and recommendations about therapists who have experience with your particular problem. When you call these professionals, ask them several important questions:

What kind of therapy do you practice?
What sort of experience have you had with my kind of problem?
How long is treatment usually necessary?
What do you charge?
Do you have hours available to see me when it is convenient for
    me to come to you?

The third step is to select two or three who seem most suited to your nature and needs, and to schedule appointments to see each of them. You should be candid with the therapist. Explain that this is an interview, and that you are trying to find a person you can work with. You should tell the therapist that you are investigating several different people to see where you feel the best fit. Be sure to explore whether your spiritual world view is compatible with the therapist's.

It will be very helpful to find a therapist who has experience in the kind of depression you are undergoing. For example, if you need help in dealing with the grief of no longer being capable of pregnancy, seek the help of a therapist with experience in grieving processes. Finally, you should consider the relative importance for you of a female therapist. Although some women find this irrelevant, others find that a female therapist offers a similarity of perceptions that cannot be achieved in even the most compassionate male.

Then take some time to decide whether any of the people you have seen seem likely to be able to help you. If so, you might want to think about entering into therapy for your depression. If not, seek out more names and begin the process again. Your final decision will probably be based partly on objective evaluation and partly on your intuition. Trust that intuition.

Once in therapy, you should feel free to terminate it at any point at which you feel it is not helping. Appropriate therapy feels right and you know it—both immediately and as you continue. Many women find that some therapy to help them get through the posthysterectomy depression is very helpful.

Women who undergo hysterectomy are particularly susceptible to depression and need to understand their heightened vulnerability. Once you begin to understand the causes of the depression and take action to combat it, the snowball effect comes into play, and your actions pick up a momentum of their own. It is helpful to realize that depression can be caused by many factors. If one approach does not produce the results you seek, another form of treatment probably will.

# Overcoming
# Urinary Incontinence

🌿 Urinary incontinence, the inability to contain the urine and control urination, is a problem that afflicts a great number of women. Fortunately, although incontinence affects as many as 60 percent of women 45 to 64 years old[77] and increases with age, the condition is usually treatable without surgery and without drugs, thanks to new research that is finally coming to light.

The blanket term *urinary incontinence* defines several related problems:

- *Urinary stress incontinence* refers to a leakage of urine during a mild physiological stress, such as a cough or a jump.
- *Urinary urge incontinence* refers to the urge to urinate more frequently than seems reasonable. Often this form of incontinence derives from the fear of leakage, causing a woman to want to urinate at the first signal of urine in the bladder. This response can set in motion a vicious cycle of more and more frequent urination.
- *Mixed incontinence* is the term used when a woman suffers from both stress and urge incontinence. It can result when a woman copes with stress incontinence by developing urge incontinence as well.

Stress incontinence plagues many healthy women. In one study of 1,000 women, 31 percent acknowledged stress incontinence; most had developed the problem during pregnancy.[51] Other studies have produced similar results. In one, 34 percent of women acknowledged stress incontinence.[626] In another, 63 percent of a postmenopausal population acknowledged the problem; 26 percent were afflicted with troublesome stress incontinence in another group.[77]

Urge incontinence afflicts perhaps 20 percent of fit, healthy women over the age of 30. A problem that increases with age, about 57 percent of women over the age of 64 acknowledge it.[872a] In advanced age, the problem becomes even more common.[765] A vast number of women past the age of 65 live with substantial limitations to their daily activities because of an inability to control their bladder and the resulting embarrassment.[338]

Although incontinence is common, many women will not tell their doctors about such problems, even when directly asked.[765] Perhaps because of women's reluctance to discuss urine problems with their physicians, as well as the gradual progression of the condition, the problems tend to get worse. Yet if you suffer from incontinence, you can be helped.

## CAUSES OF URINARY INCONTINENCE

Correcting incontinence means finding the cause and planning for a treatment for the specific problem at hand. A woman can suffer from one or more of the five common causes of incontinence:

- Tumors that press against the urinary bladder, creating pressure to urinate
- Atrophy (deterioration) of tissues of the genital-urinary system
- Surgery that disconnects necessary nerves or muscles
- PC muscle and sphincter muscle weakness (as a result of the stress of pregnancy or from hormone deficiencies)
- Generalized effects of aging, including atrophy of tissues, intellectual disorientation, and degenerative diseases

Hysterectomy can create urinary problems. Hormone deficiencies are exacerbated by pelvic surgery, and these deficiencies accelerate atrophy of the tissue and loss of muscle strength.

Surgery may disrupt the nerves that control the muscles necessary for urinary continence. It may be six to twelve months after
surgery before symptoms of incontinence emerge.[457]

One investigator reviewed data from twenty-two of his patients who had cervical cancer and for whom he provided a
radical hysterectomy, removing the other reproductive organs
and a wide margin of the vagina at the same time. In this group
of women, who ranged in age from 18 to 65, he reported several
alterations in bladder physiology, including a decreased awareness of distention of the bladder. When, as a result, the women
retained urine longer than normal, they tended to produce a
stress incontinence, which often increased with time.[264]

Radical hysterectomy can be expected to cause the greatest
incidence of incontinence; total hysterectomy causes a lower
incidence; and subtotal the least—and most hysterectomized
women can be helped.

## THE PHYSIOLOGY OF URINARY CONTINENCE

In order for a woman to be "continent"—to contain the
urine—a number of different anatomic and physiologic functions must work properly. Figure 21 depicts a side view of the
organs in the female pelvic regions, revealing the relationship
between the pubic bone; the urinary bladder; the urethra,
through which the urine passes; and the uterus and vagina,
which sit behind the bladder and urethra. The rectum, leading
to the anus, is behind the vagina. The lower spinal bones are also
shown.

Figure 22 shows a different view of the same area. The pubic
bone is at the top of the drawing, and the muscles, nerves, and
glands that control the urinary genital system are depicted. Two
versions are shown. "A" is the surface view. "B" depicts the openings, tissues, and muscles about one inch below the skin surface;
these form the structural underlay of the urinary system. If you
compare these two figures with Figure 18 (page 240), which

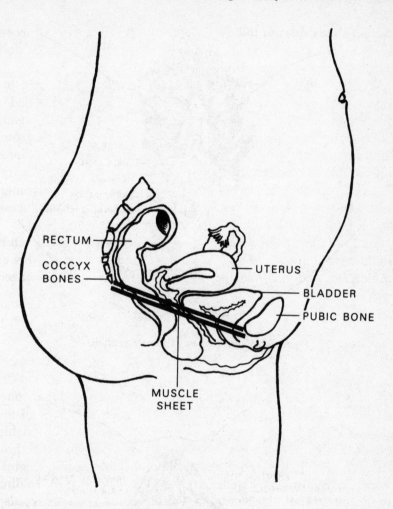

Figure 21. Pubococcygeal muscle sheet connecting coccyx and pubic bones

focuses on the PC muscles, a more complete perspective can be gained.

In order for the urinary system to function in a proper, controlled way, the muscles must be strong, the nerves must be working in good order, and the bladder itself must be in good

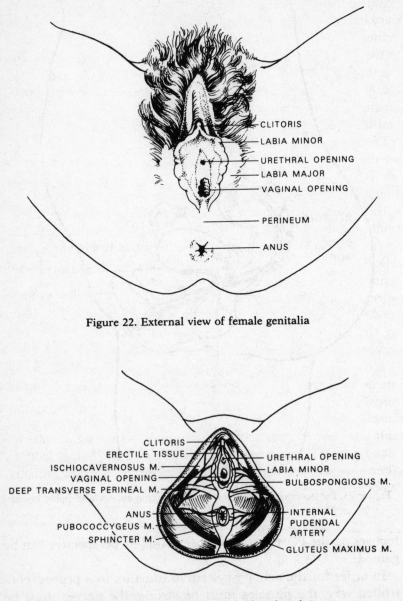

Figure 22. External view of female genitalia

Figure 22b. Cross-section of the female pelvis

physical condition. Figure 23 shows the construction of the urinary bladder, which one can think of as a holding container for urine. Composed of mainly smooth muscle with a hollow space in the center, the bladder has two principal parts: the body and the trigone. The body is composed mainly of the *detrusor* muscle. At the *trigone,* a small triangular area near the mouth of the bladder, the two ureters enter, bringing urine from the kidney, and the urethra exits, taking urine out of the bladder.

The bladder fills through the two ureters. It empties through the urethra whenever two circumstances coincide: (1) the detrusor muscle contracts, and (2) the sphincter muscle relaxes enough to let the urine pass through the tiny urethra.

This process works very much the way a turkey baster works when you squeeze the bulb to eject fluid through the tube. The detrusor muscle is comparable to the bulbous end of the baster, reflexively contracting when nerves fire in the muscle. Urination is normally under the control of reflex actions that usually require no conscious thought process. As the bladder begins to fill, the detrusor muscle begins to stretch, and sensory nerves touching that muscle are triggered to fire impulses into the central nervous system. A subsequent series of nervous impulses fire directly onto the detrusor muscle, causing it to reflexively squeeze itself into contraction. Very strong sphincter muscles normally create so much tension that, even when the detrusor muscle contracts, the urine is contained. Healthy sphincters prohibit the passage of fluid into the urethra—until you decide to relax those muscles, permitting the urine to leave the bladder. When a woman is incontinent, one or more of these mechanisms has broken down.

## WHAT CAN BE DONE ABOUT INCONTINENCE

When a woman suffers from incontinence, her water intake should *not* be restricted. Eight to ten 8-ounce portions of fluid per day are a necessary minimum in order to prevent

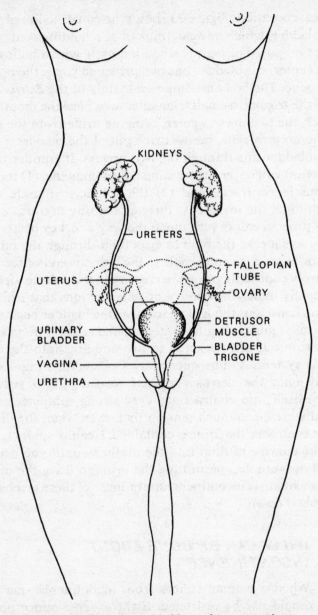

**Figure 23. The urinary bladder and its connections**

formation of a highly concentrated urine (little water, much acid), which irritates the bladder, thereby exacerbating the problems.

Although as often as 98 percent of the time women with incontinence are not sick, screening to rule out various medical diseases should be part of a complete physical exam. Possible causes based in other systems of the body, such as neurologic disease and multiple sclerosis, must be ruled out. A thorough examination also includes a detailed history of a woman's obstetric and gynecologic experience. Most incontinence is caused by inadequate muscle strength.

### Treatment of Fibroid Tumors

For the many nonhysterectomized women who suffer urinary incontinence because a uterine fibroid tumor is pressing against the bladder, the removal of either the tumor or the uterus often produces a cure. Fibroid tumors can be removed surgically, without the removal of the entire uterus. (See Chapter 4.)

### Hormonal Replacement Therapy

The sex hormones play a critical role in maintaining the structural integrity of various parts of the urinary system. The lower urinary tract and the vagina are composed of very similar tissue; both depend on estrogen to maintain their full health. Estrogen depletion produces atrophy in both tissues, and when atrophy occurs, incontinence follows. Particularly sensitive to estrogen are the mucous membranes, the connective tissue, the blood vessels, and the muscles of the urethra. If you are estrogen-deficient, these tissues deteriorate, and estrogen is needed to restore them.

If urinary incontinence is caused by tissue degeneration, such as a deterioration in the urethra or in the smooth muscles, then HRT will probably help relieve the incontinence.[826, 870] Hormone therapies reduce atrophy and improve the cell structure,[765] actions that also increase one's resistance to infection. The dose will vary depending on how much gets to the site needing it. Any way of taking HRT works well to promote the recovery of deteriorating tissue.[454, 523, 757] Oral estrogen is diluted in the blood before it gets to the urinary tissue; you will therefore need to achieve a higher blood level of estrogen if you take your hormones orally than if you use a vaginal cream.

The effectiveness of the cream forms is also good news for women who have genital-urinary atrophy but are unable to take oral estrogen because of its possible effects on other tissues of the body. Experiments have shown that even the very weak estrogen called estriol, when applied in a cream form directly on the genital-urinary skin, is absorbed into the local area, where it promotes a recovery of the atrophic tissue. Yet the hormone does not get absorbed into the bloodstream in any appreciable way; no change in the blood levels of any estrogens is noted after applying estriol on the urinary tissues. Studies show that when estrogen is applied at the vagina in the form of an estriol cream or estriol suppository, even tissue as close as the endometrium receives no estrogen.[454, 523] (Don't use estrogen creams before intercourse; they rub onto the penis and take the benefit from you, who need it, and give it to your partner, who does not.)

Infections can increase the urinary incontinence problem by ulcerating the delicate urethra and bladder. Fortunately, estrogens will stop the pain of urination that is associated with an acid urine passing across ulcerated, deteriorating tissue.

If you have had an ovariectomy, are younger than 50, and suffer from incontinence caused by severe estrogen depletion, complete reversal is possible with correct HRT. If you have passed the natural age of menopause the results may be less satisfying, depending on how much atrophy has occurred. But HRT is still worthwhile because some relief from the distress will follow.

Effective as they are in helping to reverse atrophic tissue, estrogens may be unable to completely correct either urinary stress incontinence or urge incontinence. For complete results, you will most likely need estrogen combined with exercises.

### Exercising the PC Muscle System

Urinary stress incontinence always reflects dysfunction (weakness) of muscles, and exercise usually effects a cure when properly done. Dr. Arnold Kegel established a clinic in the late 1940s in order to study incontinence. After training hundreds of patients—many for several months and some for years—he concluded that more than 85 percent of stress incontinence could be cured with special exercises aided by a device he invented.

Kegel found that patients who had symptoms of incontinence dating back to childhood were easier to cure than those who developed them during adult life, especially those who developed the problem after surgical injury or disease. The principal problem for patients who had developed the problem in childhood was that they had become resigned to it and did not realize they could overcome it. Sexual problems were very common among women who had urinary stress incontinence, principally because both may result from impaired neuromuscular function.

The pubococcygeal (PC) muscles control continence. These muscles form a very important muscle band that courses through the genital region, encompassing the bladder, the vagina, and the anal region (see Figure 18, page 240). They connect to the pubic bone at one end and the coccyx at the other, and wrap around the openings of the urethra, vagina, and anus, much like a figure eight.

Strong muscles promote urinary and fecal continence and enhance the quality of orgasm. In an incontinent woman, the muscles are so weak that she can no longer voluntarily contract them. Kegel would explain to his patients that their muscles of urination were weak because they had not learned to use them properly in childhood. He explained that in order to restore control, they would have to be willing to do accurate and diligent exercising of these weak muscles.[447]

As early as 1951, Dr. Kegel published his first series of studies showing that dysfunction of the PC muscles was present in all

cases of urinary stress incontinence. He developed the perineometer (so named because it measures the strength of the muscles of the perineum, the region between the pubic bone and the
coccyx bone); a set of exercises, since termed the Kegel exercises;
and a way of teaching the patient to do them that produced cures
for around 85 percent of the women who had the problem.[447] His
results showed very successful benefits for women in their late
eighties as well as for women who had suffered from incontinence since childhood. More recently, other researchers have
shown that the lower the PC muscle strength, the higher the
likelihood of urinary stress incontinence.[272] Drs. John Perry and
Beverly Whipple measured the strength of the PC muscles
through an improved electronic perineometer that Perry developed. They showed that women with the lowest muscle strength
almost always had urinary stress incontinence.[678] They also developed techniques by which a woman could be trained to develop her muscle strength and thereby overcome incontinence.
These techniques have been further confirmed as being highly
effective.[88]

The first step in the Kegel exercises involves locating the muscles that must be exercised. If you contract your PC muscles
correctly, your stomach should not tense up at the same time. At
a gynecological exam, after inserting a single gloved finger into
the vagina, a doctor asks the woman to contract her muscles
around the finger. Most women can feel the finger and attempt
to contract around it, an action that the therapist can feel.
Sooner or later, one of these efforts produces a contraction of the
PC muscles and when this happens, the woman is told. Very
often the contraction is very puny and weak, but it does not
matter; even these weak muscles can be retrained.

The next step (or in some biofeedback centers today, the
first step) is the insertion of the tamponlike end of the perineometer into the vagina. The instrument is inserted by the
woman, usually in privacy; she replaces her clothing and simply leads the wire out through the waistband of her clothes.
She is then seated, semireclining, in front of a computer

screen that records her muscular contractions, second by second, as they occur. When a patient contracts her pelvic muscles, the perineometer instantaneously shows the amount of the contraction. (See additional discussion of PC muscle training on page 239.) Once you learn to do these exercises with the perineometer, you can then do them without it. However, several studies have shown that it is critical to use the equipment first in order to learn how to exercise properly.[88, 678] Electronic perineometers have been developed and are currently available for use in a limited number of biofeedback and gynecological centers. The refined and updated perineometer is highly accurate. A portable unit can be purchased or rented for home use (see page 245).

Although some women can improve their muscle strength by exercising without the perineometer, the feedback that women obtain with the instrument makes for substantially better results.[88] One recent study showed that only women who began with good muscle strength could hope to solve their problem without biofeedback. For women whose initial muscle strength was weak, having a doctor telling or showing them what to do in the office was not sufficient; they needed the biofeedback information from a perineometer.

In 1956 Dr. Kegel wrote the following in an article in the *Journal of the International College of Surgeons.*

> The method that produces the quickest, surest and most lasting results combines exercises with the perineometer and exercises without it. The patient is instructed to practice contractions with the aid of the instrument for twenty minutes three times daily. It is explained that exercises against the increasing resistance provided by the apparatus are necessary to develop the reserve strength of the muscles, so that no loss of urine will occur with the added strain of coughing, laughing, etc. The more she repeats these contractions, with and without the perineometer, the sooner will she establish a new habit pattern.
>
> I give my patients the following detailed instructions for exercises without the additional apparatus:

1. Before arising in the morning, contract the muscles five times, as demonstrated with the perineometer; then contract them again five times on first standing up; try to hold the muscles in a contracted position while walking to the toilet.
2. Interrupt the urinary stream several times during each voiding.
3. Repeat contractions of the same muscles five times every half hour throughout the day. (It is brought to the patient's attention that permitting the muscles to sag for long periods retards progress and that to "bear down" during [PC] exercises may aggravate her complaints.)

The early morning exercises are especially important, for the patient begins the day with the perineum in a high position, whereas previously she started out with a sagging pelvic floor and considered the associated tired feeling normal. Because so many of my patients complain of losing urine late in the day, I have come to regard stress incontinence as part of a pelvic fatigue syndrome that must be relieved if one is to obtain permanent results. With adequate exercises the woman learns to maintain the perineum in a higher position and enjoys a sense of pelvic strength, which, by many, is appreciated as much as the relief of incontinence. Those who attain this new pelvic comfort continue the exercises with confidence and enthusiasm.

When the patient is reexamined after three to six weeks of diligent exercises (both) with and without the perineometer, it will be observed that much of the slack in the supportive muscles has been taken up; the perineum, bladder and uterus have assumed a higher position, and the vagina is longer and tighter; at the same time the strength of contractions has increased.

A regular, repeated practice of contracting the PC muscles will ultimately overcome urinary stress incontinence. Many women begin to notice improvement within a few weeks. Once you learn the muscles that are involved, they will become stronger and the work will become easier. Once you have formed the habit of contracting these muscles, you will be able to do it anytime, anywhere.

Women who suffer urinary urgency—the need to urinate more frequently than they would like—have also been helped with exercises. Most women are helped by a combination of the Kegel exercises for the development of muscle strength and bladder training for decreasing the urge to urinate.

### Bladder Training

Clinical experience shows that if a woman will delay her trip to the bathroom (that is, increase the length of time between urinations), the desire to urinate so often will decrease, alleviating urge incontinence. Apparently the reflex responses are retrained, the brain now perceiving the need to urinate only when the bladder volume is higher than it had been. Relaxation techniques, in conjunction with this approach, enhance the effort. (See, for example, "Breathing to Enhance Oxygen Consumption," page 333.) Bladder training combined with pelvic muscle strengthening cures 50 to 90 percent of women within eighteen months.[338] At the Perineometer Research Institute, working in conjunction with the staff of Paoli Memorial Hospital, researchers and physicians are finding better than 90 percent cure rates.

Leslie Talcott, M.S., R.N., who directs the Institute, describes their findings:

In our experience and that reported in the other biofeedback literature, there is really very little difference between stress and urge incontinence. In both cases, the real problem is initially a weak sphincter component of the pelvic muscles. The difference is that the stress patient denies the problem, pays little attention to the bladder signals, and is surprised when a slight physical exertion forces urine out of the bladder. The urge patient, on the other hand, is preoccupied with the bladder signals, and, knowing full well that fluid could leak past her weak sphincter, rushes to the toilet at the first sign of bladder signals. The result is that the brain learns to stop inhibiting the reflexive contractions of the bladder and the patient is more or less on constant alert to urinate.

In the experience of the therapists at the Perineometer Research Institute, women who do Kegel exercises overcome both forms of urinary incontinence.

### Common Ineffective Treatments

Because the major cause of urinary incontinence is muscle weakness, exercises to strengthen these muscles usually constitute the best therapy. Nevertheless other, less effective measures are still sometimes employed. Surgery often fails to correct a urinary incontinence problem, although sometimes there is some temporary relief until the swelling due to tissue trauma subsides.[77]

Drugs generally produce no effective long-term benefit in the treatment of any of the forms of incontinence. Physicians in England have commonly prescribed imipramine and flavoxate hydrochloride, both of which have been shown to be ineffective.[338] In addition, they produce an unpleasant sensation of "cotton mouth," a dryness of the mucous membranes that is not relieved by drinking fluids.

Sanitary pads and diapers collect the urine but do not solve the problem. Although many women resort to wearing sanitary pads or the newer "adult continence products" (designed for handling a greater volume of fluid) to catch leaking urine, much better solutions are available.

Urinary incontinence is a serious problem, but by combining all the relevant therapies, most women can gain significant relief from it.

A support group of women may be very helpful in cheering you on in your efforts to overcome urinary incontinence. Look for one or form one. For free information about help for incontinent people, you might wish to write to HIP, Inc., P.O. Box 544, Union, SC 29379.

It takes work to strengthen weak muscles. It takes proper training in order to learn which muscles these are and to develop the strength that comes from regularly working them. If you have a problem with urinary incontinence, there is no harm in trying to build the muscle strength yourself before seeking professional help. However, you should bear in mind that even if you are not successful when you try to do it by yourself, the likelihood is very good that you will become successful if you go to a bonafide urinary biofeedback center.

# 13 ❧

# *Nutrition:*
## *Designing a Healthful Eating Plan*

❧❧ Putting together a healthful nutrition plan is a challenge, and the most productive way to approach it is to first learn and incorporate the basics. After a hysterectomy, a woman must be particularly alert to her need for adequate levels of calcium and vitamins $B_6$, C, D, and E. She also must watch her dietary balance of fats and cholesterol, and ensure that she takes in enough fiber. Although all women will benefit from careful nutrition planning, it is particularly critical in helping to overcome some of the vulnerabilities created by pelvic surgery.

Most doctors focus their health maintenance efforts on crisis intervention rather than on health promotion.[936] So while research studies have increasingly refined our understanding of the nutritional needs of the woman who has had a hysterectomy, most women will have to study the subject on their own. Such independent reading and learning, and the establishment of sound eating habits, will pay off in more vibrant health. The earlier we can get started the better, but it is never too late. This chapter provides a short course in nutrition for the hysterectomized woman, with discussions of calcium, protein, fats, fiber, and vitamins. Only tentative conclusions can be offered, since research studies have not yet provided all the information we need.

# THE NEED FOR CALCIUM AND VITAMIN D

Think of the bones as a bank in which calcium is stored. About 99 percent of the calcium in the body is stored in this bank, but the 1 percent that circulates in the network of blood and muscles exerts a very powerful influence on a number of body functions. Calcium is required for muscle contraction, nervous-system function, and bone metabolism. As discussed in Chapter 8, after a hysterectomy that causes early menopause or after natural menopause, your body's need for calcium increases.

How much calcium do we need each day? Probably between 750 and 1,500 milligrams. The more estrogen you have circulating in your blood, the closer to 750 milligrams your daily intake can be.[364, 501] To check whether you are in good calcium balance, you can have twice-yearly single photon absorptiometry studies of your arm bones (see page 196). Many foods, especially dairy products, are good sources of calcium. Table 7, page 185, shows the caloric content and amount of calcium in a number of calcium-rich foods.

Some women and men have a problem digesting milk, a condition known as lactose intolerance. Its symptoms include a feeling of gastric distress, pain, and cramps leading to diarrhea within a few hours of drinking the milk. For some of these people, once a habit of drinking milk regularly is reestablished (requiring three to five days of suffering through these symptoms), the diarrhea and intestinal distress disappear. But if you cannot digest milk, there are alternatives,[554] such as yogurt, a rich low-calorie source of calcium that is easily digested, and acidified milk containing intact yogurt microorganisms.

If you cannot get adequate calcium from your diet, you may choose to take one of the calcium supplements that are widely available over the counter in drugstores. But there are two problems with calcium pills. The first has to do with the best time to take them. For best calcium absorption, the noncitrate forms (calcium carbonate and hydroxyapatite) should be taken with meals, but these calcium pills reduce the retention of iron from food.[193] Calcium citrate can be taken at any time during the day. The second problem has to do with the dissolution rate of the tablets in the stomach—important because, for effectiveness, most of the calcium should dissolve within thirty minutes. Available calcium brands differ widely in their rates of dissolution (see Table 8, page 188).

It is probably ideal to take your calcium in a natural form—that is, in food—and to separate your iron sources, such as meat, from your calcium sources. Jewish dietary laws teach that milk and meat should not be eaten together, and recent research seems to validate this rule. It may make sense to consume calcium-rich foods such as milk and cheese at various times during the day in order to ensure that a good amount of the mineral will be absorbed. One study suggests that when calcium is part of the meal, it may be wise to combine foods that are rich in vitamin C (like tomatoes or potatoes) with foods that are rich in iron (such as meat), because vitamin C promotes iron absorption (see page 305).

Calcium absorption requires vitamin D (approximately 400 IU per day). You probably get this amount if you are exposed to at least fifteen minutes of sunlight a day, drink vitamin-D-fortified milk, or take a daily multivitamin. If your intake of vitamin D through milk or exposure to sunlight is low, you could take more calcium, but it would probably be wiser to take a vitamin pill that includes vitamin D to help your intestines absorb the calcium.

Several studies have evaluated whether varying doses of calcium, with and without vitamin D, might be protective to the cardiovascular system. The answer is yes, maybe. In people who have normal blood pressure, high doses of calcium in pill form (1,000 to 1,500 milligrams per day) had no effect on blood pressure.[442, 780, 905] But another investigator considered vitamin D levels and calcium levels, and showed that if either of the two was greater than a threshold amount (800 milligrams calcium per day, 400 IU vitamin D per day), then women tended not to show high systolic blood pressure.[830]

Several foods increase the need for calcium. Because fiber can prevent a significant portion of calcium molecules from being absorbed across the intestines into the bloodstream, you should probably consume your calcium several hours apart from your high-fiber meals. While soy protein increases the urinary loss of calcium, meat protein does not cause calcium loss from the body. Caffeine has a slight effect on increasing urinary loss of calcium,[361] but the amount is so trivial that it is probably not something to be concerned about. Sodium bicarbonate, which many people take, appears to lower the urinary loss of calcium.[364, 501, 525] In order to ensure that your calcium needs are met, it makes sense to consider your own dietary preferences within the framework of these nutrient interactions. Then you can choose from among nutritionally adequate options, such as milk combined with low-fiber cookies as a snack food, or milk with a high-protein meal (provided tomatoes or another high-vitamin-C food is also present, for best possible absorption of iron).

## THE NEED FOR PROTEIN

Most meals that we eat are made up of some combination of carbohydrates, fats, and proteins. We need some of each. A diet that contains a proper balance of these three substances promotes health and well-being.

Carbohydrates most often serve as the body's fuel. Fats form the membranes that surround all the cells, and in addition to serving as a stored form of fuel that can be converted into ready energy, the fat on our bodies provides insulation and is the main material of which the sex hormones are made. Protein forms the building blocks of most of the parts of our bodies, and is especially important in providing the substance of a good part of the structure of muscle.

Our bodies need a regular supply of protein. While authorities vary in their perceptions of how much is appropriate, the amount for women is generally stated as between 30 and 70 grams of protein per day. Unless you are a vegetarian, it is generally not necessary to be concerned about protein intake, because North Americans tend to consume more than enough.

Relatively high intakes of protein, calcium, and phosphorus are beneficial to bone mineralization and maintenance,[781, 837, 838] but different kinds of protein have different effects on calcium metabolism. While it appears that meat protein is beneficial to the overall calcium balance,[273] nonmeat forms of protein (for example, those high in dietary nitrogen and soy) increase the urinary loss of calcium.* The critical issue appears to be whether phosphorus and/or sulphur accompanies the protein. When one or both of those elements are present, protein appears to be beneficial to calcium balance.[368, 459, 501, 782] Meat protein is relatively high in phosphorus and therefore, for the purpose of bone metabolism, is probably a better source of protein than soy protein.[781, 837, 838] Proteins made up of amino acids containing sulphur (fish, chicken, and eggs) are also helpful.[952, 973] While there are no clear or definitive studies about the influence of a meat-free diet on calcium balance, such regimens have been shown to produce significantly lower levels of estrogen in several groups of women,[313, 808] which would indicate a parallel low level of calcium.

## CONTROLLING DIETARY FATS

After hysterectomy women need to be especially concerned about their cardiovascular health protection because hysterectomy increases the risk of cardiovascular disease three- to sevenfold over comparably aged women who have not undergone hysterectomy. Dietary fats play a major role in determining cardiovascular health. The lower the plasma cholesterol level, the lower the risk of cardiovascular disease. As you study about fats, it is important to carefully distinguish between *dietary fats*

*Studies include 11, 17, 139, 368, 369, 542.

(or lipids), *dietary cholesterol, plasma fats* (or lipids), and *plasma cholesterol.* "Dietary" refers to our eating intake; "plasma" refers to what is traveling in the blood.

Although genetics and other predisposing factors have profound influences on plasma lipids and cholesterol, the butters and oils we eat affect the concentration of fats and cholesterol traveling in our blood. We want our blood to show a high level of HDL-Ch (high-density lipoprotein cholesterol) and low levels of both plasma cholesterol and LDL-Ch (low-density lipoprotein cholesterol). (See page 207 for descriptions of the lipoprotein-cholesterol molecules.)

Table 11 shows the interaction between blood levels of total cholesterol and the beneficial lipoprotein HDL-Ch in defining what percentage of men and women in the Framingham Study showed coronary heart disease.[111] The table shows why the statement "The cholesterol level is high" (greater than 260 mg/dl) does not necessarily predict a high risk of coronary heart disease. People with a high cholesterol level that is combined with low HDL-Ch (lower than 40 mg/dl) suffer the highest incidence (13 percent) of coronary heart disease; conversely, high levels of the beneficial HDL-Ch (higher than 60 mg/dl) protect against damage by high plasma cholesterol. Controlling both your

**Table 11.** *Incidence of Coronary Heart Disease and Blood Lipid Levels*[111]*

| HDL-Ch | Total Cholesterol | | | |
|---|---|---|---|---|
| | *200 mg/dl* | *200–229 mg/dl* | *230–259 mg/dl* | *>260 mg/dl* |
| <40 mg/dl | 11% | 12% | 11% | 13% |
| 40–49 mg/dl | 3% | 5% | 11% | 7% |
| 50–59 mg/dl | 2% | 3% | 3.5% | 9% |
| >60 mg/dl | 1.8% | 2.5% | 2% | 4% |

(Percentages indicate the incidence of coronary heart disease in each category and suggest what your risk would be in each condition)
*Mg/dl = milligrams per deciliter (one tenth of a liter); < means "less than"; > means "more than."

plasma cholesterol (to make it lower) and your HDL-Ch (to make it higher) reduces the incidence of cardiovascular disease. Fortunately, you can do this through your diet.

### The Role of Dietary Fats and Dietary Cholesterol

Dietary cholesterol is different from dietary fat, and a high-cholesterol diet does not necessarily affect the cholesterol level in the blood.[310, 652, 954]

Three major categories of dietary fats are saturated fatty acids (SFAs), monounsaturated fatty acids (MUFAs), and polyunsaturated fatty acids (PUFAs). Table 12 lists examples of each of the three categories, which are distinguished by their chemical properties. As a general principle, one wants to have no more than about 25 or 30 percent of one's total calories made up of all the fats together, and also to have a relative balance that is high in the PUFAs and relatively low in the SFAs and MUFAs. When one adheres to this formula, the dietary levels of cholesterol can be relatively higher than when one does not. Table 13 lists sources of dietary cholesterol.

The kinds of fat you eat influence the cholesterol and lipoprotein (but not the triglyceride) content of your blood.[310, 651, 796, 819] Generally total plasma cholesterol and LDL-Ch increase and decrease in concert. The higher they are, the greater your risk of cardiovascular disease (see Chapter 9). The situation for the protective HDL-Ch is a little different. Sometimes it moves up and down together with the dangerous ones; at other times it moves in the opposite direction. This change appears to be the result of the particular lipid combination in your diet.

Four general principles can help in your nutrition planning:

1. The relative quantity of PUFAs and SFAs produces significant alterations in the plasma cholesterol levels. A diet that had high PUFAs reduced the plasma cholesterol levels by 16 or 20 percent, depending on whether the accompanying dietary cholesterol level was high or low.[651]

**Table 12.** *Major Sources of Dietary Fats* [865]

| Saturated | Monounsaturated | Polyunsaturated |
|---|---|---|
| Butter & butter fat | Avocado | Cottonseed oil |
| Cheese | Olives & olive oil | Corn oil |
| Chocolate & cocoa | Margarines with | Fatty fish |
| butter | hydrogenated oil | Margarines with |
| Coconut & coconut | as first ingredient | an oil from this |
| oil | Lightly | group listed as a |
| Hydrogenated solid | hydrogenated | first ingredient |
| fats | shortening | Mayonnaise |
| Lard | Nuts, such as | Safflower oil |
| Meat fat (from | almonds brazil | Salad dressing |
| beef lamb, pork, | nuts, pecans, | made from oil in |
| veal, and poultry) | filberts, | this group |
| Palm oil | macadamia nuts | Soybeans & |
| | Peanuts, peanut | soybean oil |
| | butter, & peanut | Sunflower seeds & |
| | oil | oil |
| | | Walnuts & walnut |
| | | oil |
| | | Wheat germ & |
| | | wheat germ oil |

*Note:* Fried foods, pastries, and other foods that are cooked in or made with fat are important sources of fatty acids. Which category they should be placed in depends on which fat is used in their preparation.

2. The cholesterol level in the diet has very little effect on the plasma cholesterol.

   These two principles work in all the studies so far reported, which have had as subjects young men, sedentary middle-aged healthy men,[954] men with high levels of cholesterol in their blood,[310] and middle-aged Italian people with dangerously high levels of cholesterol.[819]

3. Increasing the PUFAs improves the blood lipids (cholesterol and LDL-Ch are lowered; HDL-Ch is raised), but the MUFAs (such as olive oil) do not affect plasma lipids one way or the other.[819]

4. Reducing the total fat content appears to be even more helpful than simply altering the ratio of one fat to another.[55, 310] In most Western diets, fat consumption commonly represents about 35 percent of the total caloric intake.[880] Both normal (healthy) people and those with dangerously high plasma cholesterol levels who lower their total dietary fats generally experience a lowering of their blood pressure or dangerous plasma lipids.[543]

But diet change is not the only factor. As you increase your estrogens, you improve your lipids. The plasma cholesterol usually drops, and the HDL-Ch usually increases, as described in chapters 6 and 9. Also there appears to be both a genetic and a body-build component in the relationship between diet and plasma cholesterol. A study of men and women in India compared those with slender, slight builds to those with medium builds. Both groups experimentally increased their fat content from the Indian normal, which is about 10 percent of the caloric total, to the Western normal of about 35 percent. As the two groups increased their dietary fats, there was no effect on the plasma cholesterol level of slender people, but the people with medium builds showed a sharp increase in cholesterol levels.[796] This may partially explain why another experimenter showed that meats (which contain saturated fats) are not necessarily bad for plasma lipid levels.[725] Their body-build type may have protected the subjects. Although safflower oil (a PUFA) lowered the cholesterol level and coconut oil (an SFA) increased it, beef fat did not alter either the plasma cholesterol or the dangerous LDL-Ch in healthy people.[725] Meat, which can be helpful for your strength, is not necessarily the culprit that many believe it to be.

If blood tests show that your plasma lipid levels are healthy, you are probably eating appropriate fat balances and you probably have good blood levels of estrogen.

**Table 13.** *Cholesterol Content of High-Cholesterol Foods*

| Food | Cholesterol (milligrams per 100 grams*) |
|---|---|
| Egg yolk, dried | 2950 |
| Brains, raw | 2000 |
| Egg yolk, fresh | 1500 |
| Egg, whole | 500 |
| Kidney, raw | 375 |
| Caviar or fish roe | 300 |
| Liver, raw | 300 |
| Butter | 250 |
| Sweetbreads | 250 |
| Oysters | 200 |
| Lobster | 200 |
| Heart, raw | 150 |
| Crabmeat | 125 |
| Shrimp | 125 |
| Cheese, cream | 120 |
| Cheese, cheddar | 100 |
| Lard and other animal fat | 95 |
| Veal | 90 |
| Cheese (25 to 30% fat) | 85 |
| Milk, dried, whole | 85 |
| Beef, raw | 70 |
| Fish, steak | 70 |
| Fish, filet | 70 |
| Lamb, raw | 70 |
| Pork | 70 |
| Cheese spread | 65 |
| Margarine (2/3 animal, 1/3 vegetable fat) | 65 |
| Mutton | 65 |
| Chicken, flesh only, raw | 60 |
| Ice cream | 45 |
| Cottage cheese, creamed | 15 |
| Milk, fluid, whole | 11 |
| Milk, fluid, skim | 3 |
| Egg white | 0 |

*Most standard kitchen scales available for purchase show the gram as well as the ounce content on the scale. If you weigh the food and note its gram content, you can then compute its cholesterol content from this chart.

### Fish Oils

Although fish oils (which are PUFAs) have recently been shown to be protective against certain of the risk factors for cardiovascular disease,[624] they should not be totally accepted as the panacea offered by some advertisers.

Although fish oils do work in reducing the risk of cardiovascular disease, the potential dangers of concentrate forms have not yet been properly studied, and this mandates against routine use unless you are under the care of a knowledgeable professional. These dangers include the potential for deleterious excess intake of vitamins A and D, as well as for an increased intake of contaminants.[97, 378] Meanwhile, moderate consumption of fish is desirable. Fish is a wonderful health food—rich in nutrients, low in fat—which contributes greatly to your nutritional health.

### What About Eggs?

Although we often hear the injunction "If you do not want high cholesterol, do not eat eggs," the facts are different.[371, 453] Because high-cholesterol foods do not necessarily affect the cholesterol level in the blood, eating six eggs a day for six weeks does not necessarily increase the plasma cholesterol level.[652] Eggs provide a very rich source of nutrients at a low calorie cost (70 per egg). A concern about cholesterol does not seem to be a valid indication for eliminating them. In fact, one could mount an argument for including eggs in a well-balanced diet, provided the dietary fat composition is relatively high in the PUFAs. If you find yourself eating a lot of beef, then you probably should go easy on eggs. But if you have a high fish or other PUFA component in your diet, then you probably should include eggs or other cholesterol-rich foods.[651, 652] Why? Because diets that are low in both SFAs and cholesterol tend to reduce both the plasma cholesterol and the protective HDL-Ch levels, a condition you want to avoid.

If you are concerned about bringing your lipids into line with those shown in Table 11, then you will want to do those things that lower your cholesterol and LDL-Ch levels while not lowering your HDL-Ch level. If most of your fats are derived from the PUFA category, you will probably need to increase your level of dietary cholesterol in order to provide yourself with adequate concentrations of the protective HDL-Ch. If most of your dietary fats are composed of the saturated form, you would probably be wise to make a shift in the direction of more PUFAs and fewer SFAs.

Cholesterol readings are a standard part of a blood profile that should be part of a (yearly) physical exam after hysterectomy. If the levels are high, check each six months until you have lowered them.

## DIETARY FIBER

*Dietary fiber,* the term used for the various dietary substances derived primarily from plant cell walls,[829, 890] has come to mean those parts of ingested foods that fail to be digested and therefore pass out of the body as waste.

Fiber-depleted foods are the result of food processing that creates "refined" products by removing fiber from, for example, white flour and white rice. Fiber-depleted foods taste, look, and feel different from full-fiber foods. They cook and combine differently, and in the words of one investigator, they yield "an irresistible pressure to consume more food and more quickly." Plant foods fall into three broad categories:

- *Cereal grains,* which are low in fat and rich in starch (oatmeal, farina, Wheatena)
- *Grain legumes,* vegetables that are high in fat and rich in starch (lima beans, peas, kidney beans)
- *Fruits and other vegetables,* which are low in fat and high in water (apples, oranges, cabbage)

After hysterectomy, women are highly susceptible to a number of diseases that are caused by fiber-depleted foods. These diseases can be prevented, provided you understand the way they develop and the role fiber plays in eliminating the risk of developing them. Fiber-depleted foods have been associated with a variety of new diseases in the Western societies including: hiatal hernia,[789] diverticular disease of the colon,[89, 662] diabetes mellitus,[540, 816] lipid metabolism and cardiovascular health problems,[471] gallstones,[370] bowel cancer,[161] varicose veins and hemorrhoids,[89] deep vein thrombosis,[89] pelvic phleboliths,[89] and kidney stones.[61] To understand why these diseases have emerged, one must consider the effects of fiber on the human body.

### How Dietary Fiber Helps

Fiber-rich foods form a bulk that enters the stomach and then the intestinal tract, providing a greater sense of fullness than the same caloric amounts of fiber-depleted foods.[367] High-bulk food is better for us because it moves more quickly through the intestinal canal, drawing water from the surrounding tissue (which further increases bulk)[161] and promoting soft stools, which can be passed without strain.

Fiber is sometimes beneficial to cardiovascular health. It lowered cholesterol levels in some studies, but not others. In one group of medical students and nurses who had normal cholesterol levels, increasing fiber content to the maximum individual tolerance rate had no effect on the plasma lipids;[338] in another study, rolled oats, guar gum, and legumes helped reduce cholesterol levels.[471] Fiber-rich diets have been associated with a relative freedom from cardiovascular disease, although the mechanism through which this effect is achieved is not yet well understood.

## The Effects of a Lack of Fiber

Varicose veins and hemorrhoids—in fact, all of the diseases mentioned above—are exclusively confined to the human race and are much more prevalent in economically developed communities. The incidence of fiber-depleted-food diseases progressively increases as the population ages. Both black and white Americans suffer from these diseases, but in African nations, where there is high fiber consumption in the diet, these diseases are not apparent among blacks.

The cause for varicose veins at first glance is shown to be an incompetence of the valves. Intact valves serve an important role, ensuring one-way flow of venous blood back to the heart. The muscles around the calves and thighs help to propel the blood small distances at a time, past a series of one-way valves. This combination—the muscles forcing upward and the valves stopping the blood from pooling back downward—contributes to normal, healthy veinous return of blood to the heart. When a valve becomes incompetent, blood is able to go back down through the opened valve, leading to a swollen, painful varicose vein.

How does fiber interact with this process? Scientists have suggested that straining to pass hard feces causes pressure against the valves located near the anus and in the legs. The pressure then damages the valves, triggering the development of varicose veins.[89]

Hemorrhoids, varicosities of the anal veins, are analogous to the varicose veins in the legs. Recent studies of this tissue have shown that three blood-filled submucosal cushions surround the upper part of the anal canal, with the specific function of maintaining continence of feces and gas. Scientists now believe that hemorrhoids are caused by straining to pass feces. The straining leads to veinous engorgement of the anal cushions, which then become more vulnerable to the shearing stress exerted by the passage of a firm fecal mass.[89] A high-fiber diet promotes soft, wet stools, thereby avoiding the need to exert excess pressure.

Diverticular disease of the colon emerged in the Western world about 1900.[662] Now the most common disorder of the colon, it is found in one out of three people past the age of 60. The disease appears to be caused by an obstruction in the normal flow of feces, from constipation or other causes. When fecal passage is blocked, the pressure caused by the reflex contraction of adjacent segments of the intestinal wall causes the muscular fibers of the intestine to be strained, and sometimes to separate from one another. This separation of muscular fiber results in the protrusion of the mucus membranes into out-pouchings. The disease is characterized by long periods of calm punctuated by flare-ups of disease, which produce intense abdominal pain and sometimes fever. Apparently the flare-ups are due to infection in the out-pouchings. The incidence of diverticulitis has risen dramatically with the increase in fiber-depleted processed foods. Several studies have shown that compared to age-matched controls, people with diverticular disease eat substantially less fiber than their healthy counterparts.

A high-fiber diet abolished or relieved the diverticular disease of nearly all of the seventy patients in one study.[662] "High" was defined as the amount of fiber that would allow each person to pass, easily and without strain, one or two stools per day. For most, two teaspoons of bran three times a day was sufficient, but some needed much more. As an added bonus, patients who had previously suffered from distention after eating found that the distention disappeared. Apparently the wet bran soothes the gut. The investigator noted that surgery does not remove the underlying cause of the problem of fiber deficiency, and only sometimes, and then temporarily, does it deal with the complications of the disease.

With all of these benefits, there remains a counterbalancing risk. An excessively high-fiber diet can lead to a loss of trace minerals, particularly a reduced absorption of calcium, magnesium, iron, and zinc.[364, 925] The fiber in high-bran diets and other high-fiber diets, when taken in conjunction with milk, attaches the calcium molecules, preventing their absorption into the bloodstream and passing them out through the bowels.[159, 160, 364, 925] For this reason, green vegetables, which are high in both fiber and calcium, may not supply their calcium to the bloodstream or the bones.

### Getting Enough Fiber

It is important for the posthysterectomized woman to consume a high-fiber diet in order to prevent hemmorhoids, diverticular disease, and the other fiber-depletion diseases. Although many foods have not yet been analyzed to determine their fiber content, Table 14 lists the fiber content of some fruits, vegetables, legumes, refined grain products, and unrefined grain products.[426] In planning your own nutritionally sound eating pattern, include enough fiber in your diet to enable you to pass soft stools without strain. Each person finds her own body requirement level. In the United States, the average person tends to take in between about 15 and 30 grams per day.

There is no reason to buy fiber products in drugstores when there are such abundant natural sources of fiber. Moreover, we don't yet know why, but studies that evaluated the efficacy of drugstore bran did not show satisfactory effects upon bowel habits.[662] Perhaps the digestive system has difficulty with the highly concentrated forms of both calcium and bran. The natural forms of fiber, abundant in foods, seem to be more effective in promoting soft stools.

### Avoid Laxatives

Constipation is a straining to defecate and an inability to pass at least one soft stool daily without effort. This condition afflicts a very large proportion of maturing people, and women are particularly at risk. Fortunately, although laxatives are widely advertised and do provide effective relief, better and more natural ways of preventing and relieving the problem exist. First, be certain that you do not have a specific disease, such as diabetes,

**Table 14.** Fiber (NDF)* Content of Foods [426]

| | | Fiber (grams) | | |
| | | per serving | per 100 g | Water (%)† |
| Food | Serving Size | | | |
|---|---|---|---|---|
| *Fruits* | | | | |
| Apple, fresh | 180 g (1 medium) | 1.1 | 0.6 | 91 |
| Apple, cooked, peeled | 122 g (1/2 cup) | 0.7 | 0.6 | 91 |
| Banana | 175 g (1 medium) | 1.1 | 0.7 | 74 |
| Blueberries, frozen | 83 g (1/2 cup) | 1.5 | 1.8 | 83 |
| Cantaloupe | 136 g (1/4 melon) | 0.7 | 0.5 | 88 |
| Grapes, green seedless, fresh | 80 g (1/2 cup) | 0.4 | 0.5 | 78 |
| Orange, fresh | 160 g (1 medium) | 1.2 | 0.8 | 87 |
| Peach, fresh | 115 g (1 medium) | 0.6 | 0.6 | 91 |
| Peach, canned | 122 g (1/2 cup) | 0.7 | 0.6 | 88 |
| Peach, cooked | 122 g (1/2 cup) | 1.1 | 0.9 | 90 |
| Pear, fresh | 180 g (1 medium) | 3.6 | 2.0 | 84 |
| Pineapple, canned | 123 g (1/2 cup) | 1.2 | 1.0 | 83 |
| *Vegetables* | | | | |
| Beans, green, canned | 120 g (1/2 cup) | 1.6 | 1.3 | 92 |
| Broccoli, cooked | 73 g (1/2 cup) | 1.5 | 2.1 | 87 |
| Cabbage, fresh | 45 g (1/2 cup) | 0.5 | 1.1 | 89 |
| Carrots, fresh | 81 g (1 medium) | 0.8 | 1.0 | 88 |
| Carrots, canned | 73 g (1/2 cup) | 0.5 | 0.7 | 92 |
| Celery, fresh, diced | 67 g (1 cup) | 0.5 | 0.7 | 94 |
| Corn, whole kernel, canned | 83 g (1/2 cup) | 1.2 | 1.4 | 78 |
| Corn, whole kernel, frozen | 88 g (1/2 cup) | 1.3 | 1.5 | 68 |
| Lettuce, fresh | 70 g (1/8 head) | 0.4 | 0.6 | 95 |
| Mushrooms, fresh | 35 g (1/2 cup) | 0.6 | 1.7 | 90 |
| Onion, fresh, chopped | 43 g (1/4 cup) | 0.5 | 1.1 | 87 |
| Potatoes, boiled, peeled | 76 g (1/2 cup) | 1.2 | 1.2 | 71 |
| Spinach, frozen, cooked | 100 g (1/2 cup) | 1.2 | 1.2 | 90 |
| Squash, zucchini, fresh | 65 g (1/2 cup) | 0.5 | 0.8 | 93 |
| Tomato, fresh | 135 g (1 medium) | 0.8 | 0.6 | 95 |
| Tomato, cooked | 120 g (1/2 cup) | 1.0 | 0.8 | 94 |
| *Legumes* | | | | |
| Beans, kidney, canned | 93 g (1/2 cup) | 3.9 | 4.2 | 39 |

| Food | Serving Size | Fiber (grams) per serving | Fiber (grams) per 100 g | Water (%)† |
|------|-------------|------|------|------|
| Beans, lima, mature, cooked | 95 g (1/2 cup) | 3.3 | 3.5 | 74 |
| Peas, canned | 79 g (1/2 cup) | 2.2 | 2.8 | 83 |
| *Refined Grain Products* | | | | |
| Bread, white | 25 g (1 slice) | 0.5 | 2.0 | 31 |
| Corn Flakes | 21 g (2/3 cup) | 0.3 | 1.4 | 5 |
| Cornmeal, cooked | 120 g (1/2 cup) | 0.6 | 0.5 | 87 |
| Cream of Wheat | 163 g (2/3 cup) | 0.7 | 0.4 | 87 |
| Macaroni, cooked | 65 g (1/2 cup) | 0.5 | 0.8 | 57 |
| Rice cereal, puffed | 11 g (2/3 cup) | 0.1 | 0.9 | 4 |
| Rice, white, cooked | 100 g (1/2 cup) | 0.5 | 0.5 | 70 |
| Rice Krispies | 18 g (2/3 cup) | 0.1 | 0.6 | 5 |
| Special K | 18 g (2/3 cup) | 0.2 | 1.1 | 4 |
| White flour | 30 g (1/4 cup) | 0.3 | 1.0 | 1 |
| Popcorn | 6 g (1 cup) | 0.5 | 8.0 | 4 |
| *Unrefined Grain Products* | | | | |
| Barley, pearled, cooked | 100 g (1/2 cup) | 1.0 | 1.0 | 84 |
| Bran Buds | 28 g (1/3 cup) | 6.4 | 22.8 | 5 |
| Bran Chex | 23 g (2/3 cup) | 3.9 | 17.0 | 4 |
| Bread, rye | 25 g (1 slice) | 1.2 | 4.8 | 36 |
| Bread, wheat | 28 g (1 slice) | 1.3 | 4.5 | 8 |
| Bread, whole wheat | 25 g (1 slice) | 1.8 | 7.2 | 7 |
| Bran Flakes (40%) | 23 g (2/3 cup) | 3.2 | 13.9 | 3 |
| Granola | 28 g (1/4 cup) | 0.8 | 3.0 | 6 |
| Oatmeal, cooked | 160 g (2/3 cup) | 1.1 | 0.7 | 86 |
| Shredded Wheat | 25 g (1 biscuit) | 2.6 | 10.0 | 6 |
| Wheat bran | 30 g (1/2 cup) | 11.2 | 37.3 | 8 |

*NDF represents the neutral detergent fiber method of testing fiber. Several different methods are currently available, and each yields somewhat different values. This method appears to be a useful one.

†Foods with higher percentages of water provide bulk without calories. As the concentration of water diminishes, the concentration of calories, fiber, and nutrient tends to increase.

hypothyroidism, or bowel abnormalities[847]—the case with only a very small minority of people. For most people, adequate fiber and regular physical exercise will prevent constipation and the diseases that fiber-depleted diets create.

## VITAMINS

In the late 1980s, the health-conscious woman is beset with a bewildering array of conflicting information about vitamins. One frequent question is why we should take vitamin supplements when foods provide a natural source. First, even a carefully designed dietary regimen may not provide optimal amounts of important vitamins. Second, aging alters our needs. Although our caloric requirement decreases with age, our mineral and vitamin needs probably increase, as, for example, is the case with calcium.

Vitamins are complex organic substances that occur naturally in plant and animal tissue. While they do not provide energy or serve as substances from which body tissues are built, they are essential in small amounts for the control of metabolic processes. Our knowledge has grown in halting steps.

In 1753 a Scottish physician, Dr. James Lind, studied scurvy, a common disease that was killing sailors, and discovered that its cure was eating foods rich in vitamin C. It is now well recognized that a daily intake of 60 milligrams of the vitamin will prevent scurvy. Other diseases that have caused a tremendous amount of suffering and death—including beriberi, pellagra, pernicious anemia, and rickets—have been discovered to be the result of a vitamin deficiency and are prevented with the intake of adequate vitamins.

After pelvic surgery, when a woman has become more vulnerable to accelerated aging and to cardiovascular and bone disease, it becomes particularly important to maintain a diet rich in vitamins. As you plan appropriate vitamin intake for yourself, three important issues emerge:

How much of a particular vitamin will maximize your health?
Is there any danger in taking too much of it?
Is there any danger in taking too little of it?

In the United States, about 35 percent of the population between ages 18 and 74 take vitamin and mineral supplements
regularly, in amounts that on average are three times higher
than the recommended daily allowance (RDA).[97, 742] Is this wise?
Is it helpful? Sometimes yes, but sometimes no. A great deal
more research must be done before the experts can speak with
assurance regarding vitamin intake.

Until the past few years, the goal of setting RDAs was the
prevention of severe nutritional deficiencies. Fortunately, the
focus has now shifted. Current efforts are aimed at setting levels
that will also prevent less serious chronic diseases and conditions that have come to be linked to nutrition. And as knowledge
expands, it is becoming clearer that the RDAs are very minimum
doses and that much higher ones are likely to lead, not only to
the absence of disease, but to a high overall level of well-being.
In fact, the tenth edition of the RDA guidelines published by the
National Research Council was not issued on schedule in 1985
because public health interests had begun to shift away from
former patterns and optimal levels could not be agreed upon by
the experts.[97]

Information on vitamins forms a mosaic rather than a cohe-
sive picture. Some relevant research is available on vitamins C,
A, D, E, and $B_6$, and these studies are reviewed here.

### Vitamin C

No vitamin has had more publicity than vitamin C, partly
because of controversy about the benefits of high doses (megadoses) and partly because of its effects on a wide range of body
systems.

Although the optimal dosage levels have not yet been defined,[498] a variety of studies suggest that megadoses of vitamin

C, also known as ascorbic acid, have beneficial effects on wound healing; cardiovascular health and reduction of atherosclerotic risk; strengthening of the bones; overcoming toxic effects from benzene, phenol, alcohol, ozone, and textile dust; the prevention of certain cancers; prevention of cataracts; central-nervous-system functioning; and promotion of iron absorption.

### Helps Wound Healing

The role of vitamin C in the healing of wounds is discussed in Chapter 5. Whenever you are healing, you need more C in order to promote the collagen synthesis that is necessary for replacement of tissue.

### Promotes Cardiovascular Health

Vitamin C appears able both to reduce the cholesterol level[673] and to increase the beneficial protective lipid HDL-Ch.[412, 794] One recent study evaluated the vitamin C and E levels in blood in populations that showed likelihoods for cardiovascular death. In those groups that had a high risk of cardiovascular disease, the blood levels of vitamins C and E were very low; in those groups that had very low risk of cardiovascular disease, the blood levels of these vitamins tended to be high.[304] As early as 1970, publishing in the *American Journal of Clinical Nutrition,* Dr. Carl Shaffer concluded: "Coronary atherosclerosis . . . appears to be, in part, a possible result of deficient ingestion of ascorbic acid."[794]

### Strengthens the Bones

Vitamin C also helps women aged 35 to 65 strengthen bone, according to one four-year study that compared calcium tablets to placebo. For the women who were not taking calcium tablets, the higher the vitamin C content in their diet, the greater their bone mass.[273] This relationship was revealed when data were examined each year as well as after the four years of the study. The author concluded: "The biological basis for this apparent contribution of vitamin C in increasing bone density could be the role of vitamin C in collagen hydroxylation [related to bone tissue buildup] and osteoblast growth or in C-induced changes of calcium absorption."

## Protects the Lungs and Counteracts Toxins

In several different kinds of experiments, vitamin C appeared to play a protective role against the reflex blockage of air flow in the lungs (which occurs when poisons are inhaled). For example, it protected hamster lung tissue against the carcinogenic effects of tobacco smoke.[494] Thus, although controversy remains about the relevant dose,[825] some investigators have suggested that those people who are unable to stop smoking should, at the very least, be taking an extra 2,000 milligrams of vitamin C per day.

Ozone, a pollutant produced in cities by cars, certain factories, certain cigarette smoke, and other poisons, causes the lung passages to constrict, and vitamin C has been shown to protect against this broncho-constriction.[125, 602] In one experiment, vitamin C (1,000 milligrams per day) combined with vitamin E (800 IU per day) protected best against ozone-induced broncho-constriction.[125] Another study looked at people with asthma (a disease in which the lungs constrict) to see whether 2,000 milligrams of vitamin C (in four 500 mg doses) would improve the airway problems. The results were positive.

Other pollutants have been studied. Chronic exposure to benzene has been implicated in leukemia; ascorbic acid is protective.[970] The body's response to benzene and its metabolized product, phenol, as well as the body's ability to handle alcohol toxicity, all appear to be enhanced when vitamin C is taken. In one set of experiments in which guinea pigs were given high amounts of alcohol, vitamin C was shown to protect against liver damage. In studies of men with high blood alcohol levels, vitamin C improved motor coordination, the ability to discriminate color, and the clearance of the alcohol from the blood.[970]

## Prevents Some Cancers

Ascorbic acid deficiency has been shown to have relationships to the development and proliferation of cancers.* Relationships between ascorbic acid and serum proteins within the immune system have also been demonstrated.[902] For example, when compared to age-matched controls, women with cervical cancer were shown to have much lower levels of vitamin C both in their diet and circulating in their blood.[748, 749, 932] The authors of one study concluded that a vitamin C intake below 30 milligrams a day coincided with an incidence of cervical cancer that was ten times greater than in women who ingest more than this.[932] Women who have cancer (breast, leukemia, and other forms) generally show less than half the amount of circulating vitamin C than matched controls who are healthy.[98] Vitamin C appears to benefit the immune system by helping to promote the secretion of some of the antibodies that protect it.[902]

## Guards the Central Nervous System

Ascorbic acid is necessary for the production of enzymes that in turn are necessary for nerves to fire properly.[309] Discoveries reported in 1987 led investigators at the New York Academy of Sciences to conclude that there should soon be no doubt that inadequate levels of vitamin C within the nerves would account for many endocrine disorders.[309] The adrenal gland produces cortisone, adrenalin (also known as epinephrine), and other substances. Adrenalin is a neurotransmitter—a substance that triggers the firing of certain nerves and that in turn promotes the activation of critical elements within the nervous system. Recent studies have shown that vitamin C is necessary in order for adrenalin to be produced within the cells of the adrenal glands.[498] Other helpful adrenal gland responses to megadose levels of vitamin C have also recently been reported.[467]

*Studies include 98, 518, 592, 748, 871, 932, 964.

## Promotes Iron Absorption

Ascorbic acid promotes iron absorption. The higher one's intake of fiber or tannin (contained in red wine), the more one needs the vitamin in order to permit the absorption of iron. Why? Apparently fiber and tannin molecules, which themselves do not get absorbed, bind to iron molecules and can prevent their absorption into the body. The 1987 publication from the New York Academy of Sciences conference on vitamin C concluded that each main meal should contain 25 to 50 milligrams of vitamin C, and that if the meal was high in fiber or tannin, then at least 250 milligrams of vitamin C were needed.[345] So, if you drink a lot of red wine with your dinner, it is conservative to consume vitamin C at the same time.

## The Correct Dose

How much vitamin C should you take? Probably somewhere between 500 and 8,000 milligrams per day, depending upon your level of stress, your exposure to colds, whether you currently have a cold or virus, whether you are a smoker, and your general immune strength. Can you achieve this level through natural dietary means? Probably not. It takes four quarts of freshly squeezed orange juice to provide 500 milligrams of vitamin C. Will this level of vitamin C potentially be harmful? Not likely. Will it help? Very likely. Although we must make decisions based on limited knowledge, the weight of evidence for and against large doses of vitamin C emerges on the side of "for."

Dr. Linus Pauling, a two-time Nobel prize winner, is a well-known and powerful advocate of megadoses of vitamin C. Because his attitude has been so strongly in favor of taking large doses, it was perhaps inevitable that an equally strong view would emerge among those who did not share his great enthusiasm.

Body levels of ascorbic acid have been studied. Given equivalent dietary intake, elderly men show significantly lower blood levels than elderly women.[296] Since women live longer than men, perhaps vitamin C plays a role in longevity. But blood levels of vitamin C are only part of the picture. Different tissues of the body store vitamin C in much higher concentrations than what is found in blood.[654, 910] Thus, blood levels may not provide relevant information about the overall level of vitamin C in the body.[654]

Our current knowledge does help us know how to maximize the blood levels of vitamin C. The results of several studies seem to suggest that 500 milligrams is the most that can be added to the blood level at one time, that maximal absorption is reflected in blood about two hours after the vitamin is taken orally,[583] and that people who spread out their daily vitamin dose maintain high blood level concentrations of vitamin C.[467] Until we know more about how much vitamin has reached the tissues, it is probably best to break up doses of vitamin C supplements into a maximum of 500 milligrams each, no more often than every two hours. People vary in the amounts of vitamin C their bowels will tolerate. Mild diarrhea will signal you to cut back your dosage level.

Are there any dangers from taking high doses (more than 1,000 milligrams at a time) of vitamin C? So far, although there have been statements in medical journals that high vitamin C dosing can be dangerous, there is no substantiated proof. In spite of earlier suggestions that vitamin $B_6$ or $B_{12}$ levels might be adversely affected by high doses of vitamin C, carefully conducted recent studies have shown that vitamins $B_6$ and $B_{12}$ are not adversely affected by vitamin C megadose supplements.[410, 653]

Vitamin C is a water-soluble vitamin.* Because the body can-

---

*Vitamins are either water- or fat-soluble; that is, they dissolve in either water or in fat. Water-soluble vitamins (C, B) cannot be stored by the body; they pass out in the urine and feces when a person takes in more than the body can metabolize. Fat-soluble vitamins (A, D, E), which are stored in the fat cells of the body, tend to be the ones that produce dangerous side effects when a person takes in more than her body can use.

not store it, if you take more than you need the excess is excreted. The question of whether vitamin C might produce an increased propensity toward kidney stones has been raised, but Dr. Pauling argues quite convincingly against that likelihood, based on a rational review of the published scientific data.[673] Several studies published in 1987 confirm that vitamin C megadosing is rarely dangerous and almost always extremely beneficial, provided the person is not a recurrent kidney stone former or susceptible to iron overload.[742] The risk of megadose vitamin C appears trivial compared to its many benefits.[871] By 1987 the consensus of the experts on vitamin C research at the New York Academy of Sciences was that vitamin C is safe at levels thirty times higher than the 60 milligram RDA.

If you take vitamin C, it is important to change levels only gradually. You probably should not increase or decrease your dose by more than 500 milligrams per day.[653] Natural vitamin C in foods and synthetic forms in the drugstore seem to be absorbed equally readily into the blood.[345] Dietary vitamin C is destroyed when foods are cooked and saved. Fresh-squeezed orange juice should be consumed as soon as it is made; it should not be left out in the air. When potatoes are cooked and allowed to sit for several hours, their vitamin C is lost.[345]

## Vitamin A

Vitamin A is essential for bone development in the growing baby in the womb and for the maintenance of skin and vision in the child and adult. How much do you need? The RDA for vitamin A was previously set at 5,000 IU per day. There is some evidence that people who take combination supplements of vitamins A, E, and C have lower risks of lung cancer, cervical cancer, and other diseases.[233, 587, 748, 964]* People who take a daily supplement that includes combinations of more than 500 milligrams vitamin C and high levels of A (18,000 IU a day) seem to

---

*So many different combination tablets are used that the dosages were not systematically specified in these studies, which compared those who did to those who did not take supplements of vitamins.

do better at avoiding diseases and living longer than those who took no vitamins.[233] But it is not yet known whether raising vitamin A levels will lower the cancer risk, because the low levels of vitamins that are seen among cancer patients may reflect a result rather than a cause of the disease.[587, 964]

Some scientists recommend 20,000 to 40,000 IU of vitamin A per day.[673] It is clear that very high doses (5,000,000 IU) of this fat-soluble vitamin cause nausea and headaches. Because the side effects of megadoses of vitamin A have not yet been established, it is unwise to take them. A 20,000 to 40,000 IU dose per day appears to be an optimum choice, given the best information currently available.

### Vitamin D

Vitamin D is a fat-soluble vitamin that serves to transfer calcium from the intestines into the bloodstream (see page 283). But when D levels get too high, calcium *leaves* bone and moves into the bloodstream. You need to have enough vitamin D but should be careful not to overdose.[189, 271, 640]

Under normal circumstances, exposing your skin to sunlight for fifteen minutes every day will cause your body to manufacture all the vitamin D it needs. If you can take a sun bath through a window, try to expose as much skin as possible. Alternatively, a quart of vitamin-D-enriched milk per day provides enough. If you do not get exposure to sunshine or do not drink a quart of milk every day, you probably should take vitamin D in tablet form, perhaps 400 IU a day; almost any multivitamin contains this amount.

### Vitamin E

Vitamin E has been studied for its relationship to health, sexual desire, energy level, aging processes, and the risk of cancer and mortality. None of these studies are conclusive.

Vitamin E appears to be ineffective in treating hot flashes and other menopausal symptoms,[379, 474] but it may increase your level of energy, which in combination with exercise protects the cardiovascular system.[379] It may also help to protect against arterial disease,[304, 673, 794] although no studies have yet addressed whether posthysterectomized vitamin E users experience a cardiovascular health benefit. One study compared ninety-nine persons with lung cancer to healthy people with similar behaviors and habits; the people who did not have lung cancer had the higher levels of vitamin E in their bloodstream.[587]

In reviewing a variety of studies and describing the arguments for and against vitamin E, Dr. Linus Pauling presents a logical analysis of the scientific data; he concludes that the current RDA of 10 IU is too low and that 800 IU per day is probably optimal. Avoid higher levels because this fat-soluble vitamin is stored by the body. A study of longevity among people over age 65 showed that extreme vitamin E levels, either very high (more than 1,000 IU a day) or very low, seem to associate with a higher death rate.[232] For the woman who has not yet passed age 65, no side effects have been reported and a strong set of evidence exists that vitamin E does help to protect the cardiovascular system.[672] Saturated fats and eggs are rich in vitamin E. But if you eat a diet high in polyunsaturated fatty acids, your body's supply of vitamin E may be destroyed.[673] Supplements will help. Again and again research reveals how a delicate balance of competing influences manipulate the prognosis. Extremes of a "good thing" are often unhealthy.

### The B Vitamins

The B vitamins were discovered during investigations of diseases that were shown to be produced by deficiencies of these substances. Table 15 shows the RDA for the B vitamins, compared to the suggestions that Dr. Pauling makes.

How can you decide what to do? In the case of vitamin $B_6$, 6,000 milligrams is dangerous, Dr. Pauling recommends 100, and the RDA lists 2.2 . Consider that the RDA level is selected to prevent specifically documented deficiency diseases and that, based on studies, Dr. Pauling establishes levels that optimize good health.

**Table 15.** *B Vitamin Dosages*

| Vitamin | RDA | Dr. Pauling |
|---------|-----|-------------|
| $B_1$ (thiamine) | 1.5 mg | 50–100 mg |
| $B_2$ (riboflavin) | 1.7 mg | 50–100 mg |
| $B_3$ (niacinamide) | 18 mg | 300–600 mg |
| $B_6$ (pyridoxine) | 2.2 mg | 50–100 mg |
| $B_{12}$ (cobalamin) | 0.003 mg | 0.1–0.2 mg |

If you are taking HRT and begin to feel low, you may be helped by including about 100 milligrams of $B_6$ a day in your dietary regimen.[174] Oral contraceptive estrogen doses have been shown to deplete vitamin $B_6$ and lead to depression, an effect that is reversible with vitamin $B_6$ at 100 milligrams daily. While no studies have asked whether HRT, at its much lower hormonal doses, also produces a vitamin $B_6$ deficiency, taking a $B_6$ supplement will protect against the possibility. Because many multivitamin supplements provide only 2 to 3 milligrams of vitamin $B_6$, you may need to take a separate supplement of $B_6$.

### Iron

Iron is a necessary element in women's diets, particularly after hysterectomy, when strength and energy can lag as a result of deficient sex hormone levels in blood. One critical job of iron is to form, within the red blood cells, the core of the hemoglobin molecule, which attaches to oxygen and carbon dioxide for transport into and out of the lungs. When we become anemic, our iron is depleted and we cannot transport these critical gasses to and from our body cells. Most multivitamins contain at least 17 milligrams of iron, a quantity that appears to be sufficient. Red meat and eggs also provide a rich source of iron.

Advances in knowledge in the past fifty years have provided women with a greatly increased life span, and women who manage to avoid disease have an opportunity to enhance their health through sound nutritional choices. Unfortunately, scientific awareness of the study of vitamins and how they promote longevity is probably just beginning.

My conclusion is that vitamin supplementation helps maximize health. I also believe that we do not yet know what the optimal level of each vitamin is. For this reason, your decisions will have to be made from your own best judgment, based on limited knowledge. It does seem clear that vitamins C, B₆, D, E, and iron are necessary additions for a posthysterectomized or postmenopausal woman's optimal health care, especially when she is taking HRT.

If you want to ensure an adequate nutritional balance, it would probably be wise to do the following:

1. Buy an inexpensive dietary food scale so that you can measure the portions you eat.
2. Buy a calorie chart that includes the vitamin and mineral contents of standard portions of food.[69]
3. Record your dietary intake for one complete week.
4. Evaluate the calories, calcium, vitamins C and D, fiber, and fat content of your diet. Try also to include your intake of vitamins A, E, and B₆.
5. Determine where you are deficient and where you are overloading.
6. Make a plan of how you would like to eat.
7. Explore new ways of optimizing your own nutritional habits.

The rewards, in combination with the other recommendations in this book, should be not only the prevention of such diseases as diverticulitis, hemorrhoids, cardiovascular disease, and osteoporosis, but increased health, vitality, and well-being.

# 14

## Controllable Health Hazards:
### Obesity and Smoking

Obesity and smoking are pervasive, but controllable, health hazards for women in North America. The two conditions are particularly problematic for the posthysterectomized woman because of the burden they place on the hormonal, cardiovascular, bone, and other body systems that have already been threatened by the pelvic surgery. Combatting either condition requires a major, all-out effort. Willpower is necessary but in most cases is not enough. Actions and techniques based on a sophisticated understanding of the underlying problems will help produce good results and a strong likelihood of conquering these two threats to good health.

### OBESITY

The term *obesity* technically refers to an increase in body weight beyond the limitation of skeletal and physical requirement, as the result of excess accumulation of fat in the body.

#### The Dangers to Your Health

Obesity is dangerous to your health. Gross obesity has been associated with an increased risk for cholesterol gallstones[795] (see Appendix B).* Also at risk are people who gorge after starva-

---

*Two different mechanisms produce two different kinds of gallstones: the cholesterol gallstone, which contains more than 50 percent cholesterol, and the pigment gallstone, which contains less than 5 percent cholesterol.[795]

tion.[768] We can conclude that obesity affects the ability of the liver to function properly.

Hormonal metabolism is different among obese women than among those of normal weight. Obese women show a much higher risk of developing endometrial cancer.[334, 435, 966] In one study that evaluated postmenopausal women with endometrial cancer and those without, the endometrial cancer group was on average 50 percent heavier than the normal women. Among all of these heavy women (240 to 430 pounds), the estrogen levels were four times that of the normal-weight subjects in the control group.[529] The reverse is also true. Slender Oriental low-fat eaters have lower estrogen levels than white medium-build high-fat eaters.[312] So do vegetarian Americans.[313]

After an ovariectomy, the fatter the woman is, the higher the amount of circulating estrogen she will show in her blood-stream.[507] It may be that the excess estrogen noted among these heavy women promoted the cancer that led to ovariectomy.

Why is it that fat women have a different hormonal metabolism? Is it the fat or the genetic component? The answer may lie in the function of fat cells, which can be thought of as miniature factories. One of the activities that takes place in these factories is the conversion of circulating androstenedione (a hormone produced in the adrenal glands and in the aging ovaries) into estrone, one of the estrogens. The more fat cells there are, the more "factory space" is available for this conversion.

### The Truth About Dieting

Strict dietary regimens aimed at quick weight loss do not always work. Repeated dieting often produces slower and slower weight-loss rates, followed by increasingly rapid rates of weight gain ("rebounds") once the diet is discontinued.[97] One reason for this seesaw problem is that our bodies have a powerful adaptation mechanism that attempts to maintain balance. Once the body gets used to being heavy, it sets itself up to maintain the weight by promoting a metabolic pattern that favors obesity.[413] Most obese people eat about the same number of calories as nonobese people.[413] Similarly, when thin people are force-fed up to twice the amount of calories they normally consume, their weight soon stabilizes. After an initially short period of minor weight gain, their metabolic rate increases to accommodate the increased food without any weight change. An obese person often has the problem in reverse. When she cuts down on her food, her metabolic rate slows as her body attempts to maintain its weight.

What can you do if you are obese? It is probably ideal to lose weight, but rapid weight loss is likely to be followed by an equally rapid and maybe even greater weight gain. It is unhealthy to lose weight rapidly because that process creates a stress to which the body must attempt to adjust. In fact, rapid weight loss lowers the metabolic rate, which in turn makes the body burn fewer calories than normal. A slow but steady weight-loss plan makes more healthful sense than rapid weight loss. If you lose weight slowly, the stress is less, and you are more likely to keep a slimmer figure.

Weight loss is an inevitably painful process. Any time a long-standing habit is changed, a strong inertia must be overcome. Powerful emotional, mental, and physical mechanisms interfere with our will to withdraw from food, or from a relationship, drugs, cigarettes, or any other habit. If you decide to diet, you will probably be wise to prepare yourself to suffer in the process. It may also be helpful (and rather exciting) to consider that in establishing a new habit and a new, thinner way of being, you are undertaking a major new journey.

Since obesity is dangerous to your health, the decision to reverse it reflects your determination to enhance your health. By carefully establishing a new diet, along with a program of exercise, you will optimize your chance to form the new habits necessary to take off pounds and keep them off.

### Sensible Weight Loss

It is known that menstruating women burn different numbers of calories at different times in their cycles.[933] They burn approximately 9 percent more energy in the luteal phase, after ovulation, than in the follicular phase, before ovulation.[934] Although the specific studies have not yet been undertaken, this suggests that when a woman takes HRT that lacks progestin, she burns fewer calories and gains weight more easily than a woman who has a progestin opposed to her estrogen.

There are a number of actions and attitudes you can form that will help you to lose weight:

1. Eat high-fiber foods such as potatoes without butter, popcorn, bran, and vegetables; they fill the stomach and produce satiety. Eat fruits, which are high in fiber, instead of drinking fiber-depleted juices. Studies with whole apples and apple juice show that the fiber present in the fruits reduces the insulin response to the sugar, preventing a rebound hypoglycemia (low blood sugar). Satiety (the sense of being "full") was found to be greater following whole fruit than after equal caloric servings of the juices of oranges and grapes. And the return of hunger was slower after eating whole fruit.[225]

2. Recognize that your body has a built-in "homeostatic" mechanism of appetite and metabolism that is geared to control weight at your current level and that will thus trigger hunger. Your appetite will gradually be retrained as you reduce your intake of food and turn your diet in a more healthful direction. In the meantime, you might provide yourself with a written affirmation to read aloud when you feel tempted, for example: "I am choosing health and vigor. This pain is burning away my fat. I want it to burn away."

3. Aim for slow and steady weight loss, about 1 pound per week maximum. This will prevent the rebound phenomenon experienced by dieters who take off weight quickly and subsequently gain more back.

4. Avoid the dangers of high-fat diets that will produce weight loss but will negatively affect your blood lipids.

5. Take action for yourself and work to develop your own plan of nutrition and dieting. Use the principles discussed in Chapter 13 in creating your menu plans.

6. Measure out and record the calories of your meals before you eat them. People have a tendency to underestimate quantities of food; by measuring portions before you eat them, you can overcome this potentially self-defeating tendency. You may want to keep a personal record book in which you record the foods you eat, their nutritional values, and your weight loss over time.

7. Exercise to burn fat and to develop attractive muscle tone. You need aerobic exercise! It increases both the speed with which your body burns its fats and the overall calories burned.[58]

8. Join a support group. Weight Watchers International and TOPS (Take Off Pounds Sensibly) are two groups that provide emotional support and a nutritionally safe approach to dieting. But they cost money, typically about $25 to join the group and then $8 per weekly meeting. As an alternative, you might consider forming a support group of other women with similar problems. If you schedule regular meetings in which you review your progress, weigh yourselves, plan for the future, and discuss ways to overcome appetite problems, you can turn dieting into an exciting and sociable journey.

Do not go on a fad diet that calls for extreme behavior, such as eating only fat, protein, or carbohydrate! A healthy diet is composed of all three in the correct proportion. Because each of these food groups provides vital nutrients, your diet should avoid risking the dangers that come from deficiency states. High-carbohydrate diets are particularly valuable for the weight-conscious woman because they provide the energy needed by muscle tissue as it does its work. They also contain fiber, which provides bowel health and a sense of fullness at a low calorie cost. Protein, while necessary, does not provide the same bulk per calorie but should also be included for your strength and long-term energy. You also need some fat, but this is the food group that can be lowered the most without harming an overweight person, because her own fat can supply the needed elements.

High-fat diets are particularly dangerous. Dr. Philip James explains why:.

A high-fat reducing diet can now be seen as not only medically harmful in view of its effect on blood lipids, but potentially less effective metabolically than a high-protein or high-carbohydrate diet. The advantages of the dangerous old-fashioned low-carbohydrate diet were that patients readily accepted the injunction not to eat bread and potatoes, and saw a rapid weight loss as glycogen levels fell in muscle and liver and sodium and water diuresis ensued. As ketonaemia [excess of particular metabolites in the blood, called ketones] developed, the patients felt less hungry and thereby reduced their overall energy intake. They came to regard the constipation of dieting as a small price to pay for a slimmer figure and fortunately did not know that their hyperlipidaemia [high blood lipids] remained untreated or was exacerbated. This short-term view of dietary management, geared simply to slimming and not to other aspects of health, was encouraged by dietitians and doctors who failed to recognize the need for a permanent change in eating habits and the desirability of a substantial reduction in fat intake. It could even be argued that the medical profession has amplified the morbidity [illness] problems of obese patients by advocating diets that induce the very complications which the obese patient seeks to avoid by slimming![413]

Recent studies that have looked at semistarvation, exercise, and the body's metabolism as it responds to carbohydrate and protein diets show major differences depending on the source of the food.[940b] When exercise is combined with these diets, it burns carbohydrate calories more efficiently than protein calories. If you restrict your calories, you will probably need carbohydrates in order to maintain physical energy. Be sure to include plenty of carbohydrates when you plan how to assign your calories.

Medically supervised weight loss may or may not be healthy. If you understand the principles of healthy eating discussed here and in Chapter 13, you will be better able to discern whether the particular medically supervised program you may be considering will do more than simply ensure help in weight loss; you need an approach that will also ensure your overall health during the time that you are dieting.

Many good books are available to help you design good eating habits. Jane Brody's cookbooks, Adelle Davis's cookbooks, the Weight Watchers cookbook series, and many, many others are for sale in most book stores.

## SMOKING

It seems that whenever an investigator studies a disease or a health process and compares those who smoke to those who do not, significant differences emerge.

### A Harmful Habit

Particularly relevant for a menopausal or posthysterectomized woman are the studies showing that smoking:

- Produces earlier menopause and earlier aging
- Causes and exacerbates cancers
- Promotes bone disease
- Alters the hormonal environment in a negative way
- Increases the risk of cardiovascular disease

Among women who have not been hysterectomized, cigarette smoking produces menopause about five years earlier than among nonsmokers.[421, 505] Hysterectomy also produces menopause about five years earlier if the ovaries are retained. Thus the combination of hysterectomy and smoking is likely to profoundly increase the rate of aging.

Although it is well known that smoking causes lung cancer, it is sometimes less well appreciated that this effect is only the most direct one, because the lungs are the first place to receive the smoke and therefore they get the highest dose of it. In fact, every single one of the diseases that has yet been analyzed for the role of smoking in its development (bone, cardiovascular disease, and cancer, for example) shows the same thing: in every case, the vast majority of the victims are heavy smokers. Smoking has also been shown to have some important relationships to breast cancer tumors. The results showed that women who did not smoke had a better chance for good prognosis after the surgery.[185] The reason for this deficit among smokers has not yet been analyzed scientifically but probably relates to the fact that smoking compromises the immune system, which plays a role in the development of and recovery from cancer.

The ability to consume oxygen and take away carbon dioxide is indicated by a measurement called *maximum oxygen consumption.* This ability normally declines with age, finally reaching a point at which the body's need for oxygen is greater than the person's ability to inhale it. For those who do not die of disease or accident, this condition appears to mark the end of the ability to sustain life. For the smoker, the age-related decline is startlingly faster and steeper.

Among women with intact ovaries, smokers showed lower circulating levels of estrogen than nonsmokers.[418, 596] Another study, conducted in a menopause clinic, compared hormone levels in women who smoked with those who did not smoke.[276] Although the authors concluded that smokers and nonsmokers had equivalent levels of estrogen, the average age of the smokers was three and a half years younger than the nonsmokers (47 versus 50). As this is the period when estrogen levels are rapidly dropping, the finding that younger women smokers had the same levels of estrogen as older nonsmokers suggests that smokers are losing estrogen prematurely. The same study showed that smokers had higher levels of progesterone and higher cortisol, a stress-related hormone.

When estrogen replacement therapy is given, the nonsmoker shows substantial increases in the estrogen levels in the blood; the smoker does not.[418] Even with high doses of ERT, estrogen levels remain about half as high in smokers as in nonsmokers who take the same dose.

Bones are affected by smoking. Most osteoporotic women with

spinal fractures smoke. In one study of women of normal weight, 94 percent of those who had a spinal fracture before the age of 65 were smokers.[184] Smokers show lower bone mass than age-matched nonsmokers.[506] The risk of hip fracture is also elevated in thin smokers.[953] These results begin to emerge about ten years after menopause. The woman who has undergone a hysterectomy enters menopause earlier and is therefore more vulnerable to bone loss at a younger age. For women who did not take hormones, smokers showed a 23 percent loss of the cortical area of their bone about fifteen years after menopause; nonsmokers showed half as much bone loss (12 percent) at the same interval.[184] HRT in this same age group (women 40 to 49 years old) had produced a profound benefit for the nonsmokers, but the HRT for smokers seemed to have almost no effect.[184] Smokers who took hormones continued to lose bone.

The increased risk of cardiovascular disease in women who smoke has been well documented, especially in women past the age of 40 who smoke and take oral contraceptives[683]. Whether the combination of HRT estrogens and smoking also increases the risk of cardiovascular disease remains undefined. The likelihood is, however, that smoking is very bad for cardiovascular health when HRT is taken.

### Stopping Smoking

If you smoke, you should stop. Ultimately, the pain of nicotine withdrawal is much less than the pain of broken bones, cancers, earlier aging, and the whole host of terrible things that smoking does to the body.

If you stop smoking, you are likely to experience intense and unpleasant cravings for a cigarette. The cravings come as the oxygen begins to pour back into the cells, which had been deprived of that vital fuel and poisoned with carbon monoxide, deadening their ability to function. When you stop smoking, oxygen once again begins to reach the cells.

A simple breathing exercise can minimize the pain of these cravings. Pretending to smoke—inhaling extra air in short bursts

that mimic the inhaling one does when smoking—has been helpful to many people. Why it should work this way, when the
craving is associated with the flooding of the system with oxygen, is unclear, but this technique does help. Likewise, increasing your vitamin C content, both by taking supplements and by
drinking lots of orange juice and grapefruit juice, seems to minimize the pain from the withdrawal of cigarettes.

The first five days are probably the worst. After that, the cravings will begin to diminish, slowly and steadily; but you will still
be highly vulnerable to reigniting the addiction if you allow
yourself to smoke "just one cigarette." Cravings continue, often
for a period as long as the time you spent smoking, but they get
easier to withstand and they diminish in intensity.

If you want to enroll in one of the many smoking cessation
groups, a first place to look would be the Yellow Pages of your
phone book. Groups such as Smoke Watchers and Smoke Enders
will be listed there under "Smokers Information and Treatment
Centers" or a similar heading. Some groups have been more
helpful than others. Unfortunately, the failure rate and the re-
starting rate in smoking cessation groups tends to be very
high.[841] If you call one of these organizations, ask for references
and statistics about their one-year cure rates.

It may be helpful to know that studies have shown that people
who stop smoking on their own are successful more often than
not. It is possible that those who are able to stop without joining
a group are depending upon themselves, whereas those who go
to a group lean too heavily on the group "doing it for them" and
then relapse once they leave the group.

If you stop smoking, one compensation for the pain of the
withdrawal is the extra energy you will begin to have within a
day of quitting. Many people have found it helpful to use the
added energy to do exercise or physical work, such as cleaning,
scrubbing floors, gardening, and other jobs that will help burn
off the energy as well as the tension that detoxification produces. People do tend to gain weight, on average about 5
pounds, when they stop smoking. It makes sense for people

who are quitting smoking to become more active, in order to burn calories.

You might find it helpful to write out an affirmation, such as: "I am choosing a healthy life and an oxygen-rich body. This pain is a temporary price. I can succeed!" Repeat your affirmation out loud every time you crave a cigarette, and if you are fortunate enough to have experienced the power of prayer, you might pray, too. You are fighting for your life when you withdraw from smoking.

# 15 ❧

# *Exercise Will Keep You Going*

❧ If we look at the human body as a machine, and especially if we realize how much power each of us has over the workings of our own body, we can easily experience a sense of awe at the majesty of the design. What other machine is improved by working it, made more beautiful by exercising it, and made more vigorous through the expense of energy? Although life is terminal and our genetic heritage plays an influence, both the length and the quality of our lives are affected by our pattern of exercise.

Particularly after undergoing a surgical procedure, you need to rebuild your body's strength. And you can. Whatever your current condition, appropriate exercise will help to improve your health. Exercise affects our hormones, our bone mass, our cardiovascular system, and our sense of well-being.

Over the past decade, the media have paid a great deal of attention to exercise. A seemingly endless number of self-help books have been published, and an astounding variety of muscle-building equipment has been designed. Yet the amount of actual research data is limited. There are no good, comprehensive studies on exactly the kinds of exercise we should be doing and the kinds we should be avoiding. This chapter presents the information that is available.

## THE IMPORTANCE OF AEROBIC EXERCISE

Every cell of the body functions like a miniature factory. Although each cell has a special job to do, and the jobs of some cells are quite different from others, each requires oxygen, which it burns as a furnace burns coal or an automobile engine burns gasoline. The need for oxygen increases whenever the cells are doing more work. Each cell produces waste products, including carbon dioxide and lactic acid. Whenever the cells work harder, they produce more metabolic waste products, which must be removed.

The job of delivering the oxygen and carrying away the waste products falls to the blood circulation. Specifically, it is the red blood cell that carries oxygen to and carbon dioxide from the cells. These gasses are diffused across the very thin membranes at the deeper recesses of the lungs as we inhale and exhale. As soon as you begin to exercise, you automatically (reflexively) engage an increased flow of blood and change your breathing pattern, to increase the flow of oxygen into and carbon dioxide out of the lungs.

The ability of your body to take in and use oxygen has a profound influence on how long you will live and how healthy you will feel. This ability, called *maximum oxygen consumption*, peaks at about age 10 for most people and declines steadily thereafter.[484] With advancing age, we become less capable of consuming oxygen. All human beings show a gradual decline in the ability to consume oxygen, but for some the decline occurs more gently and over a much longer period of time than for others. The change with age occurs much more severely for the sedentary individual than for the fit person who gets regular exercise.

A certain amount of oxygen is necessary to maintain life, that is, for the cells to continue to function. As we become less able to consume oxygen, our cells become less able to thrive. All humans reach a point at which their capacity for consuming oxygen is lower than their cellular requirement for oxygen. At this point the cells die and body death follows. For women who avoid disease, the limit to life appears to be the capacity for oxygen consumption to supply the requirements of the cells of the machine.

*Aerobic* refers to the burning of oxygen as fuels are consumed by cells. *Anaerobic* refers to the burning of nonoxygen fuels, principally glycogen, a fuel that the muscles store to be burned when the oxygen is gone. The source of this glycogen is the carbohydrates we eat, some of which is converted into a storage form (glycogen) for later use. When we exercise, our muscles first call upon the oxygen; when it is used up, they break down the glycogen and burn it. This anaerobic metabolism is not as efficient and will not sustain the muscles for very long, probably because the metabolic waste product of glycogen, lactic acid, builds up in the cells, stopping them from functioning. Experiments have compared the amount of lactic acid lost in the sweat of active women to that excreted by sedentary women.[480] When they exercise, active women sweat much less lactic acid than sedentary women, indicating that active women have a much more efficient utilization of oxygen.

No studies have yet addressed the same range of exercise issues for menopausal women or for those who have undergone a hysterectomy, but one thing is clear. For the vast majority of human beings, regular, repeated, total-body-fitness exercise has a profound influence on every body system that has been studied. Both men and women are well served by habitual exercise.

## WHAT EXERCISE DOES FOR YOU

If you exercise appropriately, you will reap rich benefits for all of your body systems, including:

- Greater muscle strength
- Greater bone strength
- Improved sense of well-being
- Better cardiovascular health
- The burning of calories

- Less fatigue
- Lower functional aerobic age
- Improved breathing and lung function

Research findings illustrate how exercise works to improve your general health and well-being.

### Greater Muscle Strength

When you exercise, your muscles become stronger and better toned. One of the benefits of a well-toned body is that the likelihood of accidental falling is much lower. When women have osteoporosis or when their bones are very brittle but have not yet broken, good muscle tone can protect these fragile bones. In women more than 70 years old, it is very often a fall that leads to a hip fracture. And about half the women who suffer a hip fracture are permanently crippled. If you maintain good muscle tone, even if your bones are thin you are unlikely to fall and suffer the devastating result of being crippled. The freedom of motion that most of us enjoy—but often take for granted—can be retained longest by a program of regular exercise.

### Greater Bone Strength

Exercise appears to have certain profound influences on bone, but the relationship is a complex one. While very few pieces of information are available about exercise and bone health, some data do exist.

One group of studies has been done on young people. In one report, Olympic-caliber athletes were shown to have significantly higher bone density in their leg bones, particularly at the end of the femur (thigh bone) near the knee. It was noted that swimming did not influence this bone. In contrast, exercise that puts a heavy load on the lower limbs did cause leg bones to increase in density.[635] Baseball players also show bone changes as a result of their sport. The humerus (the bone that connects the shoulder to the elbow) was significantly enlarged in the arm used for swinging the bat.[933] These early studies showed that young athletes had a bone response in the particular limbs that bore the brunt of a heavy load. However, the spine did not appear to respond to athletic endeavors.

In general, athletic women enjoy a major bone advantage over sedentary women. A 1986 report provided data to confirm the beneficial effect of aerobic fitness on spinal bone as well as hip bone density in postmenopause. In that study, fitness was evaluated by maximum oxygen consumption. The higher the maximum oxygen consumption, the higher the bone density in both spine and hip bones. The study showed that "fitness was the only significant predictor of [improved] bone mineral density" in the hip.[694]

One word of caution is important. It has recently become quite clear that certain forms of exercise, when carried out to very high levels of conditioning, can have adverse effects on bone. Among young women, athletes who escalate their athletic training until they stop menstruating are at a disadvantage.* For example, marathon runners (average age 35) showed a variety of disruptions in their normal menstrual cycle. So did most of the young women on the U. S. Lightweight Oarswomen Team.[827] When these kinds of conditions occur, bone density often starts to decrease.[222] Fortunately it has recently been shown that when women ease up on excessive exercise to the point at which normal menstrual cycles resume, there is an increase in bone mass and a recovery of the lost bone.[222] (No reports of excessive exercise in older women yet exist.) Thus, exercises that improve oxygen consumption do increase bone mass, but when aerobic exercise approaches extreme levels, the bone mass can decrease due to adverse endocrine changes.[732] (See Chapter 8 for additional discussion of the influence of exercise on bone mass.)

### Improved Sense of Well-being

Physical fitness also serves to improve emotional stability, according to several investigations of menstruating women.[517, 813]

*Studies include 216, 700, 705, 706, 732.

One mechanism producing this improved sense of well-being may be mediated through the endogenous opiates (the beta endorphins, also known as the endorphins).[106, 222, 517, 916a] Would endorphins respond to exercise in a menopausal woman who is deficient in sex hormones? Probably not. The studies have not yet been published to answer this question directly, but work described in chapters 2 and 11 indicates that both estrogen and progestin seem to be necessary in order for the endorphins to be secreted. If you are taking estrogen and progestin hormonal therapy, then your body should be able to produce endorphins after exercise.

There are interesting gender differences in the endorphin response to exercise. Women show an endorphin response when they exercise to 60 percent of their maximum ability, whereas men need to exercise to a level of exhaustion before their endorphin levels increase.[916a] The reason for the difference is unknown.

Aerobic exercise increases the secretion of two other hormones, *growth hormone* and *prolactin*. While men reach a plateau at which their growth hormone increase will not go any higher, women do not.[85] Growth hormone has many effects on the human body: in children it promotes growth, and in both children and adults it is involved in the regulation of lipolysis (the burning of fat), the promotion of cellular uptake of amino acids, and in turning off the effects of insulin. We do not know what the effect of the growth hormone response to exercise might be. Prolactin increases after exercise when the exercise induces breast motion. Prolactin has many effects in the body, one of which is to induce the manufacture of breast milk in lactating women.[704] While we don't yet know what these responses mean to your health, the change in hormone secretion after exercise probably serves an important function yet to be discovered.

Although premenstrual syndrome reveals itself in varying degrees of intensity, most healthy premenopausal women experience a premenstrual fluctuation in mood, water retention, and anxiety. A regular conditioning program can profoundly reduce even these normal discomforts.[702, 703] Exactly how the exercise works is uncertain. It may be that the endorphin levels increase. It may be that other hormones changes are responsible. It may be that blood circulation improves. But it does not really matter what the mechanism is when your objective is to feel well and to be healthy. What matters is that conditioning exercise will make you feel better.

### Better Cardiovascular Health

A number of investigators have measured blood concentrations of various substances before and after aerobic exercise. The results have been clear.[762] Regular exercise, even in the short bursts characteristic of the exercise patterns of time-pressured individuals, lowers the cholesterol level in blood as well as in muscles, lungs, and liver.[813] Exercise also increases the fecal loss of cholesterol.[813] These physiological responses all serve to lower the risk of cardiovascular disease.

### The Burning of Calories

Every activity in which we engage consumes calories as our cells do their work to maintain life. Table 16, standardized for a 154-pound man, represents an approximation of the number of calories burned by various activities. Variables that should be considered when you interpret the numbers include size, body type, and age; differences between individuals of the same build; physical fitness and skill in the particular activity; nutritional condition; and whether environmental conditions help or hinder the individual.[437, 611] Although it is known that these variables will affect the rate of calories burned, exactly how they do so remains to be investigated. For example, scientists at the Institute of Physiology in Lausanne, Switzerland, study the effects of different levels of exercise on obese and nonobese women, before and after meals, in their attempt to define how much a woman should exercise and when she should do it in order to achieve different physiologic effects. They conclude from their data that whether you exercise before or after the meal, the rate of energy consumed will be the same, and that contrary to popular misconception, there is no benefit to performing exercise after you eat.[809]

## Less Fatigue

Exhaustion, or fatigue, means that our cells have burned all of the available oxygen, have burned the available glycogen, and

**Table 16.** *Caloric Consumption for Various Physical Activities*

| Activity | Total Calories Per Hour |
|---|---|
| Sleeping | 70 |
| Lying quietly | 80 |
| Sitting | 100 |
| Mental work, seated | 105 |
| Standing | 110 |
| Singing | 120 |
| Driving a car | 140 |
| Office work | 145 |
| Housekeeping | 150 |
| Calisthenics | 160 |
| Walking 2 mph | 170 |
| Bicycle riding 5.5 mph | 190 |
| Walking down stairs 2 mph | 200 |
| Housepainting | 210 |
| Dancing, moderate | 250 |
| Horizontal walking 2.5 mph | 290 |
| Rowing for pleasure | 300 |
| Dancing, vigorous | 340 |
| Table tennis | 345 |
| Swimming (breast stroke) 1 mph | 410 |
| Bicycle riding, rapid | 415 |
| Swimming (crawl stroke) 1 mph | 420 |
| Chopping wood | 450 |
| Skating 9 mph | 470 |
| Skiing 3 mph | 540 |
| Swimming (side stroke) 1 mph | 550 |
| Walking up stairs 2 mph | 590 |

are so full of metabolic waste products that they no longer can function. When we rest after exhaustion, our blood carries away the waste products and delivers fresh oxygen to the cells.[611] Exhaustion can also occur when our red blood cells become crippled by carbon monoxide poisoning or when the capillaries become compressed as overworked muscles contract.

Exhaustion is a much greater problem in sedentary people than in fit, trained people. One of the great benefits of developing fitness is that you will not feel exhausted or fatigued nearly as often as when you were not fit. As you become more fit, your body changes—from a sedentary physiology into a fitness physiology. In addition to being less subject to fatigue, individuals with higher aerobic capacity burn up more fat during the recovery (rest) period after exercise than do individuals who are less well conditioned.[58, 437]

### Lower Functional Aerobic Age

Conditioning exercises serve to lower your *functional aerobic age,*[484] a term that can be thought of as defining the biologic age—or, equivalently, how long we can live. The term represents the age-equivalent aerobic capacity of the entire body. Consider the average healthy 10-year-old, who is probably at her peak lifetime aerobic capacity. If she gets on a treadmill and starts to jog at a pace that gets her heart rate up to a maximum healthy peak, the amount of oxygen consumed per minute per kilogram of her body weight will be at a lifetime high. With each year that she ages, this number will go down, even if she stays vigorously healthy. If she starts to smoke, it will go down drastically. Eventually she will reach a stage at which she can no longer consume adequate oxygen for the needs of her body, but during the years that precede this, she may function at a very high level compared to others of her chronologic age. When we lower our functional aerobic age through conditioning exercises (and we can begin at any time and whatever our condition), we increase our ability to function longer and at a higher level.

### *Improved Breathing and Lung Function*

Aerobic exercise changes the way a person breathes. More air is inhaled with each breath in an aerobically fit person. More air is exhaled as well. Not only does the entire body reap the benefit of improved oxygenation of its cells and improved transport of waste gasses, but the air that pools in the lungs (which can become stagnant and promote growth of infectious organisms) is reduced. As the "tidal volume" (amount of air moved with each "tide" of the breath) increases, one result is a decreased opportunity for infections to lodge in the lungs. Even moderate exercise improved the breathing and the lung function in one experiment on people who were *not* specimens of physical fitness. Investigators compared the effects of low- and high-intensity home-based exercises on the functional capacity (ability to take in oxygen) in healthy middle-aged men. Even low-intensity exercises provided profound benefits.[319] Whatever you do will help.

## GETTING STARTED ON YOUR EXERCISE PROGRAM

Immediately after surgery, a period of recovery is necessary in order for your body to heal completely. During the healing stages, postoperative exercises will likely be prescribed. Most physicians and hospitals guide patients in a program to get them back on their feet and moving. It is important to follow these instructions because they will promote a more rapid healing.

After you have finished healing from the surgery, it is time to plan for a long-term exercise habit, but don't begin this exercise regimen until your surgeon agrees that you have healed. Whatever your current pattern of exercise, from vigorous activity to complete lassitude, a regular disciplined exercise program will improve your energy and your strength. You do not have to be a former athlete or even be in particularly good shape. And as soon as you start, you begin to improve your overall condition.

## Breathing to Enhance Oxygen Consumption

The way we breathe influences the way we live. Recognizing this, the philosophies of the East have long emphasized the fundamental importance of training people how to breathe well.

Courses in Hatha Yoga, which are frequently offered by local YMCAs or YWCAs and adult education centers, generally begin with instructions on proper breathing.

The student is usually taught to maintain an upright sitting posture and to keep the mouth closed. Once in this position, she is instructed to slowly inhale to the count of seven. As she inhales, she is told to fill up the diaphragm first, making the correct "breathing noises" as the air hits a spot at the back of the throat. The student then allows the air to flow above the diaphragm until she has filled the air passages all the way up to the throat.

The next step of the breathing instruction is to hold that breath for a slow count of three or four. The final step is to exhale deeply, beginning with the top air, and feeling the motion of the passage of air as the diaphragm region empties and flattens out.

Usually the student is instructed to repeat this cycle of inhaling, holding, and exhaling four or five times, after which she generally feels a sense of tremendous exhilaration. This great feeling results from an extraordinary burst of oxygen coming into the body and the simultaneous removal of a large amount of carbon dioxide.

This simple exercise can be repeated throughout the day whenever one begins to feel sluggish. The result is always the same. When the exercise is done correctly, the mind clears and energy increases.

Just be cautious about pushing yourself too hard. Don't endanger your bones and your muscles.

It is important to understand the principles of conditioning so that you avoid injury. Being fit feels good. Becoming fit also feels good, if the program is developed in a sensible way. Exercise does not have to be painful; in fact, it should *not* be painful.

Although no competent research has yet provided enough facts to define the ideal exercise program,[484] certain facts are clear. No matter how "out of shape" you are, appropriate exercise is good for you. Exercise should be fun, interesting, and varied. It should be easily accessible, and you should not have to depend on someone else's availability.

## Training Effects

Also known as "conditioning," *training effects* are remarkable phenomena: What may be hard to do today can be easy next month if you form the habit of exercise and gradually work into it.

Through the repeated action of a gentle exercise, such as walking or swimming, the supply of blood to the muscle tissue increases, more rapidly replacing the oxygen, minerals, and other elements depleted by exercise, and more rapidly removing carbon dioxide and other waste products from the muscles. In a trained individual, the blood circulation is more efficient at carrying the necessary substances to and from the muscles. Nutrients get in; wastes get out. A trained individual enjoys a reserve of strength that an untrained, sedentary person cannot call upon, and she functions more efficiently each time she undertakes physical activity. This resulting better health carries over; it enhances strength and metabolism throughout the day. A trained woman can do more with less effort; she tires less easily.

Exercise works this way. Within three weeks after beginning something as simple as a twenty-minute walk, three times a week, we begin to show a "conditioning effect";[482] that is, we become able to do the walk without feeling tired. We build up our muscle strength and the capacity of our cardiovascular system to pump blood to the muscles. We build up the capacity of our lungs to take in oxygen and give off carbon dioxide, necessary for fueling the cells and removing wastes from them.

The objective in developing a regular exercise program is to achieve these training effects. When we exercise appropriately, we begin a process that allows us to live longer and with greater health.[140] Even mild exercise that produces less stress than you are capable of enduring is shown to be helpful in retaining the youthful characteristics of heart and lung function.[972] Our sense of well-being improves. Because only a few studies of women's exercise physiology exist, we should stay alert for future studies that will enhance our understanding.

## Preventing the Dangers of Inappropriate Exercise

If done incorrectly, exercise can be dangerous, causing more harm than benefit. The principles are pretty simple. Most of them are good common sense. You want exercise to improve your condition; you do not want to risk injury.

Many current exercise books are illustrated with photographs of attractive actors and actresses, who tell and show us how to exercise. One must read these books with great caution. The beauty and apparent vigor of these celebrities do not necessarily mean that their advice is good for you. In fact, some of their suggestions can be downright dangerous. Likewise, if you are taking a course in aerobic instruction and your teacher is telling you to do something that feels painful to you, the sensations of pain should alert you to danger. Do not follow instructions that cause your body to hurt. Trust your natural reaction to pain and stop the painful activity.

The rhyme is catchy, but the idea "no pain, no gain" is irrational. Pain often indicates damage to your muscles, your tendons, or your nerves. Because you have to stop until you heal, damaged tissue interferes with exercising. Before beginning an exercise program, it is useful to review the dangers of inappropriate exercise so that you will not suffer these effects.

### Flexion Exercises

The first involves flexion. *Flexion* and *extension* refer to opposite directions of limb movement. In flexion, you contract muscles that bring limbs toward the body—you bend your elbow or knee. In extension, you contract muscles that take limbs away from your body's center—when you extend your leg, you straighten the knee. Results of an exercise study of postmenopausal women who had "dowager's hump" (osteoporosis) were presented in the *Mayo Clinical Proceedings* in 1984.[817] The prescribed exercises performed by these women did not prevent bone fractures. In fact, 60 percent of the osteoporotic patients who regularly did flexion or a combination of flexion and extension exercises suffered additional bone fractures while they were undergoing the exercise program. The Mayo Clinic physicians concluded that their exercise program was dangerous and wrote up their results in order to allow readers to learn from their experiment.

Avoid forward flexion exercises such as sit-ups, but feel free to do tummy-flattening exercises that involve extension, such as leg lifts while lying flat on your back. Likewise, avoid deep knee bends, a dangerous flexion exercise. Although the reasons why forward flexion exercises such as sit-ups and deep knee bends are potentially harmful are not well explained in the physiological journals, the injury data reveal clearly that this type of strain is best avoided.

### Muscle Soreness

There appear to be two kinds of muscle soreness: the immediate soreness that you may feel while exercising and the diffuse muscle soreness that you feel more than eight hours later. The immediate form, generally caused by a buildup of metabolic waste, is not dangerous and usually disappears within a few hours.[611] You can get over this soreness faster by doing light physical work, which will stimulate the blood circulation and speed up the removal of the metabolic waste products. The delayed soreness, usually occurring eight to twenty-four hours later, represents damage or local injury.[275] In one study, people who experienced soreness within two days after having exercised were shown to have damaged their muscular tendinous junction (see Figure 24). By forcing exercise, they had apparently torn the most vulnerable part of the muscle, the place where the muscle inserts into the tendon, close to where the two bones connect.[275] Note the arrangement of muscles, tendons, and bones in the illustration.

To relieve delayed soreness, you should *not* exercise. What your body needs is rest, perhaps with heat applied to the area and only enough movement to prevent adhesions (scar tissue) from forming between the injured muscle fibers. Because damaged

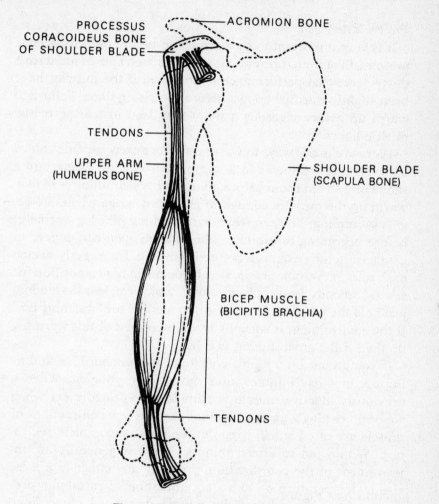

Figure 24. Muscular tendinous junction

tissues need rest to heal, you should not undertake excess exercise when you are trying to achieve fitness. Every time you do too much, every time you damage your muscles, you actually set your exercise program back by the amount of time it takes to recover and heal. To heal injured tissue, you must stop exercising. To be fit, you must keep exercising.

## Warming Up

It is very important to be warmed up before exercising your muscles, in order to prevent injury. It has been known for at least thirty years that performance is improved if the muscles have been slightly warmed up just before exercising them. Failure to warm up before vigorous activity may lead to tearing of the muscle fibers.[611]

There are many ways to warm up before exercise. One can be to spend a few minutes in a warm environment. Going into a sauna or a steam room before diving into a swimming pool may warm up the muscles enough to prevent damage when one begins swimming. You can wear extra clothing (like leg warmers) before beginning to exercise. Alternatively, you can engage in gentle stretching exercises before beginning. To properly stretch each relevant muscle group, slowly form and hold a position for several seconds. Don't bob or bounce, which can tear the tendon; just hold the position. This is the best method for "warming up." If the environment is warm, you will need less of this warming up than if the environment is cold.

If you go out on a tennis court and feel uncoordinated during the first few minutes, don't give up on yourself. When a previously inactive muscle is stimulated repeatedly (as when we begin to play a game of tennis), the first few contractions of muscle are often small, irregular, and with incomplete relaxation. Within ten to fifteen minutes, there is generally an improvement in the coordination, probably due either to a local rise in temperature or to an accumulation of metabolic products within the cells of the muscle. Increased blood flow, which takes place when muscles are exercised, delivers oxygen and warmth to the muscles.[611]

Although there is currently some controversy among researchers about whether it is absolutely necessary to warm up before we exercise, there has been no evidence to show any dangers in warming up. Meanwhile, there is probably a big benefit.

## Pacing Your Exercise

When you begin an exercise program, do not attempt to do too much before your body is trained. Pace yourself to the level that allows you to build up your strength without painful soreness afterward. As you set aside regular time for exercise, let your body tell you when you have had enough for the day. In time your ability will increase, and there is really no rush to get to the peak. You may as well enjoy the journey.

Probably the most important component in correct pacing is to set aside the time. Then, if you are unable to complete your goal, it will not be because of something else that interfered. As you continue to fill the time with exercise, you will find yourself able to achieve more physical exertion. For example, if you take up swimming, it is sufficient for the first three or four times to limit yourself to what you can do in the first five or ten minutes. Within these three or four sessions, you will probably notice that you are beginning to swim a greater distance without exhaustion. Similarly, if you take up walking, try a ⅓-mile length (about three blocks) the first day and gradually increase, perhaps by a block each day. Your body will tell you what you can handle, and in time you may be surprised to discover how much improvement you can accomplish.

### Dressing Appropriately

It is important to be sufficiently warm but not overheated when you exercise. If you go out walking during cold weather, wear enough layers of clothing that you will not feel chilled. Layers are particularly helpful because you can peel them off as you warm up. Select loose garments that will allow you to move and breathe comfortably, without any constriction. Natural fibers such as cotton or loosely woven synthetic textiles will permit your clothes to "breathe," that is, to absorb perspiration. Certain polyesters and other synthetic fibers act somewhat like the plastic wrap one uses to pack up leftover food. These prevent the exchange of gasses and sweat and can be very uncomfortable. Although fancy designer sportswear can be attractive, it serves no athletic purpose.

Appropriate shoes are extremely important. According to Pat Croce, the physical conditioning coach of the Philadelphia Flyers, "Regardless of the sport, if your sneaker's heel ridge has worn through to the mid sole, invest in a new pair. Sneaker wear causes your foot to overcompensate by slightly rotating in and your knee to slightly rotate out, thus increasing the risk of shin splints or runner's knee.

"Many foot, ankle, knee, hip, and even back injuries are a result of improper footwear or worn shoes. You need proper shoes for walking or for low-impact sports like aerobic exercise classes. To prevent these injuries, take your time when shopping for new shoes. Make sure the store where you shop has a wide variety of shoes and informed salespeople who will listen to your specific needs."

Once you know the dangers of inappropriate exercise and have confirmed with your surgeon that the healing is complete (or if more than two years have passed since your surgery), you should be ready to plan your exercise schedule.

### Planning Your Program

There are no tried and proven "rules" for how to go about the process, and whatever approach you select should fit your individual nature. You need to consider your general level of energy, fitness, and muscle tone, as well as the nature of your personality.

Some people thrive on the support of group classes. If you are one of these, be cautious about classes that suggest you "go for the burn" or endure pain as part of the price of a fit body. Pain is a warning of nerve, muscle, or tendon damage. It is unnecessary for a fitness program to hurt. If your life works best when exercise can be part of your solitude, then you might choose exercise that can be done alone.

It is important that your exercise plan have variety in it. Regular, repeated exercise can be boring if it is designed poorly. But

## *Pat Croce's Advice on Selecting Athletic Shoes**

*Timing* Make it a point to buy your shoes at the end of the day. Your feet swell by as much as half a size by late afternoon, so to ensure proper fit, this is the best time of day to select [new shoes].

*Fit* Try on several brands and models to decide which fits best. The toe of the shoe should be about one-half inch longer than your longest toe, with plenty of moving room for your toes and a snug fit throughout the remainder of the shoe.

*Wear and tear* Take a look at your former shoes and note where they are most worn. If your soles are worn on both the outside and inside edges, you can sacrifice cushioning for support. If your soles are worn predominantly on the outside edges, you need more cushioning than support.

*Surface.* Consider the surface on which you exercise. A sole with greater cushioning is needed for pavement or hard surfaces, while a thinner sole is adequate for soft surfaces. Test the shock absorption of the shoe by hopping in place on one foot.

*Balance.* Find a shoe that strikes a balance between good support and flexibility. The shoe should be sturdy enough to hold your foot firmly as it hits the ground. To test this, flex the sole, holding the shoe at both ends. It should bend easily at the ball of the foot, but not at the arch.

*Stability.* To test the stability of the shoe, stand on one foot and raise your heel so that you are on the ball of your foot. Keeping the supporting foot in place, twist your upper body and hips to the right and then again to the left. If your foot rolls outward while you are twisting, pick another pair of shoes.

*Run in place.* When you've found a pair of shoes that seem to fill the bill, run in place for several seconds to test their overall fit and comfort. You might feel strange doing this in the middle of a store, but you'll feel a lot more foolish if you've spent big bucks for shoes that cause blisters once you start exercising.

*Counter test.* Before you buy, place the shoes you have selected next to each other on the countertop and study them carefully from the rear to rule out any manufacturer's defects.

*Philadelphia Inquirer,* May 24, 1987.

you can avoid boredom, even in regular and disciplined programs, if you add music or TV to the routine.

If you try one approach and it doesn't work for you, try another. Eventually you will create a health and fitness program that does work for your unique approach to life. Respect that uniqueness and you will be rewarded with vigorous health that continues to improve. If you will respect yourself enough to set aside a regular time period for your health needs, the time you spend will be given back to you with interest, both in the increased years you will live and in the improved efficiency of your days. Most people find that once they get started, they enormously enjoy this gift they give themselves. They look forward with enthusiasm to their scheduled "fitness times."

You might choose to take one-hour walks three times a week, and to play tennis once or twice each week. You might choose to swim five days a week and to walk on the weekends. Calisthenics to exercise particular muscle groups will help tone up flabby areas and keep them toned. Exercise that gets you breathing heavily, such as brisk walking, swimming, or sports, will enhance your overall fitness. Your plan should probably include both aerobic exercise and calisthenics.

Walking is probably the easiest, cheapest, and most accessible physical activity. A 2- to 3-mile walk can be achieved in less than one hour. Although exercise classes and other expensive formats may be fun, regular walking is probably just as good for your body's health.[113]

Swim training provides an effective way to develop muscle tone and to maintain healthy heart and lung functions.[140] You will probably be able to find an inexpensive indoor pool not too far from your home. The amount of swimming that is appropriate is probably going to be defined by your own limits. Very often, beginners find it difficult to swim one length; within a month of training, they may find it quite easy to swim ten. If you take up swimming, you will probably find that fifteen or twenty minutes in the pool, as well as the showering time before and after, provides an extraordinary stimulus to your well-being. The high feeling lasts for many hours after completing the exercise.

In developing an exercise program, remember these principles:

*Exercise should be fun.* You should be able to enjoy it while you are doing it.

*Exercise should not be painful.* Remember, pain may reflect damage and set you back.

*Exercise should be regular.* You may choose three times a week or five times a week, but it should become a routine part of your life.

*Exercise should be varied.* This will enhance your enjoyment and your conditioning.

*Exercise should not be too intense.* In fact, investigators have concluded that even low-intensity exercises have profoundly beneficial effects on the ability to consume oxygen.[319]

*Maintain your health* while you are establishing your exercise routine. Do not take foolish risks with extreme exercise that can damage your muscles or your bones.

*Carbohydrate is the fuel that is burned during exercise.* If you are on a diet and are also engaged in routine exercise, according to recent studies it is probably important to have a high carbohydrate component.[940f]

*Be cautious about the advice you follow.* Be certain that the advice is given by an expert who is capable of evaluating results from scientific studies.

*Dress appropriately.* Buy good athletic shoes for sports that keep you on your feet. Choose unconstricting clothing for comfort, flexibility, and breathability.

A reasonable exercise program will increase your general fitness, help to create such strong muscle tone that you prevent injury, benefit your cardiovascular system, muscles, bones, and sense of well-being. It will increase the length of your life span and both the efficiency and the harmony of your days.

# Appendix A:
## Preservation of the Ovary

## PRESERVATION OF THE OVARY: A REEVALUATION

Celso Ramón Garcia, M.D. *Department of Obstetrics and Gynecology, Hospital of the University of Pennsylvania*
Winnifred Berg Cutler, Ph.D. *University of Pennsylvania School of Medicine, Philadelphia, Pennsylvania*

*The incidence of routine ovariectomy approximates 20% to 30% of all women at hysterectomy. The propriety of this practice is evaluated from three perspectives: (1) the review of the longevity of ovarian hormonal function throughout life, (2) the review of the low risk of subsequent disease in the retained ovary, and (3) the review of epidemiologic considerations. Because oophorectomy and the loss of its steroid contribution has such a profound influence on many body functions, with the most devastating relation to osteoporosis, and because there are no meaningful data in the literature to support the value of routine oophorectomy, removal of ovaries should only be performed when the ovaries are diseased. Fertil Steril 42:510, 1984*

The 1980s have been viewed as a time when greater efforts must be directed toward improving the health and welfare of the maturing female. A reappraisal of our attitudes concerning routine oophorectomy and its implication in the welfare of the female is mandatory. The gynecologist frequently is required to decide between ovarian preserva-

Reprinted from *Fertility and Sterility,* Vol. 42, No. 4 (October 1984).

tion versus ablation, particularly when hysterectomy is performed for benign disease. This is a significant problem, because the current incidence of hysterectomy in the United States approaches 60% by the time women reach 65 years of age. In the younger woman, the consensus is almost always favored, namely, ovarian preservation. On the other hand, in the women past 40, the reverse is usually true—routine ovariectomy. The gynecologist performing a hysterectomy is concerned with the potential of malignant transformation in the preserved ovary or ovaries, which could be a deadly prospect. Nonetheless, removing the ovaries in an ovulating woman deprives her of significant hormonal support, which often is difficult to replace adequately.

The question of the propriety of routine ovariectomy during hysterectomy is best evaluated from four perspectives: (1) the review of the longevity of ovarian function, (2) the risk of subsequent disease in the retained ovaries, (3) a consideration of current data on ovariectomy, and (4) the epidemiologic considerations.

### *Longevity of Ovarian Function*

While it has been commonly stated that ovaries become essentially nonfunctional sometime after the mid-40s, the accumulated weight of evidence supports the appropriateness of reexamining this long-held view.

As the ovary ages, it continues to contribute to the steroidal milieu of the menopausal woman, albeit in a declining fashion. As early as 1965, Novak et al.[1] had shown that postmenopausal ovaries frequently maintained a steroid capability for several decades after menses had ceased. Morphologic evidence suggests that the aging ovary is quite different from the younger ovary, particularly after the cessation of ovulation. Nonetheless, the human postmenopausal ovary is not the completely inert, nonfunctional fibrous mass that many formerly thought it to be.[2] There is a gradual diminution in ovarian mass that occurs throughout the 30s and progresses more rapidly after the age of 45.[3] The differences between the old and the young ovary, especially after age 55, are quite striking; the decreasing population density of follicular structures and a correlative increase of the stroma are evident.[4] Nonetheless, these older ovaries, replete with stroma material, are now understood to actively produce androstenedione ($\Delta^4 A$)—the hormone that, in the menopausal woman, is converted to estrone ($E_1$) in the fat depots of the body. This pathway can be significant in preventing osteoporosis.

McNatty et al.[5] have shown that postmenopausal stroma function differently than premenopausal stroma. Their in vitro analysis of the production of progesterone, androgen, and estrogen showed that, in the younger ovaries, all of the ovarian compartments were active, and stromal tissue had lower levels of cellular activity, mitotic activity, and cell hypertrophy than thecal tissue. In the postmenopausal ovaries, the situation was reversed: the level of cellular activity in the stroma was quite high, and considerable hypertrophy was observed. Other evaluations of steroid production and responsiveness to gonadotropins in isolated postmenopausal stroma tissue show that cortical stroma produces measurable amounts of $\Delta^4$A, estradiol ($E_2$), and progesterone, in vitro, while hyperplastic stromal tissue yields even greater $\Delta^4$A and $E_2$.[6] Hormone secretion of ovaries at hysterectomy was studied by Mikhail,[7] who offered that the menopausal ovarian vein was rich in dehydroepiandrosterone and $E_1$. Longcope et al.[8] also reported on a spectrum of ovarian function in postmenopausal women via venous-arterial differences in studies during hysterectomy procedures.

Combining the evidence from morphologic, histochemical, in vitro steroidogenic, and ovarian vein catheter studies leads us to confirm a lifelong ovarian developmental pattern. There is a greater appreciation of relative mass toward stromal tissue with increasing age; and, with this increase of stromal tissue, there results an increase in the capacity to synthesize $\Delta^4$A. The ovaries of women in the menopausal years, often late into the menopause, continue to secrete androgens which may support the well-being and general health of the older woman. Peripheral conversions of these androgens to estrogen are well documented. Certainly the availability of these steroids for such conversion will be terminated upon oophorectomy. Consequently, perspectives on the propriety of routine ovariectomy, in the absence of ovarian disease, are being reexamined as the evidence supporting postmenopause ovarian function accumulates. Moreover, the term "quiescent ovary," used to describe all older ovaries, is no longer justifiable.

## Posthysterectomy Ovarian Activity

The incidence of retention of ovarian cyclicity after hysterectomy remains somewhat unclear. The majority of posthysterectomy patients under age 48 continue to show an ovarian cycle, according to any of several criteria: bioassay of weekly urine samples,[9] cyclic records of premenstrual tension phenomenon,[10] plasma hormone evaluation, and studies of vaginal smears.[11] However, the phenomenon appears to be less than universal. Ranney and Abu-Ghazaleh[12] evaluated the future function and control of ovarian tissue that is retained in vivo during hysterectomy and concluded that approximately 50% of their large sample continued to show clinical signs of ovarian hormone production (i.e., vaginal tissue maintenance), but the other 50% did not. This was the only study of those just described that sampled very large groups of women; and these results, therefore, suggest that some women stop showing ovarian cyclicity shortly after hysterectomy. The nature of the influence of an intact uterus on ovarian function is currently unresolved; but with the recent discovery of uterine secretions of large quantities of prostaglandins, there is reason to study the issue.[13] Potentially, the reduction in prostaglandin after hysterectomy could be a factor in the loss of ovarian cyclicity. Alternatively, the loss of the putative reflex pathway from cervix to pituitary (as is found in lower mammals)[14] could also be responsible.

## Postoophorectomy Endocrine Activity

Studies of ovariectomized women before, immediately postoperatively, and at various time intervals after surgery have been generally consistent. Both gonadotropins predictably show a rapid rise, which, by 3 weeks, can easily have reached 10 times preoperative levels.[15, 16] Likewise, within 3 hours, estrogen drops to 60% of the presurgical level,[17] reaches a nadir by 5 days after surgery,[18] and levels off thereafter at the new lower values.

Hormone replacement therapy does somewhat reduce these gonadotropin/steroid levels. Follicle-stimulating hormone more closely approaches its preoperative levels.[15, 19] In one study, luteinizing hormone changes required a combination estrogen and progestin hormone therapy.[15] $E_2$ levels in plasma increase to preoperative levels when estrogen replacement therapies are sufficiently concentrated.[19] However, no estrogen dose is able to equilibrate both the gonadotropins and the steroids at the preoperative equivalency in women 45 to 53 years old. In order to reduce gonadotropins to preoperative levels, one must produce a hyperestrogenic state.[19] The ovarian hormones, then, probably include other substances, which are not replaced by estrogen or progestins.

Oophorectomized women frequently experience hot flushes, and studies have shown that those women who do flush postoperatively have significantly lower $\Delta^4A$ levels than those women who do not[17]—another reflection of the value of preservation of the ovaries.

Also noteworthy is the significant decline in epidermal thickness that follows oophorectomy at any age.[20] This epidermal thickness can be restored, or the decline prevented, by a weak estrogen (estriol succinate, 2 mg/day); whereas a stronger estrogen (estradiol valerate, 2 mg/day) sometimes produces the opposite effect.[21] The most critical issue, however, is loss of bone mass leading to osteoporosis, which oophorectomy is known to initiate. It is relevant to know that lowered $E_1$ and $\Delta^4A$ levels are established risk factors for osteoporosis. In contrast, $E_2$ and testosterone concentrations have not been identified as significant in assessing the osteoporosis risk factors.[22]

## Risk of Subsequent Ovarian Disease

### Benign Ovarian Tumors

Varying types of ovarian tumors may be encountered—each having its distinct anatomic and clinical properties.[23-26] A knowledge of gross anatomic disease aided by the histologic capabilities of the pathologist, particularly via frozen section, may be most helpful in deciding whether oophorectomy or simple resection of the pathologic portion—e.g., endometriosis, benign cystic teratomas, etc—is sufficient.

### Malignant Ovarian Tumors

The incidence of ovarian cancer varies markedly with age. In a study of the epithelial cancer rates of the ovary in over 2000 cases at the M. D. Anderson Hospital,[27] it was found that the peak years for this cancer are the 40s to the late 60s, paralleling the time during which estrogen levels are declining most precipitously. In that study, the wealthy had a lower survival rate, and postoperative radiation was noted to be better able to improve the survival rate than postoperative chemotherapy. As therapeutic techniques change, reevaluation will, no doubt, alter this perspective. The size of the largest remaining cancer mass in the body was more predictive of survival than the number of focal malignant sites. Interestingly enough, despite the present consensus to the contrary, the spillage of cystic contents of the mass at surgery did not lower the survival rate. Five-year survival rates were also noted to vary considerably as a function of age. Survival rates decrease with age.

The fact that ovarian cancer was so resistant to treatment led to the routine removal of perfectly healthy ovaries under the assumption that such action would prevent potential ovarian cancers. However, the presently available data do not support the logic of this course.

### Epidemiologic Considerations

The risk of ovarian cancer in women in whom hysterectomy was contemplated for benign uterine disease has now been studied in two different ways. One can look at the ovarian cancer patients and compare them with patients who have not undergone prior ovarian ablation. One can ask what the hysterectomy rate was for each population. If it were dangerous to retain the ovaries after a hysterectomy, one would expect to find a higher frequency of formerly hysterectomized women among ovarian cancer patients than among those without ovarian cancer. The opposite is true. Studies have consistently shown that ovarian cancer patients have a much *lower* incidence of hysterectomy than is found in the general population. For example, Annegers et al.[28] reported a 5% prior hysterectomy rate in ovarian cancer patients, compared with a 23% hysterectomy rate in age-matched women who had not undergone prior ovariectomy. Two other studies published in the 1950s showed a similarly low 4%[29] and 4.5%[30] rate of prior hysterectomy among the ovarian cancer patients. Unfortunately, even though these data are quite clear in showing that hysterectomy in ovarian cancer patients is disproportionately lower, misleading logic has been applied for the reverse conclusion,[31] i.e., that ovaries should be removed at hysterectomy. This incorrect conclusion has been widely cited and, thereby, a false premise perpetuated.

Another line of investigation also supports the safety of retaining the ovaries at hysterectomy. Prospective rates of ovarian cancer in ovaries retained after hysterectomy also support the absence of a risk.[32] A cohort study following 900 hysterectomized women for 20 years showed an overall rate of subsequent ovarian cancer at 0.2% in the sample.[32] The women who had both ovaries preserved showed a much lower rate (0.01%) of subsequent cancer than those who had only one ovary preserved (0.3%). There is, therefore, a consistent and clear picture when we scrutinize the data rather than analyzing the published conclusions. The goal of surgical prevention of ovarian cancer should not conclude in a decision for oophorectomy at hysterectomy. In fact, in 1982, a report of intraabdominal carcinomatosis (indistinguishable from ovarian carcinomatosis) after prophylactic oophorectomy in ovarian cancer-prone families showed the futility of such a course.[33] Oophorectomies were performed "prophylactically" on 28 members of 16 families that were at high risk of ovarian carcinoma. Three of these women subsequently developed disseminated intraabdominal malignancy.[33] The authors concluded that the development of intraabdominal carcinomatosis in oophorectomized women from ovarian cancer-prone families suggests that genetic susceptibility is not limited to ovarian carcinoma but extends to cancers arising in tissues embryologically related to the ovary. It should be pointed out that the incidence of ovarian cancer is extremely low. There appears, therefore, dubious advantage to be gained by the routine removal of healthy ovaries at hysterectomy.

In spite of what appears to be a rather clear case against routine ovariectomy during hysterectomy, current surgical practice has been different. Using data from the National Center for Health Statistics, Dicker et al.[34] evaluated women ranging in age from 25 to 44 during the interval of 1970 to 1977. They reported that ovariectomy during hysterectomy for benign causes was occurring about 25% of the time and did not change throughout the years the data were collected. Older women, the group from 40 to 44, had an approximate 50% rate of ovariectomy at hysterectomy. In light of the currently available knowledge demonstrating hormone secretion by ovaries in the 40s, 50s, and 60s (particularly $\Delta^4$A), the value of such hormones in reducing the risk of osteoporosis, and the lack of advantage in preventing ovarian cancer by oophorectomy, the routine practice of oophorectomy is challenged. While those who have inadequate sources of androgen or peripheral conversion capacity may benefit from hormonal replacement, there remain a significant (15%) number who do *not* require hormonal support. Not only will oophorectomy most often be ineffective in preventing ovarian cancer; but, more important, the loss of these ovarian secretions may play a role in producing the degenerative sequence of osteopenia and osteoporosis. This pathophysiologic sequence of osteoporosis can be more often favorably modified by estrogen hormonal replacement therapy. The osteoporotic process has recently been reviewed.[35] Nonetheless, some osteoporotic patients are resistant to these normally effective measures, as is sometimes the case in the relief of some of the other postmenopausal symptoms. The evidence continues to support the theory that ovaries should be retained unless they are diseased.

## Conclusions

In the face of the exceedingly low incidence of ovarian cancer and its questionable prevention by prophylactic oophorectomy, routine oophorectomy would deprive enormous numbers of women of the essential benefits afforded by these steroid-secreting organs. One exception might be the case of familial ovarian carcinoma syndrome.[33, 36-38] Clearly, in such an instance, the patient must be properly informed of all options and considerations, including the possibility of subsequent diseminated peritoneal carcinomatosis in some even after oophorectomy. Because oophorectomy has such profound influences at every age, particularly its devastating relation to osteoporosis, and because there are no meaningful data in the literature to support the value of routine oophorectomy, we suggest that oophorectomy only be performed when the ovaries are diseased.

## References

1. Novak ER, Goldberg B, Jones GS: Enzyme histochemistry of the menopausal ovary associated with normal and abnormal endometrium. Am J Obstet Gynecol 93:669, 1965
2. Guraya S: Histochemical observations on the corpus luteum atreticum of the human postmenopausal ovary with reference to steroid hormone synthesis. Arch Ital Anat Embriol 56:189, 1976
3. Tervila L: The weight of the ovaries after stress ending in death. Ann Chir Gynaecol Fenn 47:232, 1958
4. Nicosia SV: Morphological changes in the human ovary through life. In Comprehensive Endocrinology: The Ovary, Edited by L Martini, GB Serra. New York, Raven Press, 1983, p 57
5. McNatty KP, Makris A, DeGrazia C, Osathanondh R, Ryan KJ: The production of progesterone, androgens, and estrogens by granulosa cells, thecal tissue and stromal tissue by human ovaries in vitro. J Clin Endocrinol Metab 49:687, 1979
6. Dennefors B, Janson P, Knutson F, Hamberger L: Steroid production and responsiveness to gonadotropin in isolated stromal tissue of human postmenopausal ovaries. Am J Obstet Gynecol 136:997, 1980
7. Mikhail G. Hormone secretion by the human ovaries. Gynecol Invest 1:5, 1970
8. Longcope C, Hunter R, Franz C: Steroid secretion by the postmenopausal ovary. Am J Obstet Gynecol 138:564, 1980
9. Beavis ELG, Brown JB, Smith MA: Ovarian function after hysterectomy with conservation of the ovaries in premenopausal women. J Obstet Gynaecol Br Commonw 76: 969, 1969
10. Backstrom CT, Boyle H: Persistence of premenstrual tension symptoms in hysterectomized women. Br J Obstet Gynaecol 88:530, 1981

11. DeNeef JC, Hollenbeck ZJR: The fate of ovaries preserved at the time of hysterectomy. Am J Obstet Gynecol 96:538, 1966

12. Ranney B, Abu-Ghazaleh S: The future function and control of ovarian tissue which is retained in vivo during hysterectomy. Am J Obstet Gynecol 128:626, 1977

13. Charbonnel B, Kremer M, Gerozissis K, Dray F: Human cervical mucus contains large amounts of prostaglandins. Fertil Steril 38:109, 1982

14. Cutler WB, García CR: The psychoneuroendocrinology of the ovulatory cycle of woman. Psychoneuroendocrinology 5:89, 1980

15. Wallach EE, Root AW, Garcia C-R: Serum gonadotropin responses to estrogen and progestogen in recently castrated human females. J Clin Endocrinol Metab 31:376, 1970

16. Yen SSC, Tsai OC: The effect of ovariectomy on gonadotropin release. J Clin Invest 50:1149, 1971

17. Barlow DH, Macnaughton MC, Mowat J, Coutts JRT: Hormone profiles in the menopause. In Functional Morphology of the Human Ovary, Edited by JRT Coutts. Baltimore, University Park Press, 1981, p 223

18. Hunter DJ, Julier D, Franklin M, Green E: Plasma levels of estrogen, luteinizing hormone, and follicle-stimulating hormone following castration and estradiol implant. Obstet Gynecol 49:180, 1977

19. Utian W, Katz M, Davy D, Carr P: Effect of premenopausal castration and incremental dosages of conjugated equine estrogens on plasma follicle-stimulating hormone, luteinizing hormone and estradiol. Am J Obstet Gynecol 132:297, 1978

20. Punnonen R, Raurama L: The effect of long-term oral oestriol succinate therapy on the skin of castrated women. Ann Chir Gynaecol 66:214, 1977

21. Punnonen R: Effect of castration and peroral estrogen therapy on the skin. Acta Obstet Gynecol Scand 21:1, 1972

22. Crilly R, Horsman A, Marshall DH, Nordin BEC: Prevalence, pathogenesis and treatment of postmenopausal osteoporosis. Aust NZ J Med 9:24, 1979

23. Reed MJ, Hutton JD, Beard RW, Jacobs HS, James VH: Plasma hormone levels and oestrogen production in a postmenopausal woman with endometrial carcinoma and an ovarian thecoma. Clin Endocrinol (Oxf) 11:141, 1979

24. Rome RM, Fortune DW, Quinn MA, Brown JB: Functioning ovarian tumors in postmenopausal women. Obstet Gynecol 57:705, 1981

25. Sternberg WH: The morphology, androgenic function, hyperplasia, and tumors of the human ovarian hilus cells. Am J Pathol 25:493, 1947

26. Gordon A, Rosenstein N, Parmley T, Bhagavan B. Benign cystic teratomas in postmenopausal women. Am J Obstet Gynecol 138:1120, 1980

27. Smith JP, Day TG: Review of ovarian cancer at the University of Texas Systems Cancer Center MD Anderson Hospital and Tumor Institute. Am J Obstet Gynecol 135:984, 1979

28. Annegers JF, Strom H, Decker DG, Dockerty MD, O'Fallon WM: Ovarian cancer: reappraisal of residual ovaries. Am J Obstet Gynecol 97:124, 1967

29. Smith GV: Ovarian tumors. Am J Surg 95:336, 1958

30. Counseller VS, Hunt W, Haigler FH: Carcinoma of the ovary following hysterectomy. Am J Obstet Gynecol 69:538, 1955

31. Grogan RH: Reappraisal of residual ovaries. Am J Obstet Gynecol 97:124, 1967

32. Randall CL: Ovarian conservation. In Progress in Gynecology, Edited by JV Meigs, SH Sturgis. New York, Grune & Stratton. 1963, p 457

33. Tobachman JK, Tucker MA, Kase R, Greene MH, Costa J, Fraumen JF: Intraabdominal carcinomatosis after prophylactic oophorectomy in ovarian cancer prone families. Lancet 2:795, 1982

34. Dicker R, Greenspan J, Strauss L, Cowart M, Scally M, Peterson H, DeStefano F, Rubin G, Ory H: Complications of abdominal and vaginal hysterectomy among women of reproductive age in the United States. Am J Obstet Gynecol 144:841, 1982

35. Cutler WB, García CR: Osteoporosis. In The Medical Management of Menopause and Premenopause: Their Endocrinologic Basis. Philadelphia, J. B. Lippincott Co., 1984, p 49

36. Barber HRK: Epidemiology of cancer of the ovary. In Ovarian Carcinoma, Second edition. New York, Masson Publishing, 1982, p 25

37. Lynch H, Albano W, Lynch J, Lynch P, Campbell A: Surveillance and management of patients at high genetic risk for ovarian carcinoma. Obstet Gynecol 59:589, 1982

38. Piver MS, Barlow JJ, Sawyer DM: Familial ovarian cancer: increasing in frequency? Obstet Gynecol 60:397, 1982

## PRESERVATION OF THE OVARY

*To the Editor:*

We would like to thank Doctors García and Cutler for their very provocative paper.[1] It certainly has caused those with interests in reproductive endocrinology and gynecologic oncology to reevaluate the management of the ovary in conjunction with a hysterectomy in women over 40 years of age.

It is a given well-established, and well-documented fact that the ovary may produce hormones well into the sixties, acting after menopause primarily as an androgen-producing organ, and causing, through peripheral conversion, the production of estrone. We know, though, because osteoporosis and other stigmata develop in postmenopausal women because of the relatively insufficient quantities of estrogen, that this hormonal production is virtually ineffective. Therefore, one must conclude that there is no strong reason to leave the ovary intact at the time of hysterectomy with the aim being production of effective hormonal substances in the menopausal years.

The question, with regard to castrating the woman in her fifth decade, is not whether her ovaries will function effectively in the post-menopausal years, but whether they will function in the years between castration and menopause. There is definite controversy as to whether the ovary continues to function normally after hysterectomy because of a compromised blood supply.[2, 3] Nevertheless, the critical question is whether leaving the ovary in at the time of hysterectomy has sequelae with regard to future benign and malignant ovarian disease.

Ovarian cancer is the major cancer health hazard for the female pelvic reproductive organs. There will be more deaths this year from ovarian cancer than total deaths from cervical and endometrial cancer combined. Recent epidemiologic studies suggest that the patient at highest risk for developing ovarian cancer is a middle or upper class white woman who is nulliparous or of low parity.

In evaluating García and Cutler's[1] proposed evidence to support leaving the ovaries behind in women undergoing hysterectomy, one can only wonder how many of the women cited in their supporting references and operated on in the 1930s to 1950s actually fell into the high risk group for ever developing ovarian cancer. One must be skeptical about white nulligravidas or women of low parity constituting the overwhelming majority of these patients. Unfortunately, this sort of epidemiologic data is not available in the studies quoted by the authors. Pure familial ovarian cancer syndromes are rare. One must be very skeptical about the three cases cited by the authors as being typical of common epithelial cancer of the ovary. One of the latter patients died with brain metastases, and a second one died 2 months after diagnosis with metastases to the liver and subcutaneous tissue; clearly these are highly virulent cancers. Additional questions have been raised about whether sectioning of the ovaries from these three patients were adequate to rule out microscopic disease at the time of prophylactic oophorectomy.

The concept of leaving a visibly normal ovary behind in a woman aged 40 to 50, as suggested by the authors, when the contralateral ovary is involved with a "benign process" such as endometriosis or a benign teratoma is simply not good clinical judgment. The concept of performing frozen section analysis on the normal ovary when a benign tumor is present in the other ovary may potentially compromise ovarian function further in women aged 40 to 50. Routine use of frozen section analysis of all ovaries to be left intact at the time of hysterectomy would be extremely expensive and would involve an inherent risk of missing microscopic disease.

In conclusion, there seems to be no need to leave a perimenopausal or postmenopausal ovary in situ even though it continues to function for perhaps 10 or even 20 years. The hormonal function is ineffective in preventing postmenopausal symptoms. Ovarian neoplasm remains a major health hazard for these women. Satisfactory estrogen and progesterone replacement in women over 40 is a reality. Each adversarial side awaits more and better information.

*Alan H. DeCherney, M.D.*
*Peter E. Schwartz, M.D.*
Department of Obstetrics and Gynecology
Yale University School of Medicine
New Haven, Connecticut 06510-8063
August 20, 1985

### References

1. García CR, Cutler WB: Preservation of the ovary: a reevaluation. Fertil Steril 42:510, 1984
2. Janson PO, Jansson I: The acute effect of hysterectomy on ovarian blood flow. Am J Obstet Gynecol 127:349, 1977
3. Stone SC, Dickey RP, Mickal A: The acute effect of hysterectomy on ovarian function. Am J Obstet Gynecol 117:193, 1973

*Reply of the Authors:*

Until improvements in therapy are more evolved, our colleagues should be cognizant of the hazards and risks of ovariectomy and the all too frequent potential inability to correct for the missing ovarian hormones by replacement regimens.

A. Their statement:

"... because osteoporosis ... develop(s) in postmenopausal women ... this (ovarian postmenopausal) hormonal production is virtually ineffective. Therefore, one must conclude that there is no strong reason to leave the ovary intact ..."

In reply:

1. Removing the source of a significant production of estrone (whether through estradiol conversion into estrone in the younger woman or androstenedione conversion into estrone in the mature

ovary), (1) ignores the fact that 40% of women do not experience the development of osteoporosis and (2) increases the risk of metabolic bone disease for those 60% who are subject to osteoporosis. McNatty[1] demonstrated that stromal tissue from a menopausal ovary contains more androstenedione than stromal tissue from younger ovaries; and because androstenedione, and its conversion product, estrone, are much more relevant as risk factors than estradiol or other identified steroids correlating with the prediction of osteoporosis, even the aging ovary appears to contain a built-in mechanism to inhibit osteoporosis.

2. The use of osteoporosis as a single gauge in defining the value of aging ovaries is inappropriate. Ovarian hormones provide meaningful physiologic effects other than simply contributing to a positive bone mineral metabolism. For example, a large loss of sexual motivation (arousal, fantasy life, and desire) in oophorectomized, 46-year-old women in prospective, double-blind crossover placebo-controlled trials has been shown,[2] and the sexual motivation was found to be replaceable through androgen. Thus, although we currently do not know the precise appropriateness of androgen replacement for optimal body function, the androgen contribution of aging ovaries is acknowledged.

3. It is naive to believe that oophorectomy followed by hormonal replacement therapy does bring the patient back to the endocrine status she enjoyed prior to ovariectomy. The amount of estrogen replacement therapy currently being prescribed does not bring the gonadotropin level back to normal. Moreover, the role of ovarian androgen secretion in sexual motivation further demonstrates our currently primitive understanding of the manifold functions of the maturing ovary.

4. The degree of osteoporosis is a complex function of steroid levels (principally estrone), adequate ingestion of absorbable calcium, sufficient vitamin D, and appropriate levels of parathyroid hormone and calcitonin.

B. Their statement that *the* critical question is the risk of ovarian cancer in retained ovaries at the time of hysterectomy.

In reply:

1. There are no data that support that removing the ovaries is preventative of subsequent ovarian-type cancer.

2. Ovarian cancer deaths occur relatively infrequently (11,600 per year) in relation to deaths secondary to cardiovascular disease (485,000 per year) and during recovery from hip fracture.[3]

We agree that significant ovarian disease needs to be addressed. However, gynecologic surgeons are much too prone to remove both ovaries even when there is minimal endometriosis in the pelvis where the other ovary may have minimal benign disease that can be resected or even when the ovary is normal. Resection of the endometriosis and preservation of the normal ovary is a more preferable option in protecting the general health of women even at age 40 to 50. Physiologic age is not always compatible with chronologic age. It is obvious that it is good clinical judgement to make the correct decision about the appropriateness of retaining a normal ovary in a woman of age 40 to 50 when encountering benign disease in the pelvis. Frozen section should be used when necessary, but not routinely. However, a very superior knowledge of gross anatomic gynecologic pathology is essential. Physicians uncomfortable with their knowledge of these tissue abnormalities should not expose their patients to the increased risk of routine ovariectomy simply to ease feelings of responsibility. *All* the risks must be weighed appropriately.

Despite the decline in reproductive system circulating steroids being about equivalent for men and for women,[4] testes, perhaps because they are more accessible, are more reluctantly removed than are ovaries. Removal of ovaries occurs less frequently at vaginal hysterectomy than abdominal hysterectomy even with similar benign pelvic disease.

We remind those who would consider whether or not to remove an organ that is healthy that the burden-of-proof question ought to rest with the remover and that we should remember the dictum "Above all, do not harm."

Celso Ramón García, M.D.
Winnifred Berg Cutler, Ph.D.
Department of Obstetrics and Gynecology
Hospital of the University of Pennsylvania
Philadelphia, Pennsylvania 19104
March 17, 1986

# References*

1. McNatty KP, Hunter WM, McNeilly AS, Sawers RS: Changes in the concentration of pituitary and steroid hormones in the follicular fluid of human Graafian follicles throughout the menstrual cycle. J Endocrinol 64:555, 1975
2. Sherwin BB, Gelfand MM, Brender W: Androgen enhances sexual motivation in females: a prospective crossover study of sex steroid administration in surgical menopause. Psychosom Med 47:339, 1985
3. Vital Statistics of the United States: Death statistic references
4. Cutler WB, García CR: Sexuality and hormones. In The Medical Management of Menopause and Premenopause: Their Endocrinologic Basis. Philadelphia, J. B. Lippincott, 1984, p 92

*A complete list of 300 references is available by request.

# Appendix B:
## Gallstones

Cholesterol gallstones are more common in women than in men in every geographical region so far studied (Malmo, Sweden; Prague, Czechoslovakia; and the United States, including American Indians).[452] Because women get the disease more often than men, estrogen is a likely factor, and in fact, several epidemiologic studies have shown that when gallstone patients are compared with patients in control groups, there is always a higher incidence of hormone use among the gallstone patients than among the controls. But this fact should not be given more weight than it deserves, for the reasons that follow.

Cholesterol gallstones occur when the cholesterol quantity in the bile exceeds its normal range.[452] When the cholesterol exceeds 10 percent of the total concentration of substances in the bile, it tends to precipitate, creating seeds or crystals that form the stones. We now know that there are two different kinds of gallstone patients, with two completely different mechanisms that cause disease.[795] In extremely obese women, the gallstones are caused by an increased manufacture of cholesterol. In women who are not obese, the gallstones are caused not by cholesterol but by a reduced rate of production of bile salts and other substances.[795] In fact, one investigator showed that in men who were enrolled in an atherosclerosis-prevention program, the very diets that caused a reduction in their cholesterol levels caused an increase in the formation of gallstones.[863] It therefore appears that the prevention of one disease can increase the risk of the other disease. For that reason, it is very important to understand how rarely the disease actually occurs and whether by increasing the statistical risk, there is much actual risk to you of having that disease.

Among postmenopausal women, nonusers of estrogen developed medically diagnosed gallbladder disease at the rate of fewer than 1 in 1,000 women. Among estrogen users, the incidence is higher—about 2 women per 1,000. When we compare these rates to the cardiovascular disease rates (600 per 1,000), the risk of HRT stimulating gallbladder disease is very slight. Nonetheless, it must be considered if you are at high risk for gallbladder disease due to obesity or family history.

Changes in gallbladder function after estrogen therapy have been incompletely studied but seem to be more a reflection of how fat a woman is than how much estrogen she takes. For example, in one study that did show an increased risk of gallbladder disease in women on ERT versus age-matched control subjects,[390] a close look revealed that 10 percent of the gallbladder patients were estrogen replacement users, as opposed to 2 percent of the controls. HRT use was higher in gallstone patients. Yet, although HRT was more common among gallstone patients (10 percent versus 2 percent of controls), obesity was found in a startling 71 percent of the gallstone patients; that is, seven times as many gallstone patients were obese as used HRT. If obese women were removed from the data analysis, it is likely that hormone therapy would have shown a much less pronounced impact on gallstone risk.

The conclusions that can be drawn currently are incomplete. A superficial look at the data suggests that oral ERT may increase the risk of gallstones from a very low level to a somewhat higher but *still very low level*. When we look more closely, it appears that obesity is a much more critical factor and that for women who are not obese, ERT will probably not have any effects, even when taken orally. For obese women, the question of whether HRT will increase the risk of gallstones remains unanswered. The liver will respond to oral estrogen, and the greatest risk appears to be for those who take a synthetic estrogen such as ethinyl estradiol.[553, 784] Synthetic hormones appear to be less optimal for health than natural ones. (See Chapter 7.)

# Acknowledgments

🌿 When, in 1979 under a postdoctoral fellowship, I formed the Stanford Menopause Study to evaluate what happens to healthy women as they approach menopause, nineteen women who had undergone hysterectomies also offered to be studied. Hysterectomy was not intended to be part of the research project, but the fact that a group was asking to be studied led me to include them. In other words, I decided to accept the gift they offered (because to a research scientist data are a gift). In the process of evaluating their data, I began to be aware that hysterectomy was not the innocuous procedure that these nineteen women had expected it to be.

Since the publication of *Menopause: A Guide for Women and the Men Who Love Them* (coauthored with Drs. Celso R. García and David A. Edwards) and a more specialized textbook for scientists and physicians, *The Medical Management of Menopause and Premenopause: Their Endocrinologic Basis* (coauthored with Dr. García), I have received many letters from women describing their experience with hysterectomy and requesting a guide to help women before *and after* hysterectomy. It is entirely appropriate to say that these women planted the seed that led me to this work.

I thought it would be easily done. My personal research database, which had been in a continual state of upgrading, was on hand. I knew what I wanted to say. But as I began to outline the book, it became clear that additional branches of knowledge needed to be pursued.

And now, sitting down to read the final draft of *Hysterectomy: Before and After,* I find myself in a repeat position to that of 1981, when I had finished writing the first draft of *Menopause.* Then my perceptions as a trained scientist had led me to conclusions which were at variance with current teachings in the two medical schools, (University of Pennsylvania and Stanford University), where I had been working. Dr. Celso R. García at Penn and Dr. David A. Edwards at Emory University had agreed to coauthor the work with me and then set about critiquing and refining what I had said. By 1988, most of the 1981 conclusions had gained orthodoxy in medical school curricula.

With *Hysterectomy: Before and After*, much of what I conclude through my experience as a scholar, a reproductive scientist, and a woman derives straight from my serious attempt at a measured and rational interpretation of scientific data. Much of the data have been published since 1985 and are in such diverse fields that their synthesis here is new.

Thanks to active scientific work, critical reading of early drafts of the book—by a number of interested clinicians, academic physicians, research scientists, women who have already endured a hysterectomy, and those who have not—and helpful feedback, I learned which points could be refined and which expanded. I am particularly grateful to the following individuals.

To the members of the Metabolic Bone Disease Conference at the Hospital of the University of Pennsylvania (Dr. Frederick Kaplan, chief of metabolic bone disease; Dr. John Haddad, chief of endocrinology; Dr. Maurice Attie, associate professor of medicine; Dr. Jim McLeod, endocrinologist; Dr. Alan Wasserstein, kidney physiologist; and Dr. Michael Fallon, pathologist specializing in bone) for their continuing interaction with me through that weekly scientific conference. Through them I continue to learn the current medical opinion on the subjects related to bone endocrinology.

To Dr. Abass Alavi, chief of nuclear medicine at the University of Pennsylvania, for providing (at his expense) the costly dual-photon recordings of spinal bone of the first forty-one patients who went through the Women's Wellness Program at Penn in order to test my theory that spinal bone loss could be screened by the cheaper readings at the arm. His action gave me the opportunity to write a research paper in 1988 demonstrating the potentially critical role of *any* pelvic surgery on bone loss. Drs. Joel Karp, physicist, and Robert Stine, statistician, were collaborators and coauthors on that project (see ref. 163, page ).

Also to Dr. Celso R. García, professor of gynecology at the University of Pennsylvania, my former mentor and cofounder of the Women's Wellness Program at the Hospital of the University of Pennsylvania, whose significant comments are included in Chapter 4 (page 90) on pelvic surgery alternatives.

I thank Frits E. Riphagen, M.D., Ph.D., the director general of the International Health Foundation in Geneva, for supplying the data which showed that the U.S. has five times the hysterectomy rate of six European countries.

I am grateful to Willard F. Nagle, M.D., associate director of medical services at Rorer Pharmaceutical Corporation, (a manufacturer of calcitonin hormone) for his critical reading of Chapter 8 (page 173).

Dr. Sabine Swierenga, of the Drug Toxicology Division in Ottowa, Canada, was a tireless reviewer of the entire manuscript. She supplied literally hundreds of important comments which helped to refine the material. She also provided the lengthy computer printouts that permitted me to assemble Table 6 (page 152) on Canadian HRT options.

To Dr. John Perry, inventor of the electronic perineometer and discoverer of the role of the female homologue of the prostate, which he named the Grafenberg Spot. He critiqued, expanded, and then engaged in several hours of interesting colloquy with me on the subjects of chapters 10 and 12 (pages 225 and 266). His comments helped to improve those chapters.

Sue Silverton, M.D., Ph.D., at the University of Pennsylvania, gave a tireless reading of the entire first draft and many helpful criticisms.

Elizabeth Genovese, M.D., of the Penn Diagnostic Center in Philadelphia, provided a critical reading of the entire manuscript and particularly important were her criticisms of Chapter 9 (page 203).

Dr. Millicent Zacher, gynecological surgeon and director of the Donor Insemination Program at Albert Einstein Medical Center in Philadelphia, provided critical feedback and guidance on chapters 3 and 4 (pages 45 and 74).

Leslie Talcott, M.S., R.N., gave helpful comments on urinary incontinence and permitted me to experience personally what the vaginal perineometer is and what it can do for a woman's capacity to train strong pubococcygeal muscles.

To Dr. Alan DeCherney, director of reproductive endocrinology at Yale University, for engaging in a spirited (recorded) debate in Washington, D.C., with me as he took the opposite position to mine on preservation of the ovaries. It was through this experience that I came to more clearly understand the need for a book like this one—to provide scientific documentation on the importance and the value of preserving the reproductive organs of women and to help women after their surgery.

To Felicia Stewart, M.D., coauthor of *Understanding Your Body*, for her critical reading of chapters 3 and 4 and her encouragement of this project.

To Dr. R. Don Gambrell, at the Medical College of Georgia where he serves as clinical professor of ob/gyn, physiology, and endocrinology, for his frequent, gracious, and competent collegial interaction.

To Jerilynn Prior, M.D., FRCP, on the faculty of medicine at the University of British Columbia, for sharing her excellent prepublication manuscripts on exercise physiology and its interaction with female reproductive endocrinology, and for cogent criticism of Chapter 15 (page 323).

To Scott Harman, M.Ed., the aquatics director at St. Joseph's University in Philadelphia, for his critique of Chapter 15.

To Philip M. Sarrel, M.D., associate professor of obstetrics, gynecology, and psychiatry and director of the Mid-Life Study Program at Yale University, for his extraordinary range of scientific investigations of women's wellness issues, and his willingness to educate me through his comprehensive written replies to my questions.

To Louise Smith, director of technical policy planning at Research and Development, SmithKline and French Laboratories, for her efforts throughout the writing of the entire manuscript and her special perceptions of technology assessment.

I especially appreciate the women whose enthusiastic support and interest in the project mandated the book. Particularly those who read the manuscript and helped me to know where it needed greater clarity: Mary Joyce, in Haverford, PA; Sherley Hollos, director of both the Women's Center in Paoli and the Birth Center in Bryn Mawr, PA; Louise Ochroch, in Philadelphia.

To Pamela Thompson Sinkler, normally devoted to her work as a fine artist, a special thanks for agreeing to set aside time from her painting in order to draw the art. She patiently worked with me, sketching out the figures, trying different perspectives, suggesting alternatives geared to clarifying the exquisite symmetry of anatomical and physiological interpretation of human biology.

To Tom Quay, Esq., who serves as general counsel at Rorer, U.S., for our continuing dialogue throughout my eighteen months on this work and his role in educating me to understand why the word "ethical" precedes the word "pharmaceuticals." He showed me a new vision of the pivotal role that ethical pharmaceutical corporations contribute as part of a free-enterprise system in the development of improved health care.

I also acknowledge with great respect the thousands of scholars all over the world who have published the studies that permit others (like me) to evaluate and to synthesize, which thereby permits the rational growth of our knowledge. It is through the synthesis of the work of many that improvements in biomedical science inevitably take place.

The efforts of Harper & Row people are gratefully acknowledged. Janet Goldstein—for her vision in selecting the manuscript, in knowing what was needed to make it readable, her continuing excellent and tactful ability to improve the delivery of the information, her professional acumen, and her selection of other excellent editing people. To Pat Fogarty who worked—nonstop for close to two months—to take the text from my normal, scientific language and help me put it into the English that nonscientists use. To Katherine Ness for her fine copyediting work. To Barbara Moulton, Ms. Goldstein's assistant, and to the many others at Harper & Row who have each contributed to the book. Peter Livingston, my literary agent, is also appreciated for his skills in bringing the book to market.

I work to improve the quality of health care for women. *Much* remains to be done. I hope that this book will contribute to that effort. Please write to me, to articulate questions which were not answered, to contribute a different perspective, or to plant future seeds.

Winnifred B. Cutler, Ph.D.
May 1988

# References

1. Abbasi R, Hodgen GD (1986): Predicting the predisposition to osteoporosis: gonadotropin-releasing hormone antagonist for acute estrogen deficiency test. *JAMA* 255:12:1600–1604.

2. Abdalla HI, Hart DM, Lindsay R, Leggate I, Hooke A (1985): Prevention of bone mineral loss in postmenopausal women by norethisterone. *Obstet Gynecol* 66:6:789–792.

3. Abdalla HI, Beastall G, Fletcher D, Hawthorn JS, Smith J, Hart DM (1987): Sex steroid replacement in post-menopausal women: effects on thyroid hormone status. *Maturitas* 9:1:49–54.

4. Abraham GE, Lobotsky J, Lloyd CW (1969): Metabolism of testosterone & androstenedione in normal and ovariectomized women. *J Clin Invest* 48:696–703.

5. Adams PW, Rose DP, Folkard J, et al (1973): Effect of vitamin $B_6$ upon depression associated with oral contraception. *Lancet* 1:897–904.

6. Adinoff A, Hollister JR (1983): Steroid-induced fractures & bone loss in patients with asthma. *NEJM* 309:365–368.

7. Aitken JM, Hart DM, Lindsay R (1973): Oestrogen replacement therapy for prevention of osteoporosis after oophorectomy. *Br Med J* 3:515–518.

8. Aitken JM, Lindsay R, Hart DM (1976): Long-term oestrogens for prevention of post-menopausal osteoporosis. *Postgrad Med J* 52:6: 18–25.

9. Aitken JM, Lorimer AR, Hart DM, Lawrie TDV, Smith DA (1971): The effects of oophorectomy and long term mestranol therapy on the serum lipids of middle aged women. *Clinical Sciences* 41:597–603.

10. Aleem FA, McIntosh TK (1986): Menopausal syndrome: plasma levels of $\beta$-endorphin in post-menopausal women measured by a specific radioimmunoassay. *Maturitas* 7:4:329–334.

11. Allen LH, Oddoye EA, Margen S (1979): Protein-induced hypercalciurea: a longer term study. *Am J Clin Nutr* 32:741–749.

12. Allen T, Adler NT, Greenberg JH, Reivich M (1981): Vaginal cervical stimulation selectively increases metabolic activity in the rat brain. *Science* 211:1070–1072.

13. Allen T, Adler NT (1978): Localized uptake of (14) deogyglucose by the preoptic area of female rats in response to vaginocervical stimulation. *Neuroscience Abstracts* 4.

14. Altman N, Sachar EJ, Gruen PH, Halpern FS (1975): Reduced plasma LH concentration in postmenopausal depressed women. *Psychosom Med* 37:3:274–276.

15. Amias AG (1975): Sexual life after gynaecological operations-I. *Br Med J* 2:5971:608–609.

16. Amico JA, Seif SM, Robinson AG (1981): Elevation of oxytocin and the oxytocin-associated neurophysin in the plasma of normal women during midcycle. *J Clin Endocrinol Metab* 53:1229–1232.

17. Anand CR, Linkswiler HM (1974): Effect of protein intake on calcium balance of young men given 500 mg calcium daily. *J Nutr* 104:695–700.

18. Ananth J (1978): Hysterectomy and depression. *Obstet Gynecol* 52:724–730.

19. Anderson C, Mason W (1977): Hormones and social behavior of squirrel monkeys. *Hormones & Behavior* 8:100–106.

20. Anderson DC (1976): The role of sex hormone binding globulin in health and disease, in James VHT, Serio M, Giusti G (eds): *The Endocrine Function of the Human Ovary*. London, Academic Press, 141–158.

21. Annegers JF, Strom H, Decker DG, Dockerty MB, O'Fallon WM (1979): Ovarian cancer incidence and case-control study. *Cancer* 43:2:723–729.

22. Arey LB (1939): The degree of normal menstrual irregularity. *Am J Obstet Gynecol* 37:12.

23. Arey LB (1939): The degree of normal menstrual irregularity. *Am J Obstet Gynecol* 37:12.

24. Arnold JS (1973): Amount & quality of trabecular bone in osteoporotic vertebral fractures. *Clinics in Endocr & Meta* 2:2:221–238.

25. Askel S, Schomberg DW, Tyrey L, Hamond CB (1976): Vasomotor symptoms serum estrogens and gonadotropin levels in surgical menopause. *Am J Obstet Gynecol* 126:165–169.

26. Awbry BJ, Jacobson PC, Grubb SA, McCartney WH, Vincent LM, Talmage RV (1984): Bone density in women: A modified procedure for measurement of distal radial density. *Journal of Orthopaedic Research* 2:314–321.

27. Aylward M, Maddock J, Parker A, Protherde DA, Ward A (1978): Endometrial factors under treatment with oestrogen and oestrogen/progestogen combinations. *Postgrad Med J* 54:2:74–81.

28. Aylward M (1978): Coagulation factors in opposed and unopposed oestrogen treatment at the climacteric. *Postgrad Med J* 54:2:31–37.

29. Bachmann GA, Leiblum SR, Sandler B, Ainsley W, Narcessian R, Shelden R, Nakajima HH (1985): Correlates of sexual desire in postmenopausal women. *Maturitas* 7:211–216.

30. Backstrom T, Boyle H (1981): Persistence of premenstrual tension symptoms in hysterectomized women. *Br J Obstet Gynaecol* 88:530–536.

31. Bailar JC (1988): Mammography before age 50 years? *JAMA* 259:10:1548–1549.

32. Bain C, Willett W, Hennekens CH, Rosner B, Belanger C, Speizer FE (1981): Use of postmenopausal hormones & risk of myocardial infarction. *Circulation* 64:1:42–46.

33. Baker HWG, Burger HG, deKretser DM, Hudson B, O'Connor S, Wange C, Mirovics A, Court J, Dunlop M, Rennie GC (1976): Changes in the pituitary-testicular system with age. *Clin Endocrinol* 5:349–372.

34. Ballinger CB (1975): Psychiatric morbidity and the menopause: screening of general population sample. *Br Med J* 3:5979:344–346.

35. Banner AS, Carrington CB, Emory WB, Kittle F, Leonard G, Ringus J, Taylor P, Addington WW (1981): Efficacy of oophorectomy in lymphangioleiomyomatosis and benign metastatisizing leiomyoma. *NEJM* 305:204–209.

36. Bar AA, Hurwitz S (1979): The interaction between dietary calcium and gonadal hormones in their effect on plasma calcium, bone, 25-hydroxycholecalciferol-1 hydroxylase & duodenal calcium-binding protein, measured by a radioimmunoassay in chicks. *Endocrine Society* 104:5:1455–1459.

37. Baran DT, Bergfeld MA, Teitelbaum SL, Avioli LV (1978): Effect of testosterone therapy on bone formation in an osteoporotic hypogonadal male. *Calcif Tiss Res* 26:103–106.

38. Barber HRK (1982): Epidemiology of cancer of the ovary. *Ovarian Carcinoma* 25–38.

39. Barker MG (1968): Psychiatric illness after hysterectomy. *Br Med J* 2:91–95.

40. Barlow DH, Macnaughton MC, Mowat J, Coutts JRT (1981): Hormone profiles in the menopause, in Coutts JRT (ed): *Functional Morphology of the Human Ovary*. Baltimore, University Park Press.

41. Barlow J, Emerson K, Saxen NA (1969): Estradiol production after ovariectomy for carcinoma of the breast. *NEJM* 28:633–637.

42. Barrett-Connor E, Brown V, Turner J, et al (1979): Heart disease risk factors and hormone use in postmenopausal women. *JAMA* 20:2167–2169.

43. Barrett-Connor E, Khaw KT, Yen SSC (1986): A prospective study of dehyproepiandrosterone sulfate, mortality & cardiovascular disease. *NEJM* 315:24:1519–1524.

44. Barzel US (1984): Vitamin D deficiency and osteomalacia in the elderly. *Hospital Practice* 19:10:129–134.

45. Batra S, Losif S (1987): Progesterone receptors in vaginal tissue of post-menopausal women. *Maturitas* 9:1:87–94.

46. Baum MJ, Slob AK, DeJong FH, Westbroek DL (1978): Persistence of sexual behavior in ovariectomized stumptail macaques following dexamethasone treatment or adrenalectomy. *Hormones & Behavior* 11:323–347.

47. Bauman J, Kolodny RC, Webster SK (1982): Vaginal organic acids and hormonal changes in the menstrual cycle. *Fertil Steril* 38:572–579.

48. Baylink DJ (1984): reply in correspondence to Dr. Mazess in *NEJM* 310:321–322.

49. Baylink DJ (1983): Glucocorticoid-induced osteoporosis. *NEJM* 309:306–308.

50. Beavis ELG, Brown JB, Smith MA (1969): Ovarian function after hysterectomy with conservation of the ovaries in premenopausal women. *J Obstet Gynecol Br Commonw* 76:969–978.

51. Beck RP, Hsu N (1965): Pregnancy, childbirth & menopause related to development of stress incontinence. *Am J Obstet Gynecol* 91:820–823.

52. Bengtsson C, Lindquist O (1977): Coronary heart disease during the menopause, in Greenblatt R, Studd J (eds): *Coronary Heart Disease in Young Women*. Philadelphia, Saunders, 234–242.

53. Bengtsson C, Lindquist O, Redvall L (1979): Is the menopausal age rapidly changing? *Maturitas* 1:159–164.

54. Bennink HJTC, Schreurs WHP (1974): Disturbance of tryptophan metabolism and its correction during hormonal contracepiion. *Contraception* 9:347.

55. Berry EM, Hirsch J, Most J, McNamara DJ, Thornton J (1986): The relationship of dietary fat to plasma lipid levels as studied by factor analysis of adipose tissue fatty acid composition in a free-living population of middle-aged American men. *Am J Clin Nutr* 44:220–231.

56. Beynen AC, Katan MB (1985): Why do polyunsaturated fatty acids lower serum cholesterol? 1, 2. *Am J Clin Nutr* 42:560–563.

57. Bhattacharya AN, Dierschke DJ, Yamaji T, Knobil E (1972): The pharmacologic blockade of the circh oral mode of LH secretion in the ovariectomized rhesus monkey. *Endocrinology* 90:778.

58. Bielinski R, Schutz Y, Jequier E (1985): Energy metabolism during the post-exercise recovery in man 1, 2. *Am J Clin Nutr* 42:69–82.

59. Bingham S (1985): Dietary fibre intakes: intake studies, problems, methods & results, in Trowell H, Burkett D, Heaton K (eds): *Dietary Fibre, Fibre-Depleted Foods and Disease.* New York, Academic Press, 77–104.

60. Birnholz JC (1984): Ultrasonic visualization of endometrial movements. *Fertil Steril* 41:1:157–158.

61. Blacklock N (1985): Renal stone. In Trowell H, Burkett D, Heaton K (eds): *Dietary Fibre, Fibre-Depleted Foods and Disease.* New York, Academic Press, 345–359.

62. Blandau RJ, Moghissi K (1973): *The Biology of the Cervix.* Chicago, University of Chicago Press.

63. Blondin J, Baragi V, Schwartz ER, Sadowski JA, Taylor A (1987): Dietary vitamin C delays UN-induced eye lens protein damage. Third Conference on Vitamin C. *Ann NY Acad Sci* 498:460–463.

64. Bohlen JG (1981): Sleep erection monitoring in the evaluation of male erectile failure. *Urol Clin North Am* 8:119–134.

65. Bo-Linn GW, Davis GR, Buddrus DJ, Morawski SG, Santa Ana C, Fordtran JS (1984): An evaluation of the importance of gastric acid secretion in the absorption of dietary calcium. *J Clin Invest* 73:640–647.

66. Bolton CH, Ellwood M, Hartog M, Martin R, Rowe AS, Wensley RT (1975): Comparison of the effects of ethinyl oestradiol and conjugated

equine oestrogens in oophorectomized women. *Clin Endocrinol* (Oxf) 4:2:131–138.

67. Borglin NE, Staland B (1975): Oral treatment of menopausal symptoms with natural oestrogens. *Acta Obstet et Gynecol Scand Suppl* 43:3–11.

68. Boston Collaborative Drug Surveillance Program (1974): Surgically confirmed gallbladder disease, venous thromboembolism, and breast tumors in relation to postmenopausal estrogen therapy. A report from Boston University Medical Center. *NEJM* 290:15–19.

69. Bowes & Church (1970): *Food Values of Portions Commonly Used*, 11th ed. Revised by Charles F. Church & Helen N. Church. Philadelphia, Lippincott, 1–80.

70. Boyle IT (1981): Treatment for postmenopausal osteoporosis. *Lancet* 1376.

71. Bradley DD, Wingerd J, Petitti DB (1978): Serum high density lipoprotein cholesterol in women using oral contraceptives estrogens and progestins. *NEJM* 299:17–20.

72. Brenner PF (1982): The pharmacology of progestogens. *J Repro Med* 27:8 supp:490–497.

73. Brewer JI, Miller WH (1954): Postmenopausal uterine bleeding. *Am J Obstet Gynecol* 67:988–1013.

74. Brincat M, Versi E, O'Dowd T, Moniz CF, Magos A, Kabalan S, Studd JWW (1987): Skin collagen changes in post-menopausal women receiving oestradiol gel. *Maturitas* 9:1:1–6.

75. Brody J (1981): *Jane Brody's Nutrition Book.* New York, Bantam.

76. Brody S, Carlstrom K, Lagrelius A, Lunnell NO, Mollerstrom G (1987): Adrenal steroids in post-menopausal women: relation to obesity and to bone mineral content. *Maturitas* 9:1:25–32.

77. Brown ADG (1977): Postmenopausal urinary problems. *Clinics in Obstetrics & Gynaecology* 4:181–206.

78. Bucci L (1972): Drug induced depression and tryptophan metabolism. *Diseases of the Nervous System* Feb 105:108.

79. Buchi K, Keller PJ (1980): Estrogen receptors in normal and myomatous human uteri. *Gynecol Obstet Invest* 11:59–60.

80. Buchman MI, Kramer E, Feldman GB (1978): Aspiration curettage for asymptomatic patients receiving estrogen. *Obstet Gynecol* 51:339–341.

81. Buckley T (1982): Menstruation and the power of Yurok women: methods in cultural reconstruction. *Am Ethnological Soc* 47–60.

82. Bullamore JR, Gallagher JC, Wilkinson R (1970): Effect of age on calcium absorption. *Lancet* 2:535–537.

83. Bullock JL, Massey FM, Gambrell RD Jr (1975): Use of medroxyprogesterone acetate to prevent menopausal symptoms. *Obstet Gynecol* 46:2:165–168.

84. Bunker JP (1976): Elective hysterectomy: pro & con: public health rounds at the Harvard School of Public Health. *NEJM* 295:264–268.

85. Bunt JC, Boileau RA, Bahr JM, Nelson RA (1986): Sex and training differences in human growth hormone levels during prolonged exercise. *American Physiological Society* 1796–1801.

86. Burch JC, Byrd BF, Vaughn WK (1975): The effects of long-term estrogen administration to women following hysterectomy. *Front Horm Res* 3:208–214.

87. Burger H, Rose N (1979): Sexual impotence. *Med J Aust* 2:24–26.

88. Burgio KL, Robinson JC, Engel BT (1986): The role of biofeedback in Kegel exercise training for stress urinary incontinence. *Am J Obstet Gynecol* 154:58–64.

89. Burkett D (1985): Varicose veins, haemorrhoids, deep-vein thrombosis & pelvic phleboliths, in Trowell H, Burkett D, Heaton K (eds): *Dietary Fibre, Fibre-Depleted Foods and Disease.* New York, Academic Press, 317–329.

90. Burnier AM, Martin PL, Yen SSC, Brooks P (1981): Sublingual absorption of micronized 17β-estradiol. *Am J Obstet Gynecol* 140:146–150.

91. Burns B, Curry R, Bell MEA (1979): Morphologic features of prognostic significance in uterine smooth muscle tumors: a review of eighty-four cases. *Am J Obstet Gynecol* 135:109–114.

92. Burns DD, Mendels J (1979): Serotonin and affective disorders, in Easman WB, Valzelli L (eds): *Current Developments in Psychopharmacology,* Vol 5. New York, SP Medical & Scientific Books, 293–359.

93. Bush TL, Cowan LD, Barrett-Connor E, Criqui MH, Karon JM, Wallace RB, Tyroler HA, Rifkind BM (1983): Estrogen use and all cause mortality. *JAMA* 249:903–906.

94. Bye PB (1978): Review of the status of oestrogen replacement therapy. *Postgrad Med J* 54:2:7–10.

95. Byrd BF Jr, Burch JC, Vaughn WK (1977): The impact of long term estrogen support after hysterectomy. A report of 1016 cases. *Ann Surg* 185:5:574–580.

96. Callantine MR, Martin PL, Bolding OT, Warner PO, Greaney MO Jr (1975): Micronized 17 Beta-estradiol for oral estrogen therapy in menopausal women. *Obstet Gynecol* 46:1:37–41.

97. Callaway CW (1986): Nutrition. *JAMA* 256:15:2097–2099.

98. Cameron E, Pauling L, Lebowitz B (1979): Ascorbic acid and cancer. *Cancer Res* 29:663–681.

99. Campbell S, Whitehead M (1977): Oestrogen therapy and the menopausal syndrome. *Clinics in Obstetrics & Gynecology* 4:1:31–47.

100. Campbell S, Minardi J, McQueen J, Whitehead M (1978): Endometrial factors: the modifying effect of progestogen on the response of the post menopausal endometrium to exogenous estrogens. *Postgrad Med J* 54:59–64.

101. Caniggia A, Nuti R, Lore F, Vattimo A (1981): Pathophysiology of the adverse effects of glucoactive corticosteroids on calcium metabolism in man. *J Steroid Biochem* 15:153–161.

102. Cann CE, Genant KH, Ettinger B, Gordan GS (1980): Spinal mineral loss by quantitative computed tomography in oophorectomized women. *JAMA* 144:2056–2059.

103. Carlson LA, Bottiger LE, Ahfeldt PE (1979): Risk factors for myocardial infarction in the Stockholm prospective study. *Acta Med Scand* 206:351–360.

104. Carlson RR, Defeo VJ (1965): Role of the pelvic nerve vs. the abdominal sympathetic nerves in the reproductive function of the female rat. *Endocr* 77:1014–1022.

105. Carr BR, MacDonald PC, Simpson ER (1982): The role of lipoproteins in the regulation of progesterone secretion by the human corpus luteum. *Fertil Steril* 38:303–311.

106. Carr DB, Bullen BA, Skrinar GS, Arnold MA, Rosenblatt M, Beitens IZ, Martin JB, McArthur JW (1981): Physical conditioning facilitates the exercise-induced secretion of beta endorphin and beta lipotropin in women. *NEJM* 305:560.

107. Casper RF, Alapin-Rubillovita S (1985): Progestins increase endogenous opioid peptide activity in postmenopausal women. *J Clin Endocrinol Metab* 60:1:34–36.

108. Caspi E, Perpinial S, Reif A (1977): Incidence of malignancy in Jewish women with postmenopausal bleeding. *Isr J Med Sci* 13:299–304.

109. Cassileth BR, Lusk EJ, Strouse TB, Miller DS, Brown LL, Cross PA, Tenaglia AN (1984): Psychosocial status in chronic illness: a comparative analysis of six diagnostic groups. *NEJM* 311:506–511.

110. Castelli WP, Doyle JT, Gordon T (1977): HDL cholesterol and other lipids in coronary heart disease. *Circulation* 55:767–772.

111. Castelli W, Garrison R, Wilson P, Abbott R, Kalousdian S, Kannel W (1986): Incidence of coronary heart disease and lipoprotein cholesterol levels: the Framingham Study. *JAMA* 256:2835–2838.

112. Cattanach J (1985): Oestrogen deficiency after tubal ligation. *Lancet* April 13:847–849.

113. Cauley JA, LaPorte RE, Sandler RB, Schramm MM, Kriska AM (1987): Comparison of methods to measure physical activity in postmenopausal women, 1–3. *Am J Clin Nutr* 45:14–22.

114. Centers for Disease Control Surgical Sterilization Surveillance (1981): Hysterectomy in women aged 15–44. US Department of Health & Human Services, Centers for Disease Control, Center for Health Promotion & Education, Family Planning Evaluation Division, Atlanta, Georgia.

115. Centers for Disease Control (1981): Morbidity and Mortality Weekly Report, April 24. Hysterectomy in women aged 15–44, United States 1970–1978.

116. Centerwall BS (1981): Premenopausal hysterectomy and cardiovascular disease. *Am J Obstet Gynecol* 139:58–61.

117. Chakravarti S, Collins WP, Newton JR, Oram DH, Studd JWW (1977): Endocrine changes and symptomatology after oophorectomy in premenopausal women. *Br J Obstet Gynecol* 84:769–775.

118. Chakravarti S, Collins WP, Thom MH, Studd JWW (1979): Relation between plasma hormone profiles, symptoms and response to oestrogen treatment in women approaching the menopause. *Br Med J* 1:6169:983–985.

119. Chetkowski RJ, Meldrum DR, Steingold KA, Randle D, Lu JK, Eggena P, Hershman JM, Alkjaersig NK, Fletcher AP, Judd HL (1986): Biologic effects of transdermal estradiol. *NEJM* 314:25:1615–1620.

120. Chalmers J, Ho KC (1970): Geographical variations in senile osteoporosis: The association with physical activity. *J Bone & Joint Surgery* 52B:667–675.

121. Chalmers TC, Celano P, Sacks HS, Smith H (1983): Bias in treatment assignment in controlled clinical trials. *NEJM* 309:1358–1361.

122. Chambless D, Stein T, Sultan F, Williams A, Goldstein A, Hazzard-Lineberger M, Lifshitz P, Kelly L (1982): The pubococcygenus and female orgasm: a correlational study with normal subjects. *Arch Sex Behav* 11:479–490.

123. Chang RJ, Judd HL (1981): The ovary after menopause. *Clin Obstet Gynecol* 24:181–191.

124. Charbonnel B, Kremer M, Gerozissis K, Dray F (1982): Human cervical mucus contains large amounts of prostaglandins. *Fertil Steril* 38: 109–111.

125. Chatham MD, Eppler JH, Sauder LR, Green D, Kulle TJ (1987): Evaluation of the effects of vitamin C on ozone-induced broncho-constriction in normal subjects. Third Conference on Vitamin C. *Ann NY Acad Sci* 498:269–279.

126. Chauhan VPS, Chauhan A, Sarkar AK (1987): Effect of acute ascorbic acid deficiency on the plasma lipids & postheparin lipolytic activity in guinea pigs. Third Conference on Vitamin C. *Ann NY Acad Sci* 498:464–466.

127. Chen TL, Arnold L, Feldman D (1977): Glucocorticoid receptors and inhibition of bone cell growth in primary culture. *Endocrinol* 100: 619.

128. Cheek DB, Davis JE (1946): Pathologic findings in genital bleeding two or one year after spontaneous cessation of menstruation. *Am J Obstet Gynecol* 52:756–764.

129. Chen KTK, Schooley JL, Flam MS (1985): Peritoneal carcinomatosis after prophylactic oophorectomy in familial ovarian cancer syndrome. *Obstet Gynecol* 66:93S–94S.

130. Chen TI, Feldman D (1979): Glucocorticoid receptors and actions in subpopulations of cultured rat bone cells. *J Clin Invest* 63:750–758.

131. Chestnut CH, Baylink DJ, Nelp WB (1979): Calcitonin therapy in postmenopausal osteoporosis: preliminary results. Abstract. *Clin Res* 27:85A.

132. Chestnut CH (1981): Treatment of postmenopausal osteoporosis: some current concepts. *Scott Med J* 26:72–81.

133. Choo YC, Mak KC, Hsu C, Wong TS, Ma HK (1985): Postmenopausal uterine bleeding of nonorganic cause. *Obstet Gynecol* 66:2:225–228.

134. Christiansen C, Christensen MS (1981): Bone mass in post-menopausal women after withdrawal of oestrogen/gestagen replacement therapy. *Lancet* Feb 28:459–461.

135. Christiansen C, Christensen MS, Larsen NE, Transbol IB (1982): Pathophysiological mechanisms of estrogen effect on bone metabolism. Dose-response relationships in early postmenopausal women. *J Clin Endocrinol Metab* 55:1124–1130.

136. Christensen MS, Hagen C, Christiansen C, Transbol I (1982): Dose response evaluation of cyclic estrogen/gestagen in postmenopausal women: placebo controlled trial of its gynecological and metabolic actions. *Am J Obstet Gynecol* 144:873–879.

137. Christiansen C, Christensen MS, Hagen C, Stocklund KE, Transbol I (1981): Effects of natural estrogen/gestagen and thiazide on coronary risk factors in normal postmenopausal women. *Acta Obstet Gynecol Scand* 60:407–412.

138. Christiansen C, Riis BJ, Rodbro P (1987): Prediction of rapid bone loss in postmenopausal women. *Lancet* May 16:1106–1110.

139. Chu JY, Margen S, Costa FM (1975): Studies in calcium metabolism: effects of low calcium and variable intake on human calcium metabolism. *Am J Clin Nutr* 28:1028–1035.

140. Clanton TL, Dixon GF, Drake J, Gadek JE (1987): Effects of swim training on lung volumes & inspiratory muscle conditioning. *American Physiological Society* 39–46.

141. Claydon JR, Bell JY, Pollard P (1974): Menopausal flushing: double blind trial of a non-hormonal medication. *Br Med J* 1:409–412.

142. Cleophas TJM (1985): Statistical concepts fundamental to investigations. *NEJM* 17:1026.

143. Collet ME, Wertenburger GE, Fiske VM (1954): The effect of age upon the pattern of the menstrual cycle. *Fertil Steril* 5:437.

144. Colp R, Colp CR (1981): One of the least understood areas of sexuality. *Arch Intern Med* 141:424–425.

145. Coope J, Williams S, Patterson JS (1978): A study of the effectiveness of propanolol in menopausal hot flushes. *Br J Obstet Gynaecol* 85:6: 472–475.

146. Cooper RA, Strauss JF III (1984): Regulation of cell membrane cholesterol, in *Physiology of Membrane Fluidity.* Boca Raton, CRC Press.

147. Coppen A, Bishop M, Beard RJ, Baran GJR, Collins WP (1981): Hysterectomy, hormones & behavior. *Lancet* 126–128.

148. Coronary Drug Project Research Group (1970): The coronary drug project: initial findings leading to modifications of its research protocol. *JAMA* 214:1303–1313.

149. Costoff A, Mahesh VB (1975): Primordial follicles with normal oocytes in the ovaries of postmenopausal women. *J Am Geriatr Soc* 23:5:193–196.

150. Cottier C, Shapiro K, Julius S (1984): Treatment of mild hypertension with progressive muscle relaxation. *Arch Intern Med* 144:1954–1958.

151. Counseller VS, Hunt W, Haigler FH (1955): Carcinoma of the ovary following hysterectomy. *Am J Obstet Gynecol* 69:538–542.

152. Coutinho E, Darze E (1976): Spontaneous contractility and response of the human uterine cervix to prostaglandins F2 and E2 during the menstrual cycle. *Am J Obstet Gynecol* 126:224.

153. Craig GA, Jackson P (1975): Letter: Sexual life after vaginal hysterectomy. *Br Med J* 3:5975:97.

154. Crane MG, Harris JJ, Winsor W III (1971): Hypertension oral contraceptive agents and conjugated estrogens. *Ann Intern Med* 74:13–21.

155. Crilly RG, Marshall DH, Nordin BE (1979): Effect of age on plasma androstenedione concentration in oophorectomized women. *Clin Endocrinol (OF)* 10:2:199–201.

156. Crilly RG, Horsman A, Marshall DH, Nordin BEC (1978): Post menopausal and corticosteroid induced osteoporosis. *Front Horm Res* 5:53–75.

157. Crona N, Enk L, Mattsson LA, Samsioe G, Silfverstolpe G (1986): Progestogens & lipid metabolism. *Maturitas* 8:141–158.

158. Cullberg J (1972): Mood changes in menstrual symptoms with different gestagen/estrogen combinations: a double blind comparison with a placebo. *Acta Psychiatrica Scandinavica* Suppl 236:1–86.

159. Cummings JH, Hill MJ, Jivraj T, Houston H, Branch WJ, Jenkins DJA (1979): The effect of meat protein and dietary fiber on colonic function and metabolism; changes in bowel habit, bile acid excretion, and calcium absorption. *Am J Clin Nutr* 32:2086–2093.

160. Cummings JH (1978): Nutritional implications of dietary fiber. *Am J Clin Nutr* 31:(10 suppl):S21–S29.

161. Cummings J (1985): Cancer of the large bowel, chapter 9 in Trowell H, Burkett D, Heaton K (eds): *Dietary Fibre, Fibre-Depleted Foods and Disease.* New York, Academic Press, 161–189.

162. Cummings SR, Black D (1986): Should perimenopausal women be screened for osteoporosis? *Ann of Intern Med* 104:6:817–823.

163. Cutler WB, Karp J, Stine R (1988): Single photon absorptiometry imaging as a screen for diminished dual photon density measures. *Maturitas* 10:2: in press.

164. Cutler WB, García CR, McCoy N (1987): Perimenopausal sexuality. *Arch Sex Behav* 16:3:225–234.

165. Cutler WB, García CR, Krieger AM (1979): Infertility and age at first coitus: a possible association. *J Biosoc Sci* 11:425–432.

166. Cutler WB, García CR, Krieger AM (1979): Luteal phase defects: a possible relationship between short hyperthermic phase and sporadic sexual behavior in women. *Hormones & Behavior* 13:214–218.

167. Cutler WB, McCoy N, Davidson JM (1983): Steroids and hot flashes are associated during the perimenopause. *Neuroendo L* 5:3:185.

168. Cutler WB, García CR, Krieger AM (1979): Sexual behavior frequency and menstrual cycle length in mature premenopausal women. *Psychoneuroendocrinology* 4:297–309.

169. Cutler WB, García CR, Krieger AM (1980): Sporadic sexual behavior and menstrual cycle length in women. *Hormones & Behavior* 14:163–172.

170. Cutler WB, Preti G, Huggins GR, Erickson B, García CR (1985): Sexual behavior frequency and biphasic ovulatory type menstrual cycles. *Physiol Behav* 34:805–810.

171. Cutler W, McCoy N, García CR (1985): Perimenopausal sexuality. *Arch Sex Behav* 16:225–234.

172. Cutler WB, García CR, Edwards DA (1985): *Menopause: A Guide for Women and the Men Who Love Them.* New York, Norton.

173. Cutler WB, Preti G, Krieger A, Huggins GR, García CR, Lawley HJ (1986): Human axillary secretions influence women's menstrual cycles: the role of donor extract from men. *Hormones & Behavior* 20: 463-473.

174. Cutler WB, García CR (1984): *Medical Management of Menopause & Premenopause: Their Endocrinologic Basis.* Philadelphia, Lippincott.

175. Cutler WB (1980): Lunar and menstrual phase locking. *Am J Obstet Gynecol* 137:834–839.

176. Cutler WB, García CR (1980): The psychoneuroendocrinology of the ovulatory cycle of women. *Psychoneuroendocrinology* 5:2:89–111.

177. Cutler WB, García CR, Huggins GR, Preti G (1986): Sexual behavior & steroid levels among gynecologically mature premenopausal women. *Fertil Steril* 45:4:496–502.

178. Cutler WB, Schleidt W, Friedmann E, Preti G, Stine R (1987): Lunar influences on the reproductive cycle in women. *Human Biology* December.

179. Dalen JE, Hickler RB (1981): Oral contraceptives and cardiovascular disease. *Am Heart J* 101:626–639.

180. Dalen N, Lamke B, Wallgren A (1974): Bone-mineral losses in oophorectomized women. *J Bone Jt Surg* 56-A:1235.

181. Dalen N, Olsson KE (1974). Bone mineral content and physical activity. *Acta Orthop Scand* 45:170–174.

182. Dalton K (1957): Discussion on the aftermath of hysterectomy and oophorectomy. In section of General Practice, Proceedings of the Royal Society of Medicine 50:415–418.

183. Dambacher MA, Ittner J, Ruegsegger P (1984): Fluoride therapy of postmenopausal osteoporosis & its complications. *Osteoporosis* 39: 603–605.

184. Daniell HW (1976): Osteoporosis in the slender smoker. *Arch Intern Med* 136:298–304.

185. Daniell HW (1980): Estrogen receptors, breast cancer & smoking. *NEJM* 302:1478.

186. Davidson JM (1985): Sexual behavior and its relationship to ovarian hormones in the menopause. *Maturitas* 7:193–201.

187. Davidson JM, Camargo CA, Smith ER (1979): Effects of androgen on sexual behavior in hypogonadal men. *J Clin Endocrinol Metab* 48: 955–958.

188. Davidson JM, Chen JJ, Crapo L, Gray GD, Greenleaf WJ, Catania JA (1983): Hormonal changes and sexual function in aging men. *J Clin Endocrinol Metab* 57:41–93.

189. Davis M, Lawson DEM (1980): Assessment of plasma 25-hydroxyvitamin D response to ultraviolet irradiation over a controlled area in young and elderly subjects. *Clin Sci* 58:235–242.

190. Davis ME, Jones RJ, Jarolim C (1961): Long term estrogen substitution and atherosclerosis. *Am J Obstet Gynecol* 82:1003–1018.

191. Davis ME, Strandjord NM, Lanzl LH (1966): Estrogens and the aging process. *JAMA* 196:219–224.

192. Daw E (1974): Luteinising hormone changes in women undergoing artificial menopause. *Curr Med Res Opin* 2:256–259.

193. Dawson-Hughes B, Seligson FH, Hughes VA (1986): Effects of calcium carbonate and hydroxyapatite on zinc and iron retention in postmenopausal women. *Am J Clin Nutr* 44:83–88.

194. DeCherney A, Polan ML (1983): Hysteroscopic management of intrauterine lesions and intractable uterine bleeding. *Obstet Gynecol* 61: 392–396.

195. DeCherney AH, Schwartz PE (1986): Letters to the editor: Preservation of the ovary. *Fertil Steril* 45:738–739.

196. Deding A, Tougaard L, Jensen MK, Rodbro P (1977): Bone changes during prednisone treatment. *Acta Med Scand* 202:253–255.

197. Deftos LJ, Weisman MH (1980): Influence of age and sex on plasma calcitonin in human beings. *NEJM* 302:1351–1353.

198. Dement WC (1974): *Some Must Watch While Others Must Sleep.* San Francisco, Freeman.

199. DeNeef JC, Hollenbeck ZJR (1966): The fate of ovaries preserved at the time of hysterectomy. *Am J Obstet Gynec* 96:1088–1097.

200. DelJunco DJ, Annegers JF, Luthra HS, Coulam CB, Kurland LT (1986): Do oral contraceptives prevent rheumatoid arthritis? *JAMA* 254:14:1938–1941.

201. Denis R, Barnett JM, Forbes SE (1973): Diagnostic suction curettage. *Obstet Gynecol* 42:301–303.

202. Dennefors B, Janson P, Knutson F, Hamberger L (1980): Steroid production and responsiveness to gonadotropin in isolated stromal tissue of human postmenopausal ovaries. *Am J Obstet Gynecol* 136: 997–1002.

203. Dennerstein L, Burrows G (1986): Psychological effects of progestogens in the post-menopausal years. *Maturitas* 8:101–106.

204. Dennerstein L, Burrows G, Hyman G (1978): Menopausal hot flushes: a double blind comparison of placebo ethinyl oestradiol and norgestrel. *Br J Obstet Gynecol* 85:852–856.

205. Dennerstein L, Burrows GD, Hyman G (1979): Hormone therapy and affect. *Maturitas* 1:247–259.

206. Dennerstein L, Wood D, Burrows G (1977): Sexual response following hysterectomy and oophorectomy. *Obstet Gynecol* 49:92–96.

207. Dennerstein L, Burrows G, Wood C, Hyman G (1980): Hormones and sexuality: effect of estrogen and progestogen. *Obstet Gynecol* 56:316–322.

208. Dennerstein L, Laby B, Burrows G, Hyman G (1978): Headache and sex hormone therapy. *Headache* 18:146–153.

209. Dennerstein L, Wood C, Hudson B, Burrows G (1978): Clinical features and plasma hormone levels after surgical menopause. *Aust NZ J Obstet Gynecol* 18:3:202–205.

210. Depue RA, Slater JF, Wolfstetter-Kausch H, Klein D, Goplerud E, Farr D (1981): A behavioral paradigm for identifying persons at risk for bipolar depressive disorder: a conceptual framework and five validation studies. Monograph. *Journal of Abnormal Psychology* 90:381–437.

211. Dequeker J, De Proft G, Ferin J (1978): The effect of long term oestrogen treatment on the development of oesteoarthrosis at the small hand joints. *Maturitas* 1:27–30.

212. Dewhurst J (1983): Postmenopausal bleeding from benign causes. *Clinical Obstet Gynecol* 26:769–776.

213. Diamond MP, Daniell JF, Feste J, Surrey MW, McLaughlin DS, Friedman S, Vaughn WK, Martin DC (1987): Adhesion reformation and de novo adhesion formation after reproductive pelvic surgery. *Fertil Steril* 47:4:864–866.

214. Dicker R, Greenspan J, Strauss L, Cowart M, Scally M, Peterson H, DeStefano F, Rubin G, Ory H (1982): Complications of abdominal and vaginal hysterectomy among women of reproductive age in the United States. *Am J Obstet Gynecol* 144:841–848.

215. Dicker RG, Scally MJ, Greenspan JR, Layde PM, Maze JM (1982): Hysterectomy among women of reproductive age. *JAMA* 248:323–327.

216. Dixon G, Eurman P, Stern BE, Schwartz B, Rebar RW (1984): Hypothalamic function in amenorrheic runners. *Fertil Steril* 42:3:377–383.

217. Dizerega SG, Barber DL, Hodgen GD (1980): Endometriosis role of ovarian steroids in initiation, maintenance, and suppression. *Fertil Steril* 33:649–653.

218. Dmowski WP (1984): Current concepts in the management of endometriosis. *Acta Obstet Gynecol Scand* 123:279–311.

219. Donahue VC (1976): Elective hysterectomy: Pro and con. *NEJM* 295:264.

220. Doyle LI, Barclay DL, Duncan GW, Kirton KT (1971): Human luteal function as assessed by plasma progestin. *Am J Obstet Gynecol* 110:92–97.

221. Drinkwater BL, Nilson K, Chestnut CH, Bremner WJ, Shainholtz S, Southworth MB (1984): Bone mineral content of amenorrheic and eumenorrheic athletes. *NEJM* 311:5:277–281.

222. Drinkwater BL, Nilson K, Ott S, Chestnut CH III (1986): Bone mineral density after resumption of menses in amenorrheic athletes. *JAMA* 256:3:380–382.

223. Dupont WD, Page DL (1985): Risk factors for breast cancer in women with proliferative breast disease. *NEJM* 312:146–151.

224. Duursma SA, Bijlsma JWJ, van Paassen HC, Slootweg MC (1986): Oestrogens and bone metabolism: a hypothesis. *Maturitas* 8:1–6.

225. Eastwood M, Brydon WG (1985): Physiological effects of dietary fibre on the alimentary tract, in Trowell H, Burkett D, Heaton K (eds): *Dietary Fibre, Fibre-Depleted Foods and Disease.* New York, Academic Press, 105–132.

226. Eddy DM, Hasselblad V, McGivney W, Hendee W (1988): The value of mammography screening in women under age 50 years. *JAMA* 259L10:1512–1519.

227. Edgren RA (1980): Progestagens, in James R. Givens (ed): *Clinical Use of Sex Steroids.* Chicago, Year Book Medical Publishers, Inc. 1–29.

228. Edgren RA (1981): On oral contraceptive safety: cariovascular problems. *Int J Fertil* 26:4:241–244.

229. Elias AN, Iyer K, Pandian MR, Weathersbee P, Stone S, Trobis J (1986): $\beta$-endorphin/$\beta$-lipotropin release and gonadotropin secretion after acute exercise in normal males. *American Physiological Society* 2045–2049.

230. Englund DE, Johansson EDB (1980): Endometrial effect of oral estriol treatment in postmenopausal women. *Acta Obstet Gynecol Scand* 59:449–451.

231. Englund DE, Johansson EDB (1977): Pharmacokinetic and pharmacodynamic studies on estradiol valerianate administered orally to postmenopausal women. *Acta Obstet Gynecol Scand* 65:27–31.

232. Esdaile J, Horwitz R (1984): Resolving contradictory results in epidemiologic studies of oral contraceptives & rheumatoid arthritis. *Arth Rheum* 27 (suppl) B10.

233. Enstrom JE, Pauling L (1982): Mortality among health-conscious elderly Californians. *Proceedings of the National Academy of Sciences,* October, 6023.

234. Enk L, Silfverstolpe G, Crona N (1987): Dose and duration effects of oestradiol valerate on serum apolipoproteins A1 and B. *Maturitas* 9:1:33–40.

235. Ettinger M (1985): The relation of radius & spinal bone mineral in a mixed patient population. Presented at the Am Soc Bone Mineral Research, Washington DC, June.

236. Ettinger B, Genant H, Cann C (1987): Postmenopausal bone loss is prevented by treatment with low dosage estrogen with calcium. *Ann Int Med* 106:40–45.

237. Ettinger M, Mazess RB, Barden HS (1986): Insensitivity or peripheral measurement to spinal osteopenia. Presented at the Am Soc Bone Mineral Research, Anaheim, Calif, June.

238. Extein I, Pottash ALC, Gold MS (1982): A possible opioid receptor dysfunction in some depressive disorders. *NYAS* 398:113–119.

239. Facchinetti F, Martignoni E, Petraglia F, Sances MG, Nappi G, Genazzani AR (1987): Premenstrual fall of plasma β-endorphin in patients with premenstrual syndrome. *Fertil Steril* 47:4:570–573.

240. Fahraeus L, Larsson-Cohn U, Wallentin L (1983): L-norgestrel and progesterone have different influences on plasma lipoproteins. *Eur J Clin Invest* 13:447.

241. Fahraeus L, Wallentin L (1983): High density lipoprotein subfractions during oral and cutaneous administration of 17β estradiol to menopausal women. *J Clin Endoc Metab* 56:797.

242. Fahraeus L, Larsson-Cohn U (1982): Oestrogens, gonadotrophin & SHBG during oral and cutaneous administration of oestradiol-17β to menopausal women. *Acta Endocrinol* (Copenh) 101:592.

243. Farish E, Fletcher CD, Hart DM, et al (1983): A long-term study of the effects of norethisterone on lipoprotein metabolism in menopausal women. *Clin Chim Acta* 132:193.

244. Fedor-Freybergh P (1977): The influence of estrogens on the well being and mental performance in climacteric and postmenopausal women. *Acta Obstet Gynecol Scand* 64 (suppl) 1–66.

245. Feigen G, Fraser R, Dix C, Flynn C, Taylor K, Peterson N, Grant R (1980): Manipulation of the immune response by Na ascorbate and estradiol 17β. Abstract of 4th International Congress of Immunology, Paris, July 21–26.

246. Feigen GA, Fraser RC, Peterson NS (1978): Sex hormones and the immune response. II Perturbation of antibody production by estradiol 17β. *Int Arch Allergy Appl Immunol* 57:488–497.

247. Feigen G, Smith B, Fraser R, Dix C, Flynn C, Peterson N (1980): Ascorbate, estradiol and the immune response in guinea pigs. *Int J Immunopharmacology* 2:227.

248. Feldman JM, Postlethwaite RW, Glenn JF (1976): Hot flashes and sweats in men with testicular insufficiency. *Arch Intern Med* 136:5: 606–608.

249. Ferin M (1983): A talk to Ob/Gyn Dept., U. of P. Medical School, Phila., Pa, February 15, on his work on endogenous opiates and the menstrual cycle. Unpublished.

250. Ferin M, Wehrenberg WB, Lam NY, Alston EJ, Vande Wiele RL (1982): Effects and site of action of morphine on gonadotropin secretion in the female rhesus monkey. *Endocrinology* 111:1652–1656.

251. Fienberg R, Cohen RB (1965): A comparative histochemical study of the ovarian stromal lipid band, stromal theca cell and normal ovarian follicular apparatus. *Am J Obstet Gynecol* 92:958–969.

252. Fisher C, Schiavi RC, Edwards A (1979): Evaluation of nocturnal penile tumescence in the differential diagnosis of sexual impotence. *Arch Gen Psychiatry* 36:431–437.

253. Fisher N (1985): Cereals, milling and fibre, in Trowell H, Burkett D, Heaton K (eds): *Dietary Fibre, Fibre-Depleted Foods and Disease.* New York, Academic Press, 377–390.

254. Fluhmann CF (1956): A Classification of Disorders of Menstruation and Abnormal Uterine Hemorrhage, chapter 16 in *The Management of Menstrual Disorders.* Philadelphia, Saunders, 191–194.

255. Fluhmann CF (1956): Anovulatory Menstruation & Hyperplasia of the Endometrium, chapter 21 in *The Management of Menstrual Disorders.* Philadelphia, Saunders, 245–272.

256. Fluhmann CF (1956): Metrorrhagia, chapter 22 in *The Management of Menstrual Disorders.* Philadelphia, Saunders, 273–277.

257. Fluhmann CF (1956): Hypomenorrhea & Hypermenorrhea, chapter 20 in *The Management of Menstrual Disorders.* Philadelphia, Saunders, 231–244.

258. Fluhmann CF (1956): Secondary Amenorrhea, chapter 18 in *The Management of Menstrual Disorders.* Philadelphia, Saunders, 203–218.

259. Fluhmann CF (1956): Polymenorrhea & Oligomenorrhea, chapter 17 in *The Management of Menstrual Disorders.* Philadelphia, Saunders, 195–202.

260. Fluhmann CF (1956): Disorders of the Ovulatory Phase, chapter 13 in *The Management of Menstrual Disorders.* Philadelphia, Saunders, 153–160.

261. Fluhmann CF (1956): Menstrual Disorders of Adolescence, chapter 8 in *The Management of Menstrual Disorders.* Philadelphia, Saunders, 88–101.

262. Fluhmann CF (1956): The Management of Pathologic Uterine Bleeding, chapter 23 in *The Management of Menstrual Disorders.* Philadelphia, Saunders, 278–286.

263. Folegatti MR, Perazzini L, Serra MM (1987): Oophorectomy between the age of 45 and 50: effect on bone mineral content (BMC), in *Abstracts of 5th International Congress on the Menopause* 16:30.

264. Forney JP (1980): The effect of radical hysterectomy on bladder physiology. *Am J Obstet Gynecol* 138:374–382.

265. Fortney J (1987): *Family Planning Perspectives* 19:1.

266. Fotherby K (1974): Metabolism of synthetic steroids by animals and man. *Acta Endocrinol* 185:119–147.

267. Fox CA, Fox B (1971): Comparative study of coital physiology. *J Reprod Fert* 24:319–336.

268. Fox CA, Ismail AAA, Love DN, Kirkham KE, Loraine JA (1972): Studies on the relationship between plasma testosterone levels and human sexual activity. *J Endocrinol* 52:51–58.

269. Francis RM, Peacock M, Aaron JE, Selby PL, Taylor GA, Thompson J, Marshall DH, Horsman A (1986): Osteoporosis in hypogonadal men; role of decreased plasma 1,25-dihydroxyvitamin D, calcium malabsorption & low bone formation. *Bone* 7:261–268.

270. Fraser RC, Pavlovic S, Kurahara CG, Murata A, Peterson NS, Taylor KB, Feigen GA (1980): The effect of variations in vitamin C intake on the cellular immune response of guinea pigs. *Am J Clin Nutr* 33:839–847.

271. Fraser DR (1980): Regulation of the metabolism of vitamin D. *Physiol Rev* 60:551–613.

272. Freese MP, Levitt EE (1984): Relationships among intravaginal pressure, orgasmic function, parity factors and urinary leakage. *Arch Sex Beh* 13:3:261–268.

273. Freudenheim JL, Johnson NE, Smith EL (1986): Relationships between usual nutrient intake and bone-mineral content of women 35–65 years of age: longitudinal and cross-sectional analysis. *Am J Clin Nutr* 44:863–876.

274. Fribourg S (1982): Hysterectomy among women of reproductive age. *JAMA* 249:9.

275. Friden J, Sfakianos PN, Hargens AR (1986): Muscle soreness and intramuscular fluid pressure: comparison between eccentric and concentric load. *American Physiological Society* 61:2175–2179.

276. Friedman AJ, Ravnikar VA, Barbieri RL (1987): Serum steroid hormone profiles in postmenopausal smokers and nonsmokers. *Fertil Steril* 47:3:398–401.

277. Friedmann E (1981): Menstrual and lunar cycles. *Am J Obstet Gynecol* June 140:350.

278. Fucik RF, Kukreja SC, Hargis GK, Bowser EN, Henderson WJ, Williams GA (1975): Effect of glucocorticoids on function of the parathyroid glands in man. *J Clin Endoc Metab* 40:152–155.

279. Furman RH, Alaupovic P, Howard RP (1967): Effects of androgens and estrogens on serum lipids and the composition and concentration of serum lipoproteins in normolipemic and hyperlipidemic states. *Prog Biochem Pharmacol* 2:215–249.

280. Gallagher JC, Nordin BEC (1975): Effects of oestrogen and progesterone therapy on calcium metabolism in postmenopausal women. *Front Horm Res* 3:150–176.

281. Gallagher JC, Melton LJ, Riggs BL, Bergstrath E (1980): Epidemiology of fractures of the proximal femur in Rochester, Minnesota, USA. *Clin Orthop* 150:163–171.

282. Gallagher JC, Riggs BL, DeLuca HF (1978): Effect of age on calcium absorption and serum 1,25 OH2D. *Clin Res* 26:680A.

283. Gambrell RD (1987): *Estrogen Replacement Therapy.* Durant, Okla, Creative Informatics.

284. Gambrell RD (1986): Role of progestogens in the prevention of breast cancer. *Maturitas* 8:169–176.

285. Gambrell RD (1986): Prevention of endometrial cancer with progestogens. *Maturitas* 8:159–168.

286. Gambrell RD, Maier RC, Sanders BI (1983): Decreased incidence of breast cancer in postmenopausal estrogen-progestogen users. *Obstet Gynecol* 62:435–443.

287. Gambrell RD Jr (1982): Role of hormones in the etiology and prevention of endometrial and breast cancer. *Acta Obstet Gynecol Scand Suppl* 106:37–46.

288. Gambrell RD, Castaneda TA, Ricci CA (1978): Management of postmenopausal bleeding to prevent endometrial cancer. *Maturitas* 1:99–106.

289. Gambrell RD (1977): Postmenopausal Bleeding in Clinics in Obstetrics & Gynecology. Vol 4, No. 1, in Greenblatt R, Studd J (vol. eds): *The Menopause.* Philadelphia, Saunders.

290. Gambrell RD Jr, Massery FM, Castaneda TA, Ugenas AJ, Ricci CA, Wright JM (1980): Use of progestogen challenge test to reduce the risk of endometrial cancer. *Obstet Gynecol* 55:732–738.

291. Garns SM (1970): *The Earlier Gain and the Later Loss of Cortical Bone in Nutritional Pespective.* Springfield, Ill, Thomas, 69–137.

292. García CR, Cutler WB (1984): Preservation of the ovary: a reevaluation. *Fertil Steril* 42:510–514.

293. García CR, Cutler WB (1986): Letters to the Editor: Reply of the authors. *Fertil Steril* 45:740–741.

294. García CR, Tureck RW (1984): Submucosal leiomyomas and infertility. *Fertil Steril* 42:16–19.

295. García CR (1986): Multiple Myomectomy: a surgical procedure by Celso-Ramón García M.D., in *Obstetrics Gynecology Illustrated.* Kalamazoo, Mich, Learning Technology and Upjohn.

296. Garry PJ, VanderJagt DJ, Hunt WC (1987): Ascorbic acid intakes and plasma levels in healthy elderly. Third Conference on Vitamin C. *Ann NY Acad Sci* 498:90–99.

297. Gath DH (1980): Psychiatric aspects of hysterectomy, in Robins L (ed): *The Social Consequences of Psychiatric Illness.* New York, Brunner/Mazel.

298. Genant HK, Cann CE, Ettinger B, Gordan GS (1982): Quantitative computed tomography of vertebral spongiosa: a sensitive method for detecting early bone loss after oophorectomy. *Ann Int Med* 97:699–705.

299. Genant HK, Cann CE (1981): Vertebral mineral determination using quantitative computed tomography, in DeLuca HF, Frost HM, Jee WSS, Johnston CC, Parfitt AM (eds): *Osteoporosis: Recent Advances in Pathogenesis and Treatment.* Baltimore, University Park Press, 37–47.

300. Genazzani AR, Facchinetti F, Ricci-Danero MG, Parrini D, Petraglia F, LaRosa R, D'Antona N (1981): Beta-lipotropin & beta-endorphin in physiological & surgical menopause. *J Endocrinol Invest* 4:375–378.

301. Gennari C (1987): The rationale for the use of calcitonin in osteoporotic women. Fifth International Congress on the Menopause, Sorrento, Italy, April.

302. Geola F, Frumar AN, Tataryn I, Lu K, Hershman J, Eggena P, Sambhi M, Hudd H (1980): Biological effects of various doses of conjugated equine estrogens in postmenopausal women. *J Clin Endocrinol Metab* 51:620–625.

303. Gibbons WE, Moyer DL, Lobo RA, Roy S, Mishell DR (1986): Biochemical & histologic effects of sequential estrogen/progestin therapy on the endometrium of postmenopausal women. *Am J Obstet Gynecol* 154:2:456–461.

304. Gey KF, Stahelin HB, Puska P, Evans A (1987): Relationship of plasma level of vitamin C to mortality from ischemic heart disease. Third Conference on Vitamin C. *Ann NY Acad Sci* 498:110–123.

305. Geusens P, Dequeker J, Verstraeten A, Nijs J, VanHolsbeeck M (1986): Bone mineral content, cortical thickness and fracture rate in osteoporotic women after withdrawal of treatment with nandrolone decanoate, 1-alpha hydroxyvitamin D₃, or intermittent calcium infusions. *Maturitas* 8:281–289.

306. Ginsburg J (1983): Flushes in women—and men. *Br Med J* 287:242–243.

307. Ginsburg J, O'Reilly B, Swinhoe J (1985): Effect of oral clonidine on human cardiovascular responsiveness: a possible explanation of the therapeutic action of the drug in menopausal flushing and migraine. *Br J Obstet/Gynecol* 92:1169–1175.

308. Ginsburg J, O'Reilly B (1983): Climacteric flushing in a man. *Br Med J* 287:262–263.

309. Glembotski CC (1987): The role of ascorbic acid in the biosynthesis of the neuroendocrine peptides a-MSH and TRH. Third Conference on Vitamin C. *Ann NY Acad Sci* 498:54–62.

310. Glueck CJ, Gordon DJ, Nelson JJ, Davis, Tyroler HA (1986): Dietary and other correlates of changes in total and low density lipoprotein cholesterol in hypercholesterolemic men: the lipid research clinics coronary primary prevention trial. *Am J Clin Nutr* 44:489–500.

311. Goebelsmann U, Mashchak A, Mishell DR (1985): Comparison of hepatic impact of oral & vaginal administration of ethinyl estradiol. *J Obstet & Gynecol* 151:868–877.

312. Goldin BR, Adlercreutz H, Gorbach SL, Woods MN, Dwyer JT, Conlon T, Bohn E, Gershoff SN (1986): The relationship between estrogen levels and diets of Caucasian American and Oriental immigrant women. *Am J Clin Nutr* 44:945–953.

313. Goldin BR, Adlercreutz H, Gorbach SL, et al (1982): Estrogen excretion patterns and plasma levels in vegetarian and omnivorous women. *NEJM* 307:1542–1547.

314. Gordon H, Logue M (1985): Perineal muscle function after childbirth. *Lancet* 123–125.

315. Gordon T, Castelli WP, Hjortland MP, Kannel WB, Dawber TR (1977): The Framingham study: High density lipoprotein as a protective factor against coronary heart disease. *Am J Med* 62:707–714.

316. Gordon T, Kanel W, Hjortland M, McNamara P (1978): Menopause and coronary heart disease: the Framingham study. *Ann Int Med* 89:157–161.

317. Gordon WE, Hermann HW, Hunter DC (1979): Treatment of atrophic vaginitis in postmenopausal women with micronized estradiol cream—a follow up study. *J Ky Med Assoc* 77: 7:337–319.

318. Gori G (1977): Diet & cancer. *J Am Diet Assoc* 71:375–379.

319. Gossard D, DeBusk RF (1986): Effects of low- and high-intensity homebased exercise training on functional capacity in healthy middle-aged men. *JAMA* 256:3:401.

320. Graber B, Kline-Graber G (1979): Female orgasm: role of the pubococcygeus muscle. *J Clin Psych* 40:348–351.

321. Greenberg M (1981): Hystrectomy, hormones & behavior. Letter. *Lancet* Feb 21: 449.

322. Greenblatt RB, Leng JJ (1972): Factors influencing sexual behavior. *J Am Geriatr Soc* 20:49–54.

323. Greenblatt RB, Perez D (1974): Problems of libido in the elderly, in Greenblatt RB, Mahesh VB, McDonough PG (eds): *The Menopausal Syndrome.* New York, Medcom Press.

324. Greene JG (1976): A factor analytic study of climacteric symptoms. *J Psychosomatic Research* 20:5:425–430.

325. Greenhill JP (1973): *The Yearbook of Obstetrics & Gynecology.* Chicago, Year Book Medical Publishers, Inc.

326. Greenspan SL, Neer RM, Ridgway EC, Klibanski A (1986): Osteoporosis in men with hyperprolactinemic hypogonadism. *Ann of Intern Med* 104:777–782.

327. Grodin JM, Siiteri PK, Macdonald PC (1973): Source of estrogen production in postmenopausal women. *J Clin Endocr Metab* 36:207.

328. Grogan RH (1967): Reappraisal of residual ovaries. *Am J Obstet Gynecol* 97:124–129.

329. Gruber HE, Ivey JL, Baylink DJ, Matthews M, Nelp WB, Sisom K, Chestnut CH (1984): Long-term calcitonin therapy in post-menopausal osteoporosis. *Metabolism Clinical & Experimental* 33:4:295–303.

330. Grubb SA, Jacobson PC, Awbrey BJ, McCartney WH, Vincent IM, Talmage RV (1984): Bone density in osteopenic women: a modified

distal radius density measurement procedure to develop an "at risk" value for use in screening women. *Journal of Orthopaedic Research* 2:322–327.

331. Gruis ML, Wagner NN (1979): Sexuality during the climacteric. *Postgrad Med J* 65:5:197–207.

332. Guraya S (1976): Histochemical observations on the corpus luteum atreticum of the human postmenopausal ovary with reference to steroid hormone synthesis. *Arch It Anat E Embriol* 56:189–202.

333. Gurpide E, Gusberg SB, Tseng L (1976): Oestradiol binding and metabolism in human endometrial hyperplasia & adenocarcinoma. *J Steroid Biochem* 7:891–896.

334. Gusberg SB (1975): A strategy for the control of endometrial cancer. *Proc Royal Soc of Med* 68:163–168.

335. Gusberg SB (1976): The individual at high risk for endometrial carcinoma. *Am J Obstet Gynecol* 126:535–542.

336. Gusberg SB, Kaplan AL (1963): Adenomatous hyperplasia as stage O carcinoma of the endometrium. *Am J Obstet Gynecol* 87:662–678.

337. Gustafson A, Svanborg A (1972): Gonadal steroid effects on plasma lipoproteins and individual phospholipids. *J Clin Endoc Metab* 35:203–207.

338. Hadley EC (1986): Bladder training and related therapies for urinary incontinence in older people. *JAMA* 256:3:372–379.

339. Hafetz ESE (1973): The comparative anatomy of the mammalian cervix, in Blandau R, Moghissi K (eds): *The Biology of the Cervix.* Chicago, University of Chicago Press.

340. Hagen C, Christiansen C, Christensen MS, Transbol I (1982): Climacteric symptoms, fat mass, and plasma concentrations of LH, FSH, Prl, Oestradiol-17$\beta$ and androstenedione in the early postmenopausal period. *Acta Endocrinol* 100:4:486–491.

341. Hagstad A, Janson PO, Lindstedt G (1985): Gynaecological history, complaints & examinations in a middle-aged population. *Maturitas* 7:115–128.

342. Hagstad A, Johansson S, Wilhelmsson C, Janson PO (1985): Gynaecology of middle aged women—menstrual & reproductive histories. *Maturitas* 7:99–113.

343. Hahn TJ, Boisseau VC, Avioli LV (1974): Effect of chronic corticosteroid administration on diaphyseal & metaphyseal bone mass. *J Clin Endoc Metab* 39:274–282.

344. Hall FM, Davis MA, Baran DT (1987): Sounding board: bone mineral screening for osteoporosis. *NEJM* 316:212–214.

345. Hallberg L, Brune M, Rossander-Hulthen L (1987): Is there a physiological role of vitamin C in iron absorption? Third Conference on Vitamin C. *Ann NY Acad Sci* 498:324–332.

346. Hallstrom T (1977): Sexuality in the climacteric. *Clinics in Obstetrics & Gynecology* 4:227–239.

347. Hammond CB, Jelovsek FR, Lee KL, Creasman WT, Parker RT (1979): Effects of long term estrogen replacement therapy. II Neoplasia. *Am J Obstet Gynecol* 133:537–547.

348. Hammond CB, Ory SJ (1982): Endocrine problems in the menopause. *Clinical Obstet Gynecol* 25:1.

349. Hammond DC (1984): Screening for sexual dysfunction. *Clinical Obstet Gynecol* 27:732–737.

350. Hamou J, Taylor PJ (1982): Panoramic, contact & microcolpohysteroscopy in gynecologic practice. *Current Problems in Obstet Gynecol* 1–71.

351. Hamptom PT, Tarnasky WG (1974): Hysterectomy and tubal ligation: a comparison of the psychological aftermath. *Am J Obstet Gynecol* 119(7):949–952.

352. Harman SM, Tsitouras PD (1980): Reproductive hormones in aging men. 1. measurement of sex steroids, basal luteinizing hormone, and leydig cell response to human chorionic gonadotropin. *J Clin Endocrinol Metab* 51:35–40.

353. Harris GW (1955): *Neural Control of the Pituitary Gland.* Plymouth, England, Latimer Trend.

354. Haspels AA, Bennink HJ, Van Keep PA, Schreurs WH (1975): Estrogens & vitamin $B_6$. *Front Horm Res* 3:199–207.

355. Haspels AA, Coelingh Bennink HJT, Schreurs WHP (1978): Disturbance of tryptophan metabolism and its correction during oestrogen treatment in postmenopausal women. *Maturitas* 1:15–20.

356. Hasselquist M, Goldberg N, Schroeter A, Spelsberg T (1980): Isolation and characterization of the estrogen receptor in human skin. *J Clin Endoc Metab* 50:76–82.

357. Hatch R, Rosenfield RL, Kim MH, Tredway D (1981): Hirsutism: implications, etiology and management. *Am J Obstet Gynecol* 140:815–830.

358. Hathcock EW, Williams GA, Englehardt SM, Murphy AL (1974): Office aspiration curettage of the endometrium. *Am J Obstet Gynecol* 120:205–213.

359. Haynes SG, Feinleib M (1982): Women, work and coronary heart disease: results from the Framingham 10-year follow up study, in Berman PW, Ramey ER (eds): *Women: A Developmental Perspective.* US Dept Health & Human Services NIH Publication No 82-2298.

360. Heaney RP, Recker RR (1986): Distribution of calcium absorption in middle-aged women. *Am J Clin Nutr* 43:299–305.

361. Heaney RP, Recker RR (1982): Effects of nitrogen, phosphorus & caffeine on calcium balance in women. *J Lab Clin Med* 99:46–56.

362. Heaney RP, Recker RR, Saville PD (1977): Calcium balance and calcium requirements in middle aged women. *Am J Clin Nutr* 30:1603–1611.

363. Heaney RP, Recker RR, Saville PD (1978): Menopausal changes in calcium balance performance. *J Lab Clin Med* 92:953–963.

364. Heaney RP, Gallagher JC, Johnston CC, Neer R, Parfitt AM, Chir E, Wheldon GD (1982): Calcium nutrition and bone health in the elderly. *Am J Clin Nutr* 36:986–1013.

365. Heaney RP (1974): Pathophysiology of osteoporosis: implication for treatment. *Tex Med* 70:37–45.

366. Heath H, Sizemore G (1977): Plasma calcitonin in normal man. *Clin Invest* 60:1135–1140.

367. Heaton K (1985): Other nutritional implications: energy and micronutrients, in Trowell H, Burkett D, Heaton K (eds): *Dietary Fibre, Fibre-Depleted Foods and Disease.* New York, Academic Press, 391–402.

368. Hegsted M, Linkswiler HM (1981): Long term effects of level of protein intake on calcium metabolism in young adult women. *J Nutr* 3:244–251.

369. Hegsted M, Schuette SA, Zemel MB, Linkswiler HM (1981): Urinary calcium and calcium balance in young men as affected by level of protein and phosphorous intake. *J Nutr* 3:553–562.

370. Heaton K (1985): Gallstones, in Trowell H, Burkett D, Heaton K (eds): *Dietary Fibre, Fibre-Depleted Foods and Disease.* New York, Academic Press, 289–304.

371. Hegsted DM (1986): Serum-cholesterol response to dietary cholesterol: a re-evaluation. *Am J Clin Nutr* 44:299–305.

372. Heimer GM & Englund DE (1986): Plasma oestriol following vaginal administration: morning versus evening insertion and influence of food. *Maturitas* 8:239–243.

373. Hellberg D, Nilsson S (1987): Pilot study to evaluate a new regimen to treat climacteric complaints with cyclic combined oestradiol valerate/medroxyprogesterone acetate (short communication). *Maturitas* 9:1:103–108.

374. Heller RF, Jacobs HS, Vermeulen A, Deslypere JP (1981): Androgens, oestrogens and coronary heart disease. *Br Med J* 282:439–440.

375. Hellhammer DH, Hubert W, Schurmeyer T (1985): Changes in saliva testosterone after psychological stimulation in men. *Psychoneuroendocrinology* 10:1:77–81.

376. Hempel Von E, Kriester A, Freesmeyer E, Walter W (1979): Prospektive studie zur osteoporose naeh bilater ovarektomie mit und ohne postoperative ostrogenprophylaxe. *Zentralblatt fur gynakologie* 101: 309–319.

377. Hendy MS, Cockrill B, Burge PS (1985): The effects of naloxone infusion & stellate ganglion blockade on hot flushes in the human male. *Maturitas* 7:169–174.

378. Herold PM, Kinsella JE (1986): Fish oil consumption and decreased risk of cardiovascular disease: a comparison of findings from animal and human feeding trials. *Am J Clin Nutr* 43:566–598.

379. Herold E, Mottin J, Sabry Z (1979): Effect of vitamin E on human sexual functioning. *Archives of Sexual Behavior* 8:397–403.

380. Higano N, Cohen WD, Robinson RW (1959): Effects of sex steroids on lipids. *Ann NY Acad Sci* 72:970–979.

381. Hillman LC, Peters SG, Fisher CA, Pomare EW (1985): The effects of the fiber components pectin, cellulose and lignin on serum cholesterol levels. *Am J Clin Nutr* 42:207–213.

382. Hirvonen E, Lipasti A, Malkonen M, Karkkainen J, Nuntila J, Timonen H, Manninen V (1987): Clinical and lipid metabolic effects of unopposed oestrogen and two oestrogen-progestogen regimens in postmenopausal women. *Maturitas* 9:1:69–80.

383. Hirvonen E, Malkonen M, Manninen V (1980): Effects of different progestogens on lipoproteins during postmenopausal replacement therapy. *NEJM* 304:560–563.

384. Hodgson SF, Dickson ER, Wahner HW, Johnson KA, Mann KG, Riggs BL (1985): Bone loss and reduced osteoblast function in primary biliary cirrhosis. *Annals of Internal Medicine* 103:6:855–860.

385. Hofmeister FJ, Barbo DM (1964): Cancer detection in private gynecologic practice: a concluding study. *Obstet Gynecol* 23:386–391.

386. Hofmeister FJ (1974): Endometrial biopsy: another look. *Am J Obstet Gynecol* 119:773–777.

387. Hoikka V, Alhava EM, Aro A, Karjalalenen V (1980): Treatment of osteoporosis with 1-alpha-hydroxy-ocholecalciferal. *Acta Med Scand* 207:221–224.

388. Holmberg S, Conradi P, Kalen R, Thorngren K (1986): Mortality after cervical hip fracture: 3002 patients followed for 6 years. *Acta Orthop Scand* 57:8–11.

389. Holst J, Cajander S, von Schoultz B (1987): Endometrial effects of a continuous percutaneous oestrogen/low dose oral progestogen regimen for climacteric complaints. *Maturitas* 9:1:63–68.

390. Honore LH (1980): Increased incidence of symptomatic cholesterol cholelithiasis in perimenopausal women receiving estrogen replacement therapy. *J Reprod Med* 15:187–190.

391. Hoon PW (1984): Physiologic assessment of sexual response in women: the unfulfilled promise. *Clin Ob/Gyn* 27:767–780.

392. Hoover R, Gray LA, Cole P, MacMahom B (1976): Menopausal estrogens and breast cancer. *NEJM* 295:8:401–405.

393. Horsman A, Gallagher JC, Simpson M, Nordin BEC (1977): Prospective trial of oestrogen and calcium in postmenopausal women. *Br Med J* 2:789–792.

394. Horsman A, Jones M, Francis R, Nordin C (1983): The effect of estrogen dose on postmenopausal bone loss. *NEJM* 309:1405–1407.

395. Horsman A, Simpson M, Kirby PA (1977): Non-linear bone loss in oophorectomized women. *Br J Radiol* 50:5:504.

396. Horwitz RI, Feinstein AR, Horwitz SM, Robboy SJ (1981): Necropsy diagnosis of endometrial cancer and detection bias in case/control studies. *Lancet,* July 11, 66–67.

397. Horwitz RI, Feinstein AR (1978): Alternative analytic methods for case control studies of estrogens and endometrial cancer. *NEJM* 299:1089–1094.

398. Houston MC (1986): Review: Sodium & Hypertension. *Arch Intern Med* 146:179–185.

399. Huffman JW, Dewhurst CJ, Capravio VJ (eds) (1981): *The Gynecology of Childhood and Adolescence.* Philadelphia, Saunders.

400. Hughes ES, Csermely TV, Jacobs RD, O'Hern PA (1974): Biochemical parameters of abnormal endometrium. *Gynecol Oncol* 2:205–220.

401. Hunt JN, Johnson C (1983): Relation between gastric secretion of acid and urinary excretion of calcium after oral supplements of calcium. *Digestive Diseases & Sciences* 28:5:417–421.

402. Hunter DJ, Julier D, Franklin M, Green E (1977): Plasma levels of estrogen, luteinizing hormone, and follicle-stimulating hormone following castration and estradiol implant. *Obstet Gynecol* 49:2:180–185.

403. Hutchinson TA, Polansky SM, Feinstein AR (1979): Post-menopausal estrogens protect against fractures of hip and distal radius, a case-control study. *Lancet* 2:705–709.

404. Imparato E, Marino L, Sallusto A (1973): Use of an estrogen-progesterone-testosterone combination in control of the menopausal syndrome: double-blind clinical studies. *Ann Obstet Ginecol Med Perinat* 94:5:361–372.

405. Inglis RM, Weir JH (1976): Endometrial suction biopsy: appraisal of a new instrument. *Am J Obstet Gynecol* 125:1070–1072.

406. Ismail AAA, Harkness RA (1967): Urinary testosterone excretion in men in normal and pathological conditions. *Acta Endocrinol* 56:469–480.

407. Iversen OE, Segadal E (1985): The value of endometrial cytology: a comparative study of the Gravlee jet-washer, Isaacs cell sampler, & Endoscann versus curettage in 600 patients. *Obstet & Gynecol Survey* 40:1:14–20.

408. Jacobs HS, Hutton JD, James VHT (1981): Hormonal changes after the menopause and during hormone replacement therapy, in Coutts JRT (ed): *Functional Morphology of the Human Ovary*. Baltimore, University Park Press.

409. Jacobs HS, Hutton JD, Murray MAF, James VHT (1977): Plasma hormone profiles in post-menopausal women before and during oestrogen therapy. *Brit J Obstet Gynaec* 84:314.

410. Jacob RA, Omaye ST, Skala JH, Leggott PJ, Rothman DL, Murray PA (1987): Experimental vitamin C depletion and supplementation in young men: nutrient interactions and dental health effects. Third Conference on Vitamin C. *Ann NY Acad Sci* 498:333–346.

411. Jacobson PC, Beaver W, Grubb SA, Taft TN, Talmage RV (1984): Bone density in women: college athletes and older athletic women. *Journal of Orthopaedic Research* 2:328–332.

412. Jacques PF, Hartz SC, McGandy RB, Jacob RA, Russell RM (1987): Vitamin C and blood lipoproteins in an elderly population. Third Conference on Vitamin C. *Ann NY Acad Sci* 498:100–109.

413. James P (1985): Obesity: the interaction of environment and agenetic predisposition, in Trowell H, Burkett D, Heaton K (eds): *Dietary Fibre, Fibre-Depleted Foods and Disease.* New York, Academic Press, 249–261.

414. Janson PO, Jansson I (1977): The acute effect of hysterectomy on ovarian blood flow. *Am J Obstet Gynecol* 127:4:349–352.

415. Jaszmann LJB (1973): Epidemiology of climacteric and post climacteric complaints. *Frontiers Hormone Research* 2:22–34.

416. Jee WSS, Clark I (1981): Glucocorticoid induced osteoporosis, in DeLuca HF, Frost HM, Jee WSS, Johnston CC, Parfitt AM (eds): *Osteoporosis: Recent Advances in Pathogenesis and Treatment.* Baltimore, University Park Press, 331–342.

417. Jennings S, Mazaik C, McKinlay S (1984): Women & work: an investigation of the association between health & employment status in middle-aged women. *Soc Sci Med* 19:4:423–431.

417a. Jensen J, Christiansen C, Rodbro P (1986): Oestrogen-progestogen replacement therapy changes body composition in early post-menopausal women. *Maturitas* 8:209–216.

418. Jensen J, Christiansen C, Rodbro P (1985): Cigarette smoking serum estrogens & bone loss during hormone replacement therapy early after menopause. *NEJM* 313:16:973–975.

419. Jick H, Dinan B, Herman R, Rothman K (1978): Myocardial infarction and other vascular diseases in young women. *JAMA* 240:2548–2552.

420. Jick H, Dinan B, Rothman K (1978): Noncontraceptive estrogens and non fatal myocardial infarctions. *JAMA* 239:1407–1408.

421. Jick H, Porter J, Morrison AS (1977): Relation between smoking and age of natural menopause: report from the Boston Collaborative Drug Surveillance Program. Boston University Medical Center. *Lancet* 1 (8026):1354–1355.

422. Jick SS, Walker AM, Jick H (1986): Conjugated estrogens and fibrocystic breast disease. *Am J Epidemiology* 124:5:746–751

423. Johansson BW, Jaij L, Kullander S, Lenner HC, Svanberg L, Astedt B (1975): On some late effects of bilateral oophorectomy in the age range of 15–20 years. *Acta Obstet Gynecol Scand* 54:449–461.

424. Johnston CC Jr, Hui SL, Witt RM, et al (1985): Early menopausal changes in bone mass & sex steroids. *J Clin Endocrinol Metab* 61:905–911.

425. Johnston CC, Norton JA, Khairi RA, Longcope C (1978): Age related bone loss. *Osteoporosis* 2:91–100.

426. Johnson EJ, Marlett JA (1986): A simple method to estimate neutral detergent fiber content of typical daily menus. *Am J Clin Nutr* 44:127–134.

427. Johnson J (1982): Tubal sterilization and hysterectomy. *Family Planning Perspectives* 14:28–30.

428. Johnson L (1986): Spermatogenesis & aging in the human. *J Androl* 7:331–354.

429. Johnson L, Petty CS, Neaves WB (1986): Age-related variation in seminiferous tubules in men: a stereologic evaluation. *J Androl* 7:316–322.

430. Jones GS (1966): Sexual difficulties after 50. *Obstet & Gynecol Survey* "Gynecologic comments" section 21:628.

431. Jones KP, Ravnikar V, Schiff I (1985): A preliminary evaluation of the effect of lofexidine on vasomotor flushes in post-menopausal women. *Maturitas* 7:135–139.

432. Judd HL, Lucas WE, Yen S (1974): Effect of oophorectomy on circulating testosterone and androstenedione levels in patients with endometrial cancer. *Am J Obstet Gynecol* 38:793–798.

433. Judd HL (1976): Hormonal dynamics associated with the menopause. *Clinical Obstetrics & Gynecology* 19:775–788.

434. Judd HL, Cleary RE, Creasman WT, Figge DC, Kase N, Rosenwaks Z, Tagatz GE (1981): Estrogen replacement therapy. *Obstet Gynecol* 3:267–275.

435. Judd HL, Davidson BJ, Frumar AM, Shamonki IM, Lagasse LD, Ballon SC (1980): Serum androgens and estrogens in post-menopausal women with and without endometrial cancer. *Am J Obstet Gynecol* 135:859–871.

436. Judd HL, Judd GE, Lucas WE, Yen SSC (1974): Endocrine function of postmenopausal ovary: concentration of androgens and estrogens in ovarian and peripheral vein blood. *J Clin Endoc Metab* 39:1020.

437. Kaminsky LA, Knowlton RG, Perkins RM, Hetzler RK (1986): Relationships of aerobic capacity and percent body fat with plasma free fatty acid following walking. *Am J Clin Nutr* 44:603–609.

438. Kannel WB, Castelli WP, Gordon T, McNamara P (1971): Serum cholesterol, lipoproteins and the risk of coronary heart disease. *Ann Intern Med* 174:1–12.

439. Kaplan E (1977): Recurrent postmenopausal bleeding. *S Afr Med J* 52:1121–1123.

440. Kaplan HS (S1980): Sexual medicine, a progress report. *Arch Intern Med* 140:1575–1576.

441. Kaplan HS (1974): *The New Sex Therapy.* New York, Brunner Mazel, 111–114.

442. Karanja N, Morris CD, Illingworth DR, McCarron DA (1987): Plasma lipids and hypertension: response to calcium supplementation. *Am J Clin Nutr* 45:60–65.

443. Katz S, Branch LG, Branson MH, Papsidero JA, Beck JC, Greer DS (1983): Active life expectancy. *NEJM* 309:1218–1224.

444. Kav-Venaki S, Zakham L (1983): Psychological effects of hysterectomy in premenopausal women. *J Psychosomatic Obstet Gynaecol* 2:76–80.

445. Kay CR (1982): Progestogens and arterial disease-evidence from the Royal College of General Practitioners' study. *Am J Obstet Gynecol* 142:762–765.

446. Kay CR (1978): Logistics of study on hormone therapy in the climacteric. *Postgrad Med J* 54:2:92–94.

447. Kegel AH (1956): Stress incontinence of urine in women: physiologic treatment. *J Int Col of Surgeons* April:487–499.

448. Kegel AM (1951): Physiologic therapy for urinary stress incontinence. *JAMA* 146:915–917.

449. Keirse MJNC (1973): Aetiology of post menopausal bleeding. *Postgrad Med J* 49:344–348.

450. Kelley RM, Baker WH (1961): Progestational agents in the treatment of carcinoma of the endometrium. *NEJM* 264:216.

451. Kerr-Wilson RHJ, Shingleton HM, Orr JW, Hatch KD (1984): The use of ultrasound & computed tomography scanning in the management of gynecologic cancer patients. *Obstet Gynecol* 18:54:656–658.

452. Kern F (1978): Cholesterol gallstones. *Clinical Conference* 75:514–522.

453. Keys A (1986): Serum cholesterol response to dietary cholesterol. *Am J Clin Nutr* 44:309–311.

454. Kicovic PM, Cortes-Prieto J, Milojevic S, Haspels AA, Aljinovic A (1980): The treatment of postmenopausal vaginal atrophy with oves-

tin vaginal cream or suppositories: clinical, endocrinological and safety aspects. *Maturitas* 2:275–282.

455. Khan-Dawood FS (1987): Human corpus luteum: immunocytochemical localization of epidermal growth factor. *Fertil Steril* 47:6:916–919.

456. Kilkku P, Gronroos M (1982): Preoperative electrocoagulation of the endocervical mucosa & later carcinoma of the cervical stump. *Acta Obstet Gynecol Scand* 61:265.

457. Kilkku P, Hirvonen T, Gronroos M (1981): Supravaginal uterine amputation vs. abdominal hysterectomy: the effects on urinary symptoms with special reference to pollakisuria, nocturia & dysuria. *Maturitas* 3:197.

458. Kilkku P (1983): Supravaginal uterine amputation vs. hysterectomy: effects on coital frequency & dyspareunia. *Acta Obstet Gynecol Scand* 62:141–145.

459. Kilkku P, Gronroos M, Hirvonen T, Rauramo L (1983): Supravaginal uterine amputation vs. hysterectomy: effects on libido & orgasm. *Acta Ob Gyn Scand* 62:147–151.

460. Kim Y, Linkswiler HM (1979): Effect of level of protein intake on calcium metabolism and on parathyroid and renal function in the adult human male. *J Nutr* 109:1399–1404.

461. Kimberg DV, Baerg RD, Gershone E, Graudusius RT (1971): Effect of cortisone treatment on the active transport of calcium by the small intestine. *J Clin Invest* 50:1309–1321.

462. Kinsey A, Pomeroy W, Martin C (1953): *Sexual Behavior in the Human Female.* Philadelphia, Saunders.

463. Klaiber EL, Broverman DM, Vogel W, Kobayashi Y, Moriarty D (1972): Effects of estrogen therapy on plasma MAO activity and EEG driving responses in depressed women. *Am J Psychiatry* 128:1492–1498.

464. Klaiber EL, Kobayashi Y, Broverman DM, Hall F (1971): Plasma monoamine oxidase activity in regularly menstruating women and in amenorrheic women receiving cyclic treatment with estrogens and a progestin. *J Clin Endocrinol Metab* 33:630–638.

465. Knopp RH, Walden CE, Wahl PW, Hoover JJ (1982): Effects of oral contraceptives on lipoprotein triglycerides and cholesterol: relationships to estrogen and progestin potency. *Am J Obstet Gynecol* 1421:725–731.

466. Knussman R, Christiansen K, Couwenbergs C (1986): Relations between sex hormone levels & sexual behavior in men. *Arch Sex Behav* 15:5:429–445.

467. Komindr S, Nichoalds GE, Kitabchi AE (1987): Bimodal effects of megadose vitamin C on adrenal steroid production in man: an in vivo study. Third Conference on Vitamin C. *Ann NY Acad Sci* 498:487–490.

468. Korenman SG, Sherman BM, Korenman JC (1978): Reproductive hormone function: the perimenopausal period and beyond. *Clin Endoc Metab* 7:3:625–643.

469. Kraaimaat FW, Veeninga AT (1984): Life stress & hysterectomy oophorectomy. *Maturitas* 6:319–325.

470. Krantz KE (1959): Innervation of the human uterus. *Ann NY Acad Sci* 75:770–784.

471. Kritchevsky D (1985): Lipid metabolism and coronary heart disease, in Trowell H, Burkett D, Heaton K, (eds): *Dietary Fibre, Fibre-Depleted Foods and Disease.* New York, Academic Press, 305–315.

472. Krolner B, Nielsen SP, Lund B, Lund BJ, Sorensen OH, Uhrenholdt A (1980): Measurement of bone mineral content (BMC) of the lumbar spine, II. Correlation between forearm BMC & lumbar spine BMC. *Scand J Clin Lab Invest* 40:665–670.

473. Krolner B, Toft B, Nielsen SP, Tondevold E (1983): Physical exercise as prophylaxis against inovultional vertebral bone loss: a controlled trial. *Clin Sci* 64:541–546.

474. Kupperman HS, Wetchler BB, Blatt MHG (1959): Contemporary therapy of the menopausal syndrome. *JAMA* 171:1627–1637.

475. Kwan M, Greenleaf WJ, Mann J, Crapo L, Davidson JM (1983): The nature of androgen action on male sexuality: a combined laboratory self report study on hypogonadal men. *JCEM* Sept:1–23.

476. Lafferty FW, Helmuth DO (1985): Post-menopausal estrogen replacement: the prevention of osteoporosis & systemic effects. *Maturitas* 7:147–159.

477. Lafferty FW, Spencer GE, Pearson OH (1964): Effects of androgens, estrogens and high calcium intakes on bone formation and resorption in osteoporosis. *Am J Med* 35:514–528.

478. LaFerla JJ (1984): Inhibited sexual desire and orgasmic dysfunction in women. *Clin Ob/Gyn* 27:738–749.

479. Lamont JA (1980): Female dyspareunia. *Am J Obstet Gynecol* 136:282–285.

480. Lamont LS (1987): Sweat lactate secretion during exercise in relation to women's aerobic capacity. *American Physiological Society* 194–198.

481. Lane G, Siddle NC, Ryder TA, Pryse-Davies J, King RJB, Whitehead MI (1986): Is Provera the ideal progestogen for addition to post-menopausal estrogen therapy? *Fertil Steril* 45:3:345–352.

482. Lapidus L, Andersson H, Bengtsson C, Bosaeus I (1986): Dietary habits in relation to incidence of cardiovascular disease and death in women: a 12-year follow-up of participants in the population study of women in Gothenburg, Sweden. *Am J Clin Nutr* 44:444–448.

483. Laros RK, Work BA (1975): Female sterilization III. Vaginal hysterectomy. *Am J Obstet Gynecol* 122:693–697.

484. Larson EB, Bruce RA (1986): Exercise and aging. *Annals of Internal Medicine* 105:5:783–785.

485. Larsson-Cohn U, Johansson ED, Kagedal B, Wallentin L (1977): Serum FSH, LH & oestrone levels in postmenopausal patients on oestrogen therapy. *Br J Obstet Gynaecol* 85:5:367–372.

486. Last P, Ritchie C (1984): Cervical cancer screening for younger women. *Lancet* November 10:1100.

487. Laufer L, DeFazio J, Lu J, Meldrum D, Eggena P, Sambhi M, Hershman J, Judd H (1983): Estrogen replacement therapy by transdermal estradiol administration. *Am J Obstet Gynecol* 146:533–540.

488. Laurian L (1987): Calcitonin: an analgesic for osteoporotic women. Fifth International Congress on the Menopause, Sorrento, Italy, April.

489. Lauritzen C (1973): The management of the premenopausal and the postmenopausal patient. *Front Horm Res* 2:2–21.

490. Lavori PW, Louis TA, Bailar JC III, Polansky M (1983): Designs for experiments—parallel comparisons of treatment. *NEJM* 309:1291–1299.

491. Lee CJ, Lawler GS, Johnson GH (1981): Effects of supplementation of the diets with calcium and calcium rich foods on bone density of elderly females with osteoporosis. *Am J Clin Nutr* 34:819–823.

492. Legros JJ, Mormont C, Servais J (1978): A psychoneuroendocrinological study of erectile "psychogenic impotence": a comparison between normal patients & patients with abnormal reaction to glucose tolerance test, in Carenza L, Pancheri P, Zichella L (eds): *Clinical Psychoneuroendocrinology in Reproduction.* New York, Academic Press, 301–319.

493. Leiblum S, Bachmann G, Kemmann E, Colburn D, Swartzman L (1983): Vaginal atrophy in the postmenopausal woman: the importance of sexual activity and hormones. *JAMA* 249:2195–2198.

494. Leuchtenberger L, Leuchtenberger R (1977): Protection of hamster lung culture of L-cysteine or vitamin C against carcinogenic effects of fresh smoke from tobacco or marijuana cigarettes. *Br J Exp Pathol* 58:625–634.

495. Lemay A (1987): Monthly implant of luteinizing hormone-releasing hormone agonist: a practical therapeutic approach for sex-steroid dependent gynecologic diseases. *Fertil Steril* 48:1:10–12.

496. Levin DL, Devesa SS, Godwin JDII, Silverman DT (1964): *Cancer Rates and Risks.* Washington, Dept. of Health, Education and Welfare, 13.

497. Levine M (1986): New concepts in the biology and biochemistry of ascorbic acid. *NEJM* 314:892–902.

498. Levine M, Hartzell W (1987): Ascorbic acid: the concept of optimum requirements. Third Conference on Vitamin C, *Ann NY Acad Sci* 498: 424–444.

499. Levine SB (1976): Marital sexual dysfunction: erectile dysfunction. *Ann Intern Med* 85:342–350.

500. Lewis D (1983): The gynecologic consideration of the sexual act. *JAMA* 250:222–227.

501. Licata AA, Bori E, Bartter FC, West F (1976): Acute effects of dietary protein on calcium metabolism in patients with osteoporosis. *J Geron* 36:1:14–19.

502. Lief WI (1968): Roundtable: sex after 50. *Medical Aspects of Human Sexuality* 2:41–45.

503. Lightman A, Rzasa PJ, Culler MD, Tarlztzis BC, Jones C, Fernandez LA, DelValle A, Caride VJ, Negro-Vilar AF, DeCherney AH, Naftolin F (1986): OVRAS: The ovarian renin-angiotensin system-biochemical, immunohistochemical & tissue culture evidence. *Fertility News* 20: 1:6.

504. Lind T, Cameron EC, Hunter WM, Leon C, Moran PF, Oxley A, Gerrard J, Lind UCG (1979): A prospective controlled trial of six forms of hormone replacement therapy given to postmenopausal women. *Brit J Obstet Gynecol* 86:3:1–29.

505. Lindquist O, Bengtsson C (1979): The effect of smoking on menopausal age. *Maturitas* 1:171–174.

506. Lindsay R (1981): The influence of cigarette smoking on bone mass and bone loss, in DeLuca HF et al (eds): *Osteoporosis: Recent Advances in Pathogenesis and Treatment.* Baltimore, University Park Press, 481.

507. Lindsay R, Coutts JR, Hart DM (1977): The effect of endogenous oestrogen on plasma and urinary calcium and phosphate in oophorectomized women. *Clin Endocrinol (Oxf)* 6:2:87–93.

508. Lindsay R, Aitken JM, Hart DM, Purdue D (1978): The effect of ovarian sex steroids on bone mineral status in the oophorectomized rat and in the human. *Postgrad Med J* 54:2:50–58.

509. Lindsay R, Aitken JM, Anderson JB (1976): Long term prevention of postmenopausal osteoporosis by estrogen. *Lancet* 1:1038–1040.

510. Lindsay R, Hart DM, Clark DM (1984): The minimum effective dose of estrogen for prevention of postmenopausal bone loss. *Obstet Gynecol* 63:6:759–763.

511. Lindsay R, Hart DM, MacLean A (1979): Bone loss during oestriol therapy in postmenopausal women. *Maturitas* 1:279.

512. Lindsay R, Hart DM (1978): Failure of response of menopausal vasomotor symptoms to clonidine. *Maturitas* 1:21–25.

513. Lindsay R, Hart DM, MacLean A, Clark AC, Kraszewski A, Garwood J (1978): Bone response to termination of oestrogen treatment. *Lancet* 1:8078:1325–1327.

514. Lobo RA, Cristo M, Crary W (1987): Effects of estrogen on psychological function in asymptomatic postmenopausal women. *Abstracts of 5th International Congress on the Menopause,* Sorrento, Italy, April. Oak Ridge, NJ, Parthenon Publishing, 87.

515. Lobo RA, McCormick M, Singer F, Roy S (1984): Depomedroxyprogesterone acetate compared with conjugated estrogens for the treatment of postmenopausal women. *Obstet Gynecol* 63:1–5.

516. Lobo RA (1982): The modulating role of obesity & 17 BE on bound & unbound E2 & adrenal androgens in oophorectomies. *J Clin Endocr Metab* 54:320–324.

517. Lobstein DD (1985): Physical fitness endorphins and emotional stability. *Research News* 8.2, *ISPNE Members' Forum* 2:30–31.

518. Lohmann W (1987): Ascorbic acid and cancer. Third Conference on Vitamin C. *Ann NY Acad Sci* 498:402–417.

519. Longcope C, Hunter R, Franz C (1980): Steroid secretion by the postmenopausal ovary. *Am J Obstet Gynecol* 138:564–568.

520. Lucas WE (1974): Causal relationships between endocrine metabolic variables in patients with endometrial carcinoma. *Obstet & Gynecol Survey* 29:507–528.

521. Ludwig H (1982): The morphologic response of the human endometrium to long-term treatment with progestational agents. *Am J Obstet Gynecol* 142:796–808.

522. Lueg MC, Anging RH (1986): Brief Review: hypercholester-olemia: new values, new strategies. *Hospital Practice* Jan 30:112–121.

523. Luisi M, Franchi F, Kicovic PM (1980): A group-comparative study of effects of ovestin cream versus premarin cream in postmenopausal women with vaginal atrophy. *Maturitas* 2:311–319.

524. Luotola H, Pyoralia T, Loikkanen M (1986): Effects of natural oestro-gen/progestogen substitution therapy on carbohydrate and lipid me-tabolism in postmenopausal women. *Maturitas* 8:245–253.

525. Lutz J (1984): Calcium balance and acid-base status of women as affected by increased protein intake and by sodium bicarbonate inges-tion. *Am J Clin Nutr* 39:281–288.

526. Lutz J (1986): Bone mineral, serum calcium and dietary intakes of mother/daughter pairs. *Am J Clin Nutr* 44:99–106.

527. Lyon LJ, Gardner JW (1977): The rising frequency of hysterectomy: its effect on uterine cancer rates. *Am J Epidemiology* 105:439–443.

528. MacLeod TL, Eisen A, Sussman GL (1987): Anaphylactic reaction to synthetic luteinizing hormone-releasing hormone. *Fertil Steril* 48:3: 500–502.

529. MacDonald PC, Edman CD, Hemsell DL, Porter JC, Siiteri PK (1978): Effect of obesity on conversion of plasma androstenedione to estrone in postmenopausal women with and without endometrial cancer. *Am J Obstet Gynecol* 130:4:448–455.

530. MacIntyre I, Evans IMA, Hobitz HHG, Joplin GF, Stevenson JC (1980): Chemistry, physiology, and therapeutic applications of cal-citonin. *Arthritis & Rheumatism* 23:1139–1147.

531. MacKenzie IZ, Bibby JG (1978): Critical assessment of D & C in 1029 females. *Lancet* 2:566–568.

532. MacMahon B (1974): Risk factors for endometrial cancer. *Gynecol Oncol* 2:122–129.

533. MacMahon B, Worcester J (1966): Age at Menopause, US 1960–1962. National Center for Health Statistics. Washington DC USPHS Publica-tion 1000, Series 11, No. 19.

534. Maddock J (1978): Effects of progestogens on serum lipids in the post-menopause. *Postgrad Med J* 54:2:38–41.

535. Madsen M (1977): Vertebral & peripheral bone mineral content by photon absorptiometry. *Investigative Radiology* 12:185–188.

536. Magos AL, Brincat M, O'Dowd T, Wardle PJ, Schlesinger P, Studd JWW (1985): Endometrial & menstrual response to subcutaneous oestradiol & testosterone implants & continuous oral progestogen therapy in postmenopausal women. *Maturitas* 7:4:297–302.

537. Maheux R, Lemay A, Merat P (1987): Use of intranasal luteinizing hormone-releasing hormone agonist in uterine leiomyomas. *Fertil Steril* 47:2:229-233.

538. Mallampati RS, Casida LE (1970): Ovarian compensatory hypertrophy following unilateral ovariectomy during the breeding season of the ewe. *Biol Reprod* 3:43–46.

539. Malkasian GD, Annegers JF, Fountain KS (1980): Carcinoma of the endometrium: stage 1. *Am J Obstet Gynecol* 136:872–888.

540. Mann J (1985): Diabetes mellitus: some aspects of aetiology and management of non-insulin-dependent diabetes, in Trowell H, Burkett D, Heaton K (eds): *Dietary Fibre, Fibre-Depleted Foods and Disease.* New York, Academic Press, 263–287.

541. Mantalenakis SJ, Papapostolon MG (1977): Genital bleeding in females aged 50 and over. *Int Surg* 62:103–105.

542. Margen S, Chu JY, Kaufmann NA, Calloway DH (1974): Studies in calcium metabolism: the calciuretic effect of dietary protein. *Am J Clin Nutr* 27:584–589.

543. Margetts BM (1986): Recent developments in the etiology and treatment of hypertension: dietary calcium, fat and magnesium. *Am J Clin Nutr* 44:704.

544. Marks R, Shahrad P (1977): Skin changes at the time of the climacteric. *Clinics in Obstetrics and Gynecology* 4:207–226.

545. Marmorston J, Madgson O, Lewis JJ, Mehl J, Moore FJ, Bernstein J (1958): Effect of small doses of estrogen on serum lipids in female patients with myocardial infarction. *NEJM* 258:583–586.

546. Marshall DH, Crilly R, Nordin BE (1978): The relation between plasma androstenedione and oestrone levels in untreated and corticosteroid treated post-menopausal women. *Clin Endocrinol (Oxf)* 9:5:407–412.

547. Marshall DH, Nordin BE (1977): The effect of lalpha-hydroxy-vitamin $D_3$ with and without oestrogens on calcium balance in postmenopausal women. *Clin Endocrinol (Oxf)* 7:159S–168S.

548. Marshall DH, Crilly RG, Nordin BE (1977): Plasma androstenedione and oestrone levels in normal and osteoporotic postmenopausal women. *Br Med J* 2:6096:1177–1179.

549. Marshall JM (1970): Andrenergic innervation of the female reproductive tract. *Rev Physiol* 62:6.

550. Martin, Purvis (1982): Unpublished data in file.

551. Martin P, Yen SSC, Burnier AM, Hermann H (1979): Systemic absorption and sustained effects of vaginal estrogen creams. *JAMA* 242: 2699–2700.

552. Martin RL, Roberts WV, Clayton PJ, Wetzel R (1977): Psychiatric illness and non cancer hysterectomy. *Diseases of the Nervous System* 38:11:974–980.

553. Mashchak CA, Lobo RA, Dozono-Takano R, Eggena P, Nakamura RM, Brenner PF, Mishell DR (1982): Comparison of pharmacodynamic properties of various estrogen formulations. *Am J Obstet Gynecol* 144:511–518.

554. Martini MC, Bollweg GL, Levitt MD, Savaiano DA (1987): Lactose digestion by yogurt B-galactosidase: influence of pH and microbial cell integrity. *Am J Clin Nutr* 45:432–436.

555. Masters WH (1959): The sexual response cycle of the human female: vaginal lubrication. *Ann NY Acad Sci* 83:301–317.

556. Masters WH, Johnson V (1966): *Human Sexual Response.* Boston, Little Brown.

557. Masters WH, Johnson V (1970): *Human Sexual Inadequacy.* Boston, Little Brown.

558. Mathur RS, Landgrebe SC, Moody LO, Semmens JP, Williamson HO (1985): The effect of estrogen treatment on plasma concentrations of steroid hormones, gonadotropins, prolactin & sex hormone-binding globulin in post-menopausal women. *Maturitas* 7:129–133.

559. Mattingly RF (1977): *Myomata Uteri in Operative Gynecology,* 5th ed. Philadelphia, Lippincott.

560. Mattingly RF, Thompson JD (1984): Psychological aspects of pelvic surgery, in *TeLinde's Operative Gynecology,* 6th ed. 2:15–23.

561. Mattingly RF, Huang WY (1969): Steroidogenesis of the menopausal and post menopausal ovary. *Am J Obstet Gynecol* 103:679–693.

562. Mattingly RF, TeLinde (1977): Presacral neurectomy, in *TeLinde's Operative Gynecology,* 5th ed. Philadelphia, Lippincott.

563. Mauvais-Jarvis P, Sitruk-Ware R, Kuttenn F (1985): Luteal phase defect and benign breast disease: relationship to breast cancer genesis. *Breast Diseases-Senologia* 1:no 1, 58–66.

564. Mazess RB (1987): Bone densitometry in osteoporosis. *Internal Medicine* 8:4.

565. McBride JM (1959): Premenopausal cystic glandular hyperplasia & endometrial carcinoma. *J Ob Gyn of the Br Commonwealth* 66:288–296.

566. McCoy N, Cutler W, Davidson JM (1985): Relationships among sexual behavior hot flashes & hormone levels in perimenopausal women. *Arch Sex Beh* 14:385–394.

567. McCoy NL, Davidson JM (1985): A longitudinal study of the effect of menopause on sexuality. *Maturitas* 7:203–210.

568. McCracken JA (1984): Update on luteolysis—receptor regulation of pulsatile secretion of prostaglandin F2a from the uterus. *Res in Reproduction* 16:2:1–2.

569. McDonald TW, Annegers JF, O'Fallon WM (1977): Exogenous estrogen and endometrial carcinoma. *Am J Obstet Gynecol* 127:572–580.

570. McKinlay SM, Jeffreys M (1974): The menopausal syndrome. *Brit J Prev Soc Med* 28:108–115.

571. McNatty KP, Makris A, DeGrazia C, Osathanondh R, Ryan KJ (1979): The production of progesterone, androgens, and estrogens by granulosa cells, thecal tissue and stromal tissue by human ovaries in vitro. *J Clin Endocrinol Metab* 49:687–699.

572. Meade TW (1982): Effects of progestogens on the cardiovascular system. *Am J Obstet Gynecol* 142:776–780.

573. Meade TW (1982): Oral contraceptives, clotting factors, and thrombosis. *Am J Obstet Gynecol* 142:758–761.

574. Meema HE, Bunker MI, Meema S (1965): Loss of compact bone due to menopause. *Obstet Gynecol* 26:333–343.

575. Meema S, Meema HE (1982): Evaluation of cortical bone mass, thickness & density by z-scores in osteopenic conditions & in relation to menopause & estrogen treatment. *Skeletal Radiol* 8:259–268.

576. Meema S, Meema HE (1976): Menopausal bone loss & estrogen replacement. *Israel J Med Sci* 12:601–606.

577. Meikle AW, Odell WD (1986): Effect of short and long-term dexamethasone on 3ox-androstanediol glucuronide in hirsute women. *Fertil Steril* 46:2:227–231.

578. Meikle S, Brody H, Pysh F (1977): An investigation into the psychological effects of hysterectomy. *J Nervous & Mental Disease* 164:36–41.

579. Meisels A (1966): The menopause: a cytohormonal study. *Acta Cytol* 10:49–55.

580. Meldrum DR, Davidson B, Tataryn I, Judd H (1981): Changes in circulating steroids with aging in postmenopausal women. *Obstet Gynecol* 57:624–628.

581. Meldrum DR, Tataryn I, Frumar A, Erlik J, Lu K, Judd H (1980): Gonadatropins, estrogens, and adrenal steroids during the menopausal hot flash. *J Clin Endocrinol Metab* 50:685–689.

582. Melton LJ, Wahner HW, Richelson LS, O'Fallon WM, Dunn WL, Riggs BL (1985): Bone density specific fracture risk: a population based study of the relationship between osteoporosis & vertebral fractures. *J Nucl Med* 26:24.

583. Melethil S, Subrahmanyam MB, Chang CJ, Mason WD (1987): Megadoses of vitamin C: a pharmacokinetic evaluation. Third Conference on Vitamin C. *Ann NY Acad Sci* 498:491–493.

584. Melton LJ, Wahner HW, Richelson LS, O'Fallon WM, Riggs BL (1986): Osteoporosis and the risk of hip fracture. *Am J Epidemiology* 124:2:254–261.

585. Menczer J, Modan M, Ezra D, Serr DM (1980): Prognosis in pre- and post-menopausal patients with endometrial adenocarcinoma. *Maturitas* 2:37–44.

586. Mendeloff AI (1986): Dietary fibre, fibre-depleted foods and disease. Book Review. *Am J Clin Nutr* 43:859.

587. Menkes M, Comstock G, Vuilleumier J, Helsing K, Rider A, Brookmeyer R (1986): Serum beta-carotene, vitamins A and E, selenium and the risk of lung cancer. *NEJM* 315:1250–1254.

588. Merrill JA (1981): Management of postmenopausal bleeding. *Clinical Obstetrics & Gynecol* 24:285–299.

589. Meunier P, Courpron P, Edourd C, Bernard J, Bringuier J, Vignon E (1973): Physiological senile involution & pathological rarefaction of bone. *Clin Endocr Metab* 2:239–256.

590. Meyer WC, Malkasian GD, Dockerty MB, et al (1971): Postmenopausal bleeding from atrophic endometrium. *Obstet Gynecol* 38:731.

591. Michael RP & Welegalla J (1968): Ovarian hormones & the sexual behaviour of the female rhesus monkey (Macaca mulatta) under laboratory conditions. *J Endocr* 41:407–420.

592. Michael RP, Zumpe D (1976): Environmental & endocrine factors influencing annual changes in sexual potency in primates. *Psychoneuroendocrinology* 1:303–313.

593. Michael RP, Keverne EB (1970): Primate sex pheromones of vaginal origin. *Nature* 225:84.

594. Michael RP, Keverne EB, Bonsall RW (1971): Pheromones isolation of male sex attractants from a female primate. *Science* 172:964.

595. Michael RP, Richter MC, Cain JA, Bonsall RW (1978): Artificial menstrual cycles, behavior and the role of androgens in female rhesus monkeys. *Nature* 275:439–444.

596. Michnovicz JJ, Hershcopf, RJ, Naganuma H, Bradlow HL, Fishman J (1986): Increased 2-hydroxylation of estradiol as a possible mechanism for the anti-estrogenic effect of cigarette smoking. *NEJM* 315:21: 1305–1309.

597. Mickal A, Torres J (1974): Adenocarcinoma of endometrium, in Greenblatt RB, Mahesh VB, McDonough PG (eds): *The Menopausal Syndrome.* New York, Medcom Press, 139–142.

598. Mikhail G (1970): Hormone secretion by the human ovaries. *Gynec Invest* 1:5–20.

599. Miller NE (1979): The evidence for the antiatherogenecity of high density lipoprotein in man. *Lipids* 13:914–919.

600. Miller NE, Hammett F, Saltissi S, Rao S, van Zeller H, Coltart J, Lewis B (1982): Relation of angiographically defined coronary artery disease to plasma lipoprotein subfractions & apolipoproteins. *Br J Med* 282:1741–1744.

601. Minkoff JR, Young G, Grant B, Marcus R (1986): Interactions of medroxyprogesterone acetate with estrogen on the calcium-parathyroid axis in postmenopausal women. *Maturitas* 8:35–45.

602. Mohsenin V, DuBois AB (1987): Vitamin C and airways. Third Conference on Vitamin C. *Ann NY Acad Sci* 498:259–268.

603. Molinas G, Bompani R, Scali G, et al (1970): Modifications induced by treatment with medroxyprogesterone acetate in the urinary excretion of the calcium after oral and intravenous load in old subject. *Giornale de Gerontologia* 18:361–372.

604. Molnar GW (1975): Body temperatures during menopausal hot flashes. *J Appl Physiol* 38:3:499–503.

605. Molnar GW (1981): Menopausal hot flashes: their cycles & relation to air temperature. *Obstet Gynecol* 57:525–555.

606. Money J (1961): Sex hormones & other variables in human eroticism, in Young WC (ed): *Sex & Internal Secretions.* Baltimore, Williams & Wilkins, Vol 2, 3rd ed, 1383–1400.

607. Montague DK, James RE, DeWolf VG, et al (1979): Diagnostic evaluation, classification & treatment of men with sexual dysfunction. *Urology* 14:545–548.

608. Moore B, Paterson M, Sturdee D (1987): Effect of oral hormone replacement therapy on liver function tests. *Maturitas* 9:1:7–16.

609. Moore J, Tolley D (1976): Depression following hysterectomy. *Psychosomatics* 17:2:86–89.

610. Morales A, Surridge HC, Marshall PG, Fenemore J (1982): Nonhormonal pharmacological treatment of organic impotence. *J Urol* 128: 45–47.

611. Morehouse LE, Miller AT (1959): *Physiology of Exercise.* St. Louis, Mosby.

612. Morley JE, Melmed S (1979): Gonadal dysfunction in systemic disorders. *Metabolism* 28:1051–1073.

613. Morrell MJ, Dixen JM, Carter CS, Davidson JM (1984): The influence of age & cycling status on sexual arousability in women. *Am J Obstet Gynecol* 148:66–71.

614. Morrison JC, Martin DC, Blair RA, et al (1980): The use of medroxyprogesterone acetate (DepoProvera) for relief of climacteric symptoms. *Am J Obstet Gynecol* 138:99–104.

615. Muckle CW (1977): Clinical anatomy of the uterus, fallopian tubes, & ovaries, in McElin T, Sciarra JJ (eds): *Gynecology & Obstetrics.* New York, Harper & Row.

616. Mueller MN (1976): Effects of corticosteroids on bone mineral in rheumatoid arthritis & asthma. Abstract. *AJR* 126:1300.

617. Murphy AA (1987): Operative laparoscopy. *Fertil Steril* 47:1:1 18.

618. Nachtigall LE, Nachtigall RH, Nachtigall RD, Beckman EM (1979): Estrogen replacement therapy II: a prospective study in the relationship to carcinoma and cardiovascular and metabolic problems. *Obstet Gynecol* 54:74–79.

619. Nachtigall LE, Nachtigall RH, Nachtigall RD, Beckman EM (1979): Estrogen replacement therapy I: a 10 year prospective study in the relationship to osteoporosis. *Obstet Gynecol* 53:277–281.

620. Nankin HR (1985): Fertility in aging men. *Maturitas* 7:259–265.

621. Neaves WB, Johnson L, Porter JC, Parker CR, Petty CS (1984): Leydig cell numbers, daily sperm production & serum gonadotropin levels in aging men. *J Clin Endoc Metab* 59:4:756–763.

622. Need AG, Chatterton BE, Walker CJ, Steurer TA, Horowitz M, Nordin BEC (1986): Comparison of calcium, calcitriol, ovarian hormones and nandrolone in the treatment of osteoporosis. *Maturitas* 8:275–280.

623. Needham J, Gwei-Djen L (1968): Sex hormones in the Middle Ages. *Endeavor* 27:130–132.

624. Nestel PJ (1986): Fish oil attenuates the cholesterol induced rise in lipoprotein cholesterol. *Am J Clin Nutr* 43:752–757.

625. Netter A, Lambert A (1953): Déclanchement de l'ovulation par l'infiltration du ganglion sympathique cervical supérieur. *Rivista di obstericia e ginecologia* 8:2:77–82.

626. Newman HF, Northup JD (1961): Female urinary stress incontinence. *Am J Surg* 102:663.

627. Newman HF, Northup JD (1981): The mechanism of human penile erection—an overview. *Urology* 17:399–408.

628. Ng ABP, Reagan JW, Storaasli JP, Wentz WB (1973): Mixed adenosquamous carcinoma of the endometrium. *Am J Clin Pathology* 59:765–781.

629. Ng ABP, Reagan JW (1970): Incidence & prognosis of endometrial carcinoma by histologic grade & extent. *Obstet Gynecol* 35:437–442.

630. NIH Consensus Conference on Osteoporosis (1987). Feb 9–11.

631. Nicosia SV (1983): Morphological changes in the human ovary through life, in Serra GB (ed): *Comprehensive Endocrinology: The Ovary*. New York, Raven Press.

632. Nielsen FH, Honore E, Kristoffersen K, Secher NJ, Pedersen GT (1977): Changes in serum lipids during treatment with norgestrel, oestradiol-valerate & cycloprogynon. *Acta Obstet et Gynecol Scand* 56:4:367–370.

633. Nilas L, Borg J, Gotfredsen A, Christiansen C (1985): Comparison of single- and dual-photon absorptiometry in postmenopausal bone mineral loss. *J Nucl Med* 26:1257–1262.

634. Nilas L, Pondenphant J, Riis BJ, Gotfredsen A, Christiansen C (1987): Usefulness of regional bone measurements in patients with osteoporotic fractures of the spine and distal forearm. *J Nucl Med* 28:960–965.

635. Nilson BE, Westlin NE (1971): Bone density in athletes. *Clin Orthopaedics & Rel Res* 77:179–182.

636. Nisker JA, Siiteri PK (1981): Estrogens & breast cancer. *Clinical Obstetrics & Gynecology* 24:301–322.

637. Nordin BEC, Baker MR, Horsman A, Peacock M (1985): A prospective trial of the effect of vitamin D supplementation on metacarpal bone loss in elderly women 1, 2. *Am J Clin Nutr* 42:470–474.

638. Nordin BEC, Robertson A, Seamark RF, Bridges A, Philcox JC, Need AG, Horowitz M, Morris HA, Deam S (1985): The relation between calcium absorption, serum dehydroepiandrosterone, and vertebral mineral density in postmenopausal women. *J Clin Endocrinol Metab* 60:4:651–657.

639. Nordin BEC, Peacock M, Crilly RG, Francis RM, Speed R, Barkwoth S (1981): Summation of risk factors in osteoporosis, in DeLuca FH, Frost HM, Jee WSS, Johnston CC, Parfitt AM (eds): *Osteoporosis: Recent Advances in Pathogenesis and Treatment.* Baltimore, University Park Press, 359–367.

640. Nordin BEC, Horsman A, Marshall DH, Simpson M, Waterhouse GM (1979): Calcium requirement and calcium therapy. *Clin Orthopaedics & Rel Res* 140:216–239.

641. Norment WB (1956): The hysteroscope. *Am J Obstet Gynecol* 71:426–432.

642. Notelovitz M (1977): Coagulation, oestrogen & the menopause. *Clinics in Obstetrics & Gynecology* 4:107–128.

643. Notelovitz M (1975): Effect of natural oestrogens on blood pressure & weight in postmenopausal women. *S Afr Med J* 49:2251–2254.

644. Notelovitz M, Southwood B (1974): Metabolic effect of conjugated oestrogens (USP) on lipids & lipoproteins. *S Afr Med J* 48:2552–2556.

645. Novak ER (1970): Ovulation after fifty. *Obstet Gynecol* 36:903–910.

646. Novak ER, Goldberg B, Jones GS (1965): Enzyme histochemistry of the menopausal ovary associated with normal & abnormal endometrium. *Am J Obstet Gynecol* 93:669–673.

647. Novak E, Richardson EH (1941): Proliferative changes in the senile endometrium. *Am J Obstet Gynecol* 42:564.

648. Nyirjesy I, Billingsley FS (1984): Detection of breast carcinoma in a gynecologic practice. *Obstet Gynecol* 64:6:747–751.

649. O'Brien WF, Buck DR, Nash JD (1984): Evaluation of sonography in the initial assessment of the gynecologic patient. *Am J Obstet Gynecol* 149:598-602.

650. O'Dca JP, Wieland RG, Hallberg MC, Llerena LA, Zorn EM, Genuth SM (1979): Effect of dietary weight loss on sex steroid binding, sex

steroids & gonadotropins in obese postmenopausal women. *J Lab Clin Med* 93:6:1007–1008.

651. Oh SY, Monaco PA (1985): Effect of dietary cholesterol and degree of fat unsaturation on plasma lipid levels, lipoprotein composition and fecal steroid excretion in normal young adult men, 1–3. *Am J Clin Nutr* 42:399–413.

652. Oh SY, Miller LT (1985): Effect of dietary egg on variability of plasma cholesterol levels and lipoprotein cholesterol, 1–3. *Am J Clin Nutr* 42:421–431.

653. Omaye ST, Skala JH, Jacob RA (1986): Plasma ascorbic acid in adult males: effects of depletion and supplementation. *Am J Clin Nutr* 44:257–264.

654. Omaye ST, Schaus EE, Kutnink MA, Hawkes WC (1987): Measurement of vitamin C in blood components by high-performance liquid chromatography: implication in assessing vitamin C status. Third Conference on Vitamin C. *Ann NY Acad Sci* 498:389–401.

655. Ott S (1986): Should women get screening bone mass measurements? *Annals of Internal Medicine* 104:6:874–876.

656. Osterholzer HO, Grillow D, Kruger PS, Dunnihoo DR (1977): The effect of oral contraceptive steroids on branches of the uterine artery. *Obstet Gynecol* 49:227–232.

657. Ottoson UB, Johansson BG, von Schoultz B (1985): Subfractions of high density lipoprotein cholesterol during estrogen replacement therapy: comparison between progestogens and natural progesterone. *Am J Obstet Gynecol* 1151:746.

658. Padwick ML, Endacott J, Matson C, Whitehad MI (1986): Absorption & metabolism of oral progesterone when administered twice daily. *Fertil Steril* 46:3:402–407.

659. Padwick ML, Pryse-Davies J, Path FRC, Whitehead MI (1986): A simple method for determining the optimal dosage of progestin in postmenopausal women receiving estrogens. *NEJM* 315:15:930–934.

660. Paffenbarger R, Hyde R, Wiag L, Steinmetz C (1984): A natural history of athleticism and cardiovascular health. *JAMA* 252:491–495.

661. Paganini-Hill A, Ross RD, Gerkins VR (1981): A case-control study of menopausal estrogen therapy & hip fractures. *Ann Intern Med* 95:28.

662. Painter N (1985): Diverticular disease of the colon, in Trowell H, Burkett D, Heaton K (eds): *Dietary Fibre, Fibre-Depleted Foods and Disease.* New York, Academic Press, 145–159.

663. Pallas KG, Holzwarth GJ, Stern MP, Lucas CP (1977): The effect of conjugated estrogen on the renin-angiotensin system. *J Clin Endocrinol Metab* 44:1061–1068.

664. Panda S, Panda SN, Sarangi RK, Habeebullah S (1977): Postmenopausal bleeding. *J Indian Med Assoc* 68:185–188.

665. Paniagua R, Martin A, Nistal M, Amat P (1987): Testicular involution in elderly men: comparison of histologic quantitative studies with hormone patterns. *Fertil Steril* 47:4:671–679.

666. Pao EM, Mickle SJ, Burk MC (1985): One-day and 3-day nutrient intakes by individuals. Nationwide Food Consumption survey findings, Spring 1977. *Am Dietetic Assoc* 85:313–323.

667. Parke A (1985): Rheumatoid arthritis & oral contraceptives. *IM* 6:5: 105–111.

668. Parkin ED, Deeny M, McLay V, Hart DM (1987): Reduced bone density in women with endometriosis. *Abstracts of 5th International Congress on the Menopause* 61, p. 80.

669. Parkin DE, Smith D, Al AzzAwi F, Lindsay R, Hart DM (1987): Effects of long-term ORG OD 14 administration on blood coagulation in climacteric women. *Maturitas* 9:1:4:95–102.

670. Parsons L, Sommers SC (1962): *Gynecology.* Philadelphia, Saunders, 629–649.

671. Pasquale SA, Murphy RJ, Norwood PK, McBride LC (1982): Results of a study to determine the effects of three oral contraceptives on serum lipoprotein levels. *Fertil Steril* 38:559–563.

672. Paterson MEL, Wade-Evans T, Sturdee DW, Thom MH, Studd JWW (1980): Endometrial disease after treatment with oestrogens & progestogens in the climacteric. *Br Med J* 96:1–8.

673. Pauling L (1986): *How to Live Long and Feel Better.* New York, Freeman.

674. Payne FL, Wright RC, Getterman HH (1959): Postmenopausal bleeding. *Am J Obstet Gynecol* 77:1216–1227.

675. Pelleter O (1968): Smoking and vitamin C levels in humans. *Am J Clin Nutr* 21:1259–1267.

676. Perl V, Marquez J, Schally AV, Comaru-Schally AM, Leal G, Zacharias S, Gomez-Lira C (1987): Treatment of leiomyomata uteri with D-Trp6-luteinizing hormone-releasing hormone. *Fertil Steril* 48:3:383–389.

677. Perry HM (1986): Thyroid replacement and osteoporosis. *Arch Intern Med* 146:41–42.

678. Perry JD, Whipple B (1982): Vaginal myography, in Graber B (ed): *Circumvaginal Musculature & Sexual Function.* Omaha, Nebraska, New York, S. Karger, 61–73.

679. Perry JD, Whipple B (1981): Pelvic muscle strength of female ejaculators: evidence in support of a new theory of orgasm. *J Sex Res* 17:22–39.

680. Persky H, Lief H, O'Brien C, Strauss D (1977): Reproductive hormone levels & sexual behaviors of young couples during the menstrual cycle, in Gemme R, Wheeler CC (eds): *Progress in Sexology.* New York, Plenum Press.

681. Persky H, Dreisbach L, Miller W, et al (1982): The relation of plasma androgen levels to sexual behaviors & attitudes of women. *Psychosom Med* 44:305–319.

682. Persky H, Lief H, Strauss D, Miller W, O'Brien C (1978): Plasma testosterone level & sexual behavior of couples. *Arch Sex Behav* 7:157–173.

683. Petitti DB, Wingerd J, Pellegrin F, Ramcharan S (1979): Risk of vascular disease in women: Smoking, oral contraceptives, non contraceptive estrogens & other factors. *JAMA* 242:1150–1154.

684. Petraglia F, Facchinetti F, M'Futa K, Ruspa M, Bonavera JJ, Gandolfi F, Genazzani AR (1986): Endogenous opioid peptides in uterine fluid. *Fertil Steril* 46:2:247–251.

685. Petraglia F, DiMeo G, DeLeo V, Nappi C, Facchinetti F, Genazzani AR (1986): Plasma B-endorphin levels in anovulatory states: changes after treatments for the induction of ovulation. *Fertil Steril* 45:2:185–190.

686. Petraglia F, Segre A, Facchinetti F, Campanini D, Ruspa M, Genazzani AR (1985): B-endorphin & met-enkephalin in peritoneal & ovarian follicular fluids of fertile & postmenopausal women. *Fertil Steril* 44:5:615–621.

687. Pfeffer RI (1978): Estrogen use, hypertension & stroke in postmenopausal women. *J Chron Dis* 31:389–398.

688. Pfeffer RI, Whipple GH, Kurosaki TT, Chapman JM (1978): Coronary risk & estrogen use in postmenopausal women. *Am J Epidemiology* 107:479–487.

689. Pfeffer RI, Van Den Noort S (1976): Estrogen use & stroke risk in postmenopausal women. *Am J Epidemiology* 103:445–456.

690. Pfeiffer E, Verwoerdt A, Davis G (1972): Sexual behavior in middle life. *Am J Psychiat* 128:1262–1267.

691. Pisantry S, Rafaely B, Polishuk W (1975): The effect of steroid hormones on buccal mucosa of menopausal women. *Oral Surg* 40:3:346–353.

692. Plant M, Krey LC, Moossy J, McCormack JT, Hess DL, Knobil E (1978): The arcuate nuclus & the control of gonadotropin and PRL secretion in the female rhesus monkey. *Endocrinology* 102:52–62.

693. Plunkett ER (1982): Contraceptive steroids, age and the cardiovascular system. *Am J Obstet Gynecol* 142:747–751.

694. Pocock NA, Eisman JA, Yeates MG, Sambrook PN, Eberl S (1986): Physical fitness is a major determinant of femoral neck and lumbar spine bone mineral density. *J Clin Invest* 78:618–621.

695. Pocock NA, Eisman JA, Yeates MG, Sambrook PN, Eberl S, Wren BG (1986): Limitations of forearm bone densitometry as an index of vertebral or femoral neck osteopenia. *J Bone & Mineral Research* 1:4:369–375.

696. Poliak A, Seegar-Jones G, Goldberg IB (1968): Effect of human chorionic gonadotropin on postmenopausal women. *Am J Obstet Gynecol* 101:731–739.

697. Polivy J (1974): Psychological reactions to hysterectomy. *Am J Obstet Gynecol* 118:417–426.

698. Preti G, Cutler WB, García CR, Huggins GR, Lawley HJ (1986): Human axillary secretions influence women's menstrual cycles: the role of donor extract of females. *Hormones & Behavior* 20:474–482.

699. Preti G, Cutler WB, Christensen CM, Lawley H, Huggins GR, García CR (1987): Human auxillary extracts: analysis of compounds from samples which influence menstrual timing. *J Chemical Ecology* 13:4:-717–731.

699b. Prinz W, Bortz R, Bragin B, Hersch M (1977): The effect of ascorbic acid supplementation on some parameters of the human immunologic defense system. *I J Vitamin Nutr Res* 47:248-256.

700. Prior JC (1985): Luteal phase defects & anovulation: adaptive alterations occurring with conditioning exercise. *Seminars in Repro Endocrinology* 3:1:27–33.

701. Prior JC, Vigna Y, Burgess R (1987): Medroxyprogesterone increases trabecular bone density in women with menstrual disorders. *Endocrine Society* June 10–12, 1987. Abstract 560.

702. Prior JC, Vigna Y, Sciaretta D, Alojado N, Schultzer M (1987): Conditioning exercise decreases premenstrual symptoms: a prospective, controlled six month trial. *Fertil Steril* 47:402–408.

703. Prior JC, Vigna Y, Alojada N (1986): Conditioning exercise decreases premenstrual symptoms—a prospective controlled three month trial. *Euro J Appl Physiol*

704. Prior JC, Jensen L, Ho Yuen B, Higgins H, Browlie L (1982a): Prolactin changes with exercise vary with breast motion—analysis of running versus cycling. *Fertil Steril* 38:2:272.

705. Prior JC, Cameron K, Yuen BH, Thomas J (1982b): Menstrual cycle changes with marathon training: anovulation and short luteal phase. *Canadian J Appl Sprt Sciences* 7:3:173–177.

706. Prior JC, Vigna Y (1985): Gonadal steroids in athletic women, contraception, complications and performance. *Sports Medicine* 2:287–295.

707. Procope BJ (1971): Aetiology of postmenopausal bleeding. *Acta Obsteteica et Gynecologica Scandinavica* 50:311–313.

708. Prosky L, Harland B (1985): Dietary fibre methodology, chapter 4 in Trowell H, Burkett D, Heaton K (eds): *Dietary Fibre, Fibre-Depleted Foods and Disease.* New York, Academic Press.

709. Punnonen R, Lammintausta R, Erkkola R, Rauramo L (1980): Estradiol valerate therapy and the renin-aldosterone system in castrated women. *Maturitas* 2:91–94.

710. Punnonen R, Rauramo L (1976): The effect of castration and oral estrogen therapy on serum lipids, in van Keep PA, Greenblatt RB, Albeaux-Fernet M (eds): *Consensus on Menopause Research.* Proc First International Congress on the Menopause held in France. Baltimore, University Park Press.

711. Punnonen R, Rauramo L (1977): The effect of long-term oral oestriol succinate therapy on the skin of castrated women. *Ann Chir Gynaecol* 66:4:214–215.

712. Punnonen R (1972): Effect of castration and peroral estrogen therapy on the skin. *Acta Obstetrica et Gynecologica Scandinavica* Suppl 21:1–44.

713. Punnonen R, Rauramo L (1976): Effect of bilateral oophorectomy and peroral estradiol valerate therapy on serum lipids. *Int J Gynaecol Obstet* 14:13–16.

714. Punnonen R, Salmi J, Tuimala R, Jarvinen M, Pystynen P (1986): Vitamin D deficiency in women with femoral neck fracture. *Maturitas* 8:291–295.

715. Pyorala T (1976): The effect of synthetic and natural estrogens on glucose tolerance, plasma insulin and lipid metabolism in postmenopausal women, in Campbell S (ed): *The Management of the*

*Menopause and Postmenopausal Years.* Lancaster, Eng, MTP Press, 195–210.

716. Rader MD, Flickinger GL, deVilla GO, Mikuta JJ, Mikhail G (1973): Plasma estrogens in postmenopausal women. *Am J Obstet Gynecol* 116:1069–1073.

717. Randall CL, Paloucek FP (1968): Frequency of oophorectomy at hysterectomy. *Am J Obstet Gynecol* 100:716–726.

718. Randall CL (1963): Ovarian conservation, in Meigs JV, Sturgis SH (eds): *Progress in Gynecology.* New York, Grune & Stratton, 457–464.

719. Ranney B, Abu-Ghazaleth S (1977): The future function and control of ovarian tissue which is retained in vivo during hysterectomy. *Am J Obstet Gynecol* 128:626–634.

720. Ranney B, Frederick I (1978): The occasional need for myomectomy. *Obstet Gynecol* 53:437–441.

721. Ravnikar V, Elkind-Hirsch K, Schiff I, Ryan KJ, Tulchinsky D (1984): Vasomotor flushes & the release of peripheral immunoreactive luteinizing hormone-releasing hormone in postmenopausal women. *Fertil Steril* 41:6:881–886.

722. Recker RR (1985): Calcium absorption and achlorhydria. *NEJM* 313: 70–73.

723. Recker RR, Saville PC, Heaney RP (1977): Effect of estrogens & calcium carbonate on bone loss in postmenopausal women. *Ann Intern Med* 87:6:649–655.

724. Reid RL (1985): Premenstrual syndrome. *Obstet Gynecol & Fertility* VII, #2:1–57.

725. Reiser R, Probstfield JL, Silvers A, Scott LW, Shorney ML, Wood RD, O'Brien BC, Gotto AM, Phil D, Insull W (1985): Plasma lipid and lipoprotein response of humans to beef fat, coconut oil and safflower oil. *Am J Clin Nutr* 42:190–197.

726. Rentoul JR (1983): Management of the hirsute woman. *Int J Dermatol* 22:265–272.

727. Reynolds SRM (1949): *Physiology of the Uterus.* New York, Hoeber, 463–490.

728. Rhoads GG, Dahlen G, Berg K, Morton NE, Dannenberg AL (1986): Lp(a) lipoprotein as a risk factor for myocardial infarction. *JAMA* 256:18:2540–2544.

729. Richards BC (1978): Hysterectomy: from women to women. *Am J Obstet Gynecol* 131:446–449.

730. Richards DH (1973): Depression after hysterectomy. *Lancet* 2:430–433.

731. Richards DH (1974): A post hysterectomy syndrome. *Lancet* 2:983–985.

732. Riggs BL, Eastell R (1986): Exercise, hypogonadism & osteopenia. *JAMA* 256:3:392.

733. Riggs BL, Wahner HW, Dunn WL, Mazess RB, Offord KP, Melton LJ (1981): Differential changes in bone mineral density of the appendicular & axial skeleton with aging. *J Clin Invest* 67:328–335.

734. Riis BJ, Christiansen C (1986): Postmenopausal bone loss: effects of oestrogens and progestogens, a review. *Maturitas* 8:267–274.

735. Ringsdorf WM, Cheraskin E (1982): Vitamin C and human wound healing. *Oral Surgery* 53:231–236.

736. Rigg LA, Hermann H, Yen SSC (1977): Absorption of estrogens from vaginal creams. *NEJM* 29:8:195–197.

737. Riggs BL, Seeman E, Hodgson SF, Taves DR, O'Fallon WM (1982): Effect of the fluoride/calcium regimen on vertebral fracture occurrence in postmenopausal osteoporosis. *NEJM* 306:446–450.

738. Riggs BL, Melton LJ III (1986): Medical Progress: Involutional osteoporosis. *NEJM* 314:1676–1686.

739. Riggs BL, Jowsey J, Goldsmith RS, Kelly PJ, Hoffman DL, Arnaud CD (1972): Short and long-term effects of estrogen and synthetic anabolic hormone in postmenopausal osteoporosis. *J Clin Invest* 51:1659–1663.

740. Riggs BL, Hodgson SF, Hoffman DL, Kelly PJ, Johnson KA, Taves D (1980): Treatment of primary osteoporosis with fluoride and calcium. *JAMA* 243:446–449.

741. Riis B, Thomsen K, Christiansen C (1987): Does calcium supplementation prevent postmenopausal bone loss: a double blind controlled clinical study. *NEJM* 316:173–177.

742. Rivers JM (1987): Safety of high-level vitamin C ingestion. Third Conference on Vitamin C. *Ann NY Acad Sci* 498:445–454.

743. Robinson RW, Cohen WD, Higano N (1958): Estrogen replacement therapy in women with coronary atherosclerosis. *Annals Int Med* 48:95–101.

744. Robinson RW, Higano N, Cohen WD (1959): Increased incidence of coronary heart disease in women castrated prior to menopause. *Arch Intern Med* 104:908–913.

745. Robinson RW, Higano N, Cohen W (1960): Effects of long-term administration of estrogens on serum lipids of postmenopausal women. *NEJM* 263:828–831.

746. Rock J, Bartlett MK (1937): Biopsy studies of human endometrium. *JAMA* 108:2022.

747. Rodin M, Moghissi KS (1973): Intrinsic innervation of the human cervix: a preliminary study, in Blandau RJ, Moghissi K (eds): *The Biology of the Human Cervix.* Chicago, University of Chicago Press.

748. Romney SL, Palan PR, Duttagupta C, et al (1981): Retinoids and the prevention of cervical dysplasia. *Am J Obstet Gynecol* 141:890–894.

749. Romney SL, Duttagupta C, Basu J, Palan PR, Karp S, Slagle S, Dwyer A, Wassertheil-Smoller S, Wylie-Rosett J (1985): Plasma vitamin C & uterine cervical dysplasia. *Am J Obstet Gynecol* 151:976–980.

750. Rosenberg L, Armstrong B, Jick H (1976): Myocardial infarction and estrogen therapy in postmenopausal women. *NEJM* 294:1256–1259.

751. Rosenberg L, Hennekens CH, Rosner B, Belanger C, Rothman KJ, Speizer RE (1981): Early menopause and the risk of myocardial infarction. *Am J Obstet Gynecol* 139:47–51.

752. Ross RK, Paganini-Hill A, Gerkins VR, Mack TM, Pfeffer R, Arthur M, Henderson BE (1980): A case control study of menopausal estrogen therapy and breast cancer. *JAMA* 243:1635–1639.

753. Ross RK, Paganini-Hill A, Mack TM, Arthur M, Henderson B (1981): Menopausal oestrogen therapy and protection from death from ischaemic heart disease. *Lancet* 1:858–860.

754. Rowe JW (1983): Systolic hypertension in the elderly. *NEJM* 309:1246–1247.

755. Rowland DL, Heiman JR, Gladue BA, Hatch JP, Doering CH, Weiler SJ (1987): Endocrine, psychological and genital response to sexual arousal in men. *Psychoneuroendocrinology* 12:2:149–158.

756. Rozenbaum H (1982): Relationship between chemical structure and biological properties of progestogens. *Am J Obstet Gynecol* 142:719–724.

757. Rud T (1980): The effects of estrogens and gestagens on the urethral pressure profile in urinary continent and stress incontinent women. *Acta Obstet Gynecol Scand* 49:265–270.

758. Rudge SR (1985): Effect of menstrual cyclicity on disease activity in rheumatoid arthritis. *IM* 6:1:111–119.

759. Ruegsegger P, Dambacher MA, Ruegsegger E, Fischer JA, Anliker M (1984) Bone loss in premenopausal & postmenopausal women. *J Bone & Joint Surgery* 66-A:7:1015–1023.

760. Rui H, Thomassen Y, Oldereid NB, Purvis K (1986): Accessory sex gland function in normal young (20–25 years) and middle-aged (50–55 years) men. *J Androl* 7:93–99.

761. Rutkow IM (1986): Obstetric & gynecologic operations in the United States, 1979–1984. *Obstet Gynecol* 67:6:755–759.

762. Sady SP, Thompson PD, Cullinane EM, Kantor MA, Domagala E, Herbert PN (1986): Prolonged exercise augments plasma triglyceride clearance. *JAMA* 256:18:2552–2555.

763. Sakhaee K, Nicar MJ, Glass K, Zerweks JEL, Pak CYC (1984): Reduction in intestinal calcium absorption by hydrochlorothiazide in postmenopausal osteoporosis. *J Clin Endocrinol Metab* 59:6:1037–1043.

764. Salmon UJ, Geist SH (1943): Effect of androgens upon libido in women. *J Clin Endocrinol* 3:235–238.

765. Samsioe G, Jansson I, Mellstrom D, Svanborg A (1985): Occurrence nature & treatment of urinary incontinence in a 70-year old female population. *Maturitas* 7:335–342.

766. Samuelsson B (1963): Isolation and identification of prostaglandins from human seminal plasma. *J Biol Chem* 238:3229.

767. Sakhaee K, Nicar MJ, Glass K, Pak CYC (1985): Postmenopausal osteoporosis as a manifestation of renal hypercalciuria with secondary hyperparathyroidism. *J Clin Endocrinol Metab* 61:2:368–373.

768. Sarles H, Gerolami A, Cros RC (1978): Diet and cholesterol gallstones: a further study. *Digestion* 17:128–134.

769. Sarrel PM, Whitehead MI (1985): Sex & menopause: defining the issues. *Maturitas* 7:217–224.

770. Saunders DM, Hunter JC, Shutt DA, O'Neill BJ (1978): The effect of oestradiol valerate therapy on coagulation factors and lipid and oestrogen levels in oophorectomized women. *Aust NZ J Obstet Gynaecol* 18:3:198–201.

771. Schaumburg H, Kaplan J, Windebank A, Vick N, Rasmus S, Pleasure D, Brown M (1983): Sensory neuropathy from pyridoxine abuse: a new megavitamin syndrome. *NEJM* 309:445–448.

772. Schiavi R, Davis D, Fogel M, White D, Edwards A, Igel G, Szechterr R, Fisher C (1977): Luteinizing hormone and testosterone during nocturnal sleep: relation to penile tumescent cycles. *Arch Sex Behav* 6:97–104.

773. Schiff I, Regestein Q, Tulchinsky D, Ryan KJ (1979): Effects of estrogens on psychological state of hypogonadal women. *JAMA* 242:2405–2407.

774. Schiff I, Ryan K (1980): Benefits of estrogen replacement. *Obstet & Gynecol Survey* 35:400–411.

775. Schiff I, Tulchinsky D, Cramer D (1980): Oral medroxyprogesterone in the treatment of postmenopausal symptoms. *JAMA* 244:1443–1445.

776. Schiff I, Tulchinsky D, Ryan KJ (1977): Vaginal absorption of estrone and 17B estradiol. *Fertil Steril* 213:1063–1066.

777. Schlaen I, Bocanera R, Figueroa-Casas P (1986): Endometrial cancer and its precursors: a comparison of histological and clinical features. *Maturitas* 8:335–344.

778. Schlenker RA (1976): Percentages of cortical & trabecular bone mineral mass in the radius & ulna. *AJR* 126:1309–1312.

779. Schneider MA, Brotherton PL, Hailes J (1977): The effect of exogenous oestrogens on depression in menopausal women. *Med J Aust* 2:5:162–163.

780. Schramm MM, Cauley JA, Black Sandler R, Slemenda CW (1986): Lack of an association between calcium intake and blood pressure in postmenopausal women. *Am J Clin Nutr* 44:505–511.

781. Schuette SA, Linkswiler HM (1982): Effects of Ca and P metabolism in humans by adding meat, meat plus milk, or purified proteins plus Ca and P to a low protein diet. *J Nutr* 112:338–349.

782. Schuette SA, Zemel MB, Linkswiler HM (1980): Studies on the mechanism of protein-induced hypercalciuria in older men and women. *J Nutr* 110:305–315.

783. Schwartz D, Mayaux M-J, Spira A, Moscato M-L, Jouannet P, Czyglik F, David G (1983): Semen characteristics as a function of age in 833 fertile men. *Fertil Steril* 39:4:530–535.

784. Schwartz U, Schneller E, Moltlz L, Hammerstein J (1982): Vaginal administration of ethinyl estradiol: effects on ovulation and hepatic transcortin synthesis. *Contraception* 25:253.

785. Segraves KA, Segraves RT, Schoenberg HW (1987): Use of sexual history to differenetiate organic from psychogenic impotence. *Arch Sex Behavior* 16:2:125–137.

786. Segraves RT, Schoenberg HW, Zarins CK, et al (1981): Characteristics of erectile dysfunction as a function of medical care system entry point. *Psychosom Med* 43:227–234.

787. Seibel M (1980): Carcinoma of the cervix and sexual function. *Obstet Gynecol* 55:484–487.

788. Seeman E, Wahner HW, Offord KP, Kumar R, Johnson WJ, Riggs BL (1982): Differential effects of endocrine dysfunction on the axial and the appendicular skeleton. *J Clin Invest* 69:1302–1309.

789. Segal I (1985): Hiatal hernia and gastro-oesophageal reflux, in Trowell H, Burkett D, Heaton K (eds): *Dietary Fibre, Fibre-Depleted Foods and Disease.* New York, Academic Press, 241–247.

790. Semmens JP (1983): In reply to Wulf Utian's Letter to the editor. *JAMA* 249:195.

791. Semmens JP, Wagner G (1982): Estrogen deprivation and vaginal function in postmenopausal women. *JAMA* 248:445–448.

792. Sengupta BS, Wynter HH, Matadial L, Halfen A (1978): Myomectomy in infertile Jamaican women. *Int J Gynaecol Obstet* 15:397–399.

793. Sessums JV, Murphy DP (1932): Hysterectomy and the artificial menopause. *Surg Gynec & Obstet* 55:286–289.

794. Shaffer CF (1970): Ascorbic acid and atherosclerosis. *Am J Clin Nutr* 23:127–30.

795. Shaffer EA, Small DM (1977): Biliary lipid secretion in cholesterol gallstone disease. *J Clin Invest* 59:828–840.

796. Shanmugasundaram KR, Visvanathan A, Dhandapani K, Srinivasan N, Rasappan P, Gilbert R, Alladi S, Kancharla S, Vasanthi N (1986): Effect of high-fat diet on cholesterol distribution in plasma lipoproteins, cholesterol esterifying activity in leucocytes and erythrocyte membrane components studied: importance of body weight. *Am J Clin Nutr* 44:805–815.

797. Shapiro M, Schoenbaum S, Tager I, Munoz A, Polk F (1983): Benefit-cost analysis of antimicrobial prophylaxis in abdominal and vaginal hysterectomy. *JAMA* 249:10:1290–1294.

798. Shapiro S, Venet W, Strax P, Venet L, Roeser R (1982): Ten to fourteen year effect of screening on breast cancer mortality. *JNCI* 69:349–355.

799. Sharma SP, Misra SD, Mittal VP (1979): Endometrial changes—a criterion for the diagnosis of submucous uterine leiomyoma. *Indian J Pathol Microbiol* 22:33–36.

800. Shaw RW, Kerr-Wilson RHJ, Fraser HM, McNeilly AS, Howie PW, Sandow J (1985): Effect of an intranasal LHRH agonist on gonadotropins & hot flushes in post-menopausal women. *Maturitas* 7:161–167.

801. Sheldon AER (1984): Effect of estrogen dose on postmenopausal bone loss. *NEJM* 311:604.

802. Sherman AI, Brown S (1979): The precursors of endometrial carcinoma. *Am J Obstet Gynecol* 135:947–956.

803. Sherman HC (1920): Calcium requirements of maintenance in man. *J Biol Chem* 44:21–27.

804. Sherwin BB, Gelfand MM (1985): Sex steroids & affect in the surgical menopause: a double-blind, cross-over study. *Psychoneuroendocrinology* 10:3:325–335.

805. Sherwin BB, Gelfand MM, Brender W (1985): Androgen enhances sexual motivation in females: a prospective, crossover study of sex steroid administration in the surgical menopause. *Psychosom Med* 474:339–351.

806. Short RV (1977): The discovery of the ovaries, in Zuckerman L, Weir J (eds): *The Ovary,* I. New York, Academic Press.

807. Shoupe D, Mont FJ, Lobo RA (1985): The effects of estrogen and progestin on endogenous opioid activity in oophorectomized women. *J Clin Endocrinol Metab* 60:1:178–183.

808. Shultz TD, Leklem JE (1983): Nutrient intake and hormonal status of premenopausal vegetarian Seventh Day Adventists and premenopausal nonvegetarians. *Nutr Cancer* 4:247–259.

808a. Schurz B, Metka M, Heytmanek G, Wimmer-Greinecker G, Reinold E (1988): Sonographic changes in the endometrium of climacteric women during hormonal treatment. *Maturitas* 9:367-374.

809. Schutz Y, Bessard T, Jequier (1987): Exercise & postprandial thermogenesis in obese women before and after weight loss. *Am J Clin Nutr* 45:1423–1432.

810. Siddle N, Sarrel P, Whitehead M (1987): The effect of hysterectomy on the age at ovarian failure: identification of a subgroup of women with premature loss of ovarian function and literature review. *Fertil Steril* 47:1:94–100.

811. Silfverstolpe G, Gustafson A, Samsioe G, Svanborg A (1979): Lipid metabolic studies in oophorectomized women: effects of three different progestogens. *Acta Obstet Gynecol Scand* Suppl 88:89–95.

812. Silman A, Marr J (1985): A better Western diet: what can be achieved? in Trowell H, Burkett D, Heaton K (eds): *Dietary Fibre, Fibre-Depleted Foods and Disease.* New York, Academic Press, 403–418.

813. Simko V (1978): Physical exercise and the prevention of atherosclerosis and cholesterol gallstone. *Postgrad Med J* 54:828:270–277.

814. Simmons K (1985): Scientists ponder diet's behavioral effects. *JAMA* 254:24:3407–3408.

815. Simon JA, diZerega GS (1982): Physiologic estradiol replacement following oophorectomy: failure to maintain precastration gonadotropin levels. *Obstet Gynecol* 59:511–513.

816. Simpson HCR, Mann JI (1982): Effect of high-fibre diet on hemostatic variables in diabetes. *Br Med J* 284:1608.

817. Sinaki DR (1984): Postmenopausal spinal osteoporosis: physical therapy and rehabilitation principles. *Mayo Clinical Proceedings* 57:669–703.

818. Sintchak G, Geer JH (1975): A vaginal plethysomograph system. *Psychophysiology* 12:113–115.

819. Sirtori CR, Tremoli E, Gatti E, Montanari G, Sirtori M, Colli S, Gianfranceschi G, Maderna P, Dentone CZ, Testolin G, Galli C (1986): Controlled evaluation of fat intake in the Mediterranean diet: comparative activities of olive oil and corn oil on plasma lipids and platelets in high-risk patients. *Am J Clin Nutr* 44:635–642.

820. Sitruk-Ware R, deLignieres B, Mauvais-Jarvis P (1986): Progestogen treatment in post-menopausal women. *Maturitas* 8:95–100.

821. Skrabanek P (1985): False premises and false promises of breast cancer screening. *Lancet* 10:316–320.

822. Slag MF, Morley JE, Elson MK, Trence DL, Nelson CJ, Nelson AE, Kinlaw WB, Beyer HS, Nuttall FQ, Shafer RB (1983): Impotence in medical clinic outpatients. *JAMA* 249:1736–1740.

823. Sloan D (1978): The emotional & psychosexual aspects of hysterectomy. *Am J Obstet Gynecol* 131:598.

824. Smith GV (1958): Ovarian tumors. *Am J Surg* 95:336–340.

825. Smith JL, Hodges RE (1987): Serum levels of vitamin C in relation to dietary & supplemental intake of vitamin C in smokers and nonsmokers. Third Conference on Vitamin C. *Ann NY Acad Sci* 498:144–152.

826. Smith P (1972): Age changes in the female urethra. *Brit J Urol* 44:667–676.

827. Snyder AC, Wenderoth MP, Johnston CC, Hui SL (1986): Bone mineral content of elite lightweight amennorheic oarswomen. *Human Biology* 48:6:863–869.

828. Soules MR, Clifton DK, Steiner RA, Cohen NL, Bremner WJ (1987): Gonadotropin-releasing hormone-induced changes in testosterone secretion in normal women. *Fertil Steril* 48:3:423–427.

829. Southgate D, Englyst H (1985): Dietary fibre: chemistry, physical properties and analysis, chapter 3 in Trowell H, Burkett D, Heaton K (eds): *Dietary Fibre, Fibre-Depleted Foods and Disease.* New York, Academic Press, 31–55.

830. Sowers MFR, Wallace RB, Lemke JH (1985): The association of intakes of vitamin D and calcium with blood pressure among women, 1–3. *Am J Clin Nutr* 42:135–142.

831. Sowers MFR, Wallace RB, Lemke JH (1986): The relationship of bone mass and fracture history to fluoride and calcium intake: a study of three communities. *Am J Clin Nutr* 44:889–898.

832. Sox HC (1986): Probability theory in the use of diagnostic tests. *Annals of Internal Medicine* 104:60–66.

833. Spark RF, White RA, Connolly PB (1980): Impotence is not always psychogenic: newer insights into hypothalamic-pituitary-gonadal dysfunction. *JAMA* 243:750–755.

834. Spellacy WN (1982): Carbohydrate metabolism during treatment with estrogen, progestogen and low dose oral contraceptives. *Am J Obstet Gynecol* 142:732–734.

835. Spellacy WN, Birk SA (1972): The effect of intrauterine devices, oral contraceptives, estrogens and progestogens on blood pressure. *Am J Obstet Gynecol* 112:912–919.

836. Spellacy WN, Buhi WC, Birk SA (1972): The effect of estrogens on carbohydrate metabolism: glucose, insulin and growth hormone studies on one hundred and seventy-one women ingesting Premarin, mestranol and ethinyl estradiol for six months. *Am J Obstet Gynecol* 114: 378–392.

837. Spencer H, Kramer L, DeBartol M, Norris C, Osis D (1983): Further studies of the effect of a high protein diet as meat on calcium metabolism. *Am J Clin Nutr* 37:924–929.

838. Spencer H, Kramer L, Osis D, Norris C (1978): Effect of a high protein (meat) intake on calcium metabolism in man. *Am J Clin Nutr* 31: 2167–2180.

839. Stadel BV, Weiss N (1975): Characteristics of menopausal women: a survey of King and Pierce Counties in Washington, 1973–1974. *Am J Epidemiology* 102:3:209–216.

840. Stahelin HB, Gey KF, Brubacher G (1987): Plasma vitamin C and cancer death: the prospective Basel study. Third Conference on Vitamin C. *Ann NY Acad Sci* 498:124–131.

841. Stamford BA, Matter S, Fell RD, Papanek P (1986): Effects of smoking cessation on weight gain, metabolic rate, caloric consumption and blood lipids. *Am J Clin Nutr* 43:486–494.

842. Stamler J, Wentworth D, Neaton JD (1986): Is the relationship between serum cholesterol and risk of premature death from coronary heart disease continuous and graded? *JAMA* 256:20:2823–2827.

843. Stampfer MJ, Willett WC, Colditz GA, Rosner B, Speizer FE, Hennekens CH (1985): A prospective study of postmenopausal estrogen therapy and coronary heart disease. *NEJM* 313:17:1044–1049.

844. Stangel JJ, Innerfield I, Reyniak JV (1976): The effects of conjugated estrogens on hh coagulability in menopausal women. *Obstet Gynecol* 49:314–316.

845. Steege JF, Stout AL, Carson CC (1986): Patient satisfaction in Scott and Small Carrion penile implant recipients: a study of 52 patients. *Arch Sex Behav* 15:5:393–399.

846. Steingold KA, Cefalu W, Pardridge W, Judd HL, Chaudhuri G (1986): Enhanced hepatic extraction of estrogens used for replacement therapy. *J Clin Endoc Metab* 62:4:761–766.

847. Stephen A (1985): Constipation, chapter 7 in Trowell H, Burkett D, Heaton K (eds): *Dietary Fibre, Fibre-Depleted Foods and Disease.* New York, Academic Press, 133–144.

848. Stevenson JC, Hillyard CJ, Abeyasekara G, Phang KG, MacIntyre I, Campbell S, Young O, Townsend PT, Whitehead MI (1981): Calcitonin and the calcium-regulating hormones in postmenopausal women: effect of estrogens. *Lancet* 693–695.

849. Stevenson JC, MacIntyre I (1985): Prevention of postmenopausal osteoporosis. *Lancet* 334–335.

850. Stevenson JC (1980): The structure end function of calcitonin. *Investigations Cell Pathology* 3:187–193.

851. Stevenson JC, Whitehead MI (1982): Calcitonin secretion and postmenopausal osteoporosis. *Lancet* April 3, 804.

852. Stevenson JC (1987): The use of estrogen replacement therapy on calcitonin in the prevention of postmenopausal bone loss. Fifth International Conference on the Menopause, Sorrento, Italy, April.

853. Steward F, Guest F, Stewart G, Hatcher R (1987): *Understanding Your Body.* New York, Bantam.

854. Stone SC, Dickey RP, Mickal A (1975): The acute effect of hysterectomy on ovarian function. *Am J Obstet Gynecol* 121:2:193–197.

855. Stone SC, Mickal A, Rye PH (1975): Postmenopausal symptomatology, maturation index, and plasma estrogen levels. *Obstet Gynecol* 45:6:625–627.

856. Strathy JH, Coulam CB, Spelsburg TC (1982): Comparison of estrogen receptors in human premenopausal and postmenopausal uteri: indication of biologically inactive receptor in postmenopausal uteri. *Am J Obstet Gynecol* 142:372–382.

857. Strauss EB (1950): Impotence from a psychiatric standpoint. *Br Med J* 1:697–699.

858. Strickler RC, Warren JC (1979): Hirsutism: diagnosis and management. *J Clin Endocrinol Metab* 45:1039–1048.

859. Studd JWW, Collins WP, Chakravarti S, Newton JR, Oram D, Parsons A (1977): Oestradiol and testosterone implants in the treatment of psychosexual problems in the postmenopausal woman. *Brit J Obst & Gynecol* 84:314–316.

860. Studd J, Thom M, White PJ (1978): Menopausal therapy and endometrial pathology. *Br Med J* 2:1369.

861. Studd J, Dubiel M, Kakkar VV, Thom M, White PJ (1978): The effect of hormone replacement therapy on glucose tolerance, clotting factors, fibrinolysis and platelet behaviour in postmenopausal women, in Cooke ID (ed): *The Role of Estrogen/Progestogen in the Management of the Menopause.* Baltimore, University Park Press, 41–60.

862. Sturdee DW, Wade-Evans T, Paterson ME, Thom M, Studd JW (1978): Relations between bleeding pattern, endometrial histology and oestrogen treatment in menopausal women. *Br Med J* 1:6127:1575–1577.

863. Sturdevant RAL, Pearce ML, Dayton S (1973): Increased prevalence of cholelithiasis in men ingesting a serum-cholesterol-lowering diet. *NEJM* 288:24–27.

864. Subcommittee on Postdoctoral Training, Committee on Education and Training of the American Society for Clinical Nutrition (1986): A report of the Conference on Clinical Nutrition Training for Physicians. *Am J Clin Nutr* 44:135–153.

865. Suitor CJW, Crowley MF (1986): *Nutrition Principles and Application in Health Promotion,* 2nd ed. Philadelphia, Lippincott.

866. Supinski GS, Levin S, Kelsen SG (1986): Caffeine effect on respirator muscle endurance and sense of effort during loaded breathing. *American Physiological Society* 2040–2047.

867. Suzuki Y, Ichikawa Y, Saito E, Homma M (1983): Importance of increased urinary calcium excretion in the development of secondary

hyperparathyroidism of patients under glucocorticoid therapy. *Metabolism* 32:151–156.

868. Symmonds RE, Pettit DPM (1979): Ovarian remnant syndrome. *Obstet Gynecol* 154:174–177.

869. Taggart H, Ivey JL, Sison K, Chestnut III CH, Baylink DJ, Huber MB, Roos BA (1982): Deficient calcitonin response to calcium stimulation in postmenopausal osteoporosis. *Lancet* 27:475–478.

870. Tamaya T, Motoyama T, Ohono Y, Ide N, Tsurusaki T, Okada H (1979): Estradiol-17$\beta$-progesterone and 5a-dihydrotestosterone receptors of uterine myometrium and myoma in the human subject. *J Ster Biochem* 10:615–622.

871. Tannenbaum SR, Wishnok JS (1987): Inhibition of nitrosamine formation by ascorbic acid. Third Conference on Vitamin C. *Ann NY Acad Sci* 498:354-363.

871a. Tapp AJS, Cardozo L (1986): The postmenopausal bladder. *Br J Hospital Med* Jan.

872. Taylor H, McAuley P, Engle ET (1951): The morphologic basis of ovarian function. *Am J Obstet Gynecol* 61:5:1056–1064.

873. Taylor RW (1979): Gynecolical malignancy. *Practitioner* 222:1328: 195–201.

874. Teichmann AT, Wieland H, Cremer P, Hinney B, Kuhn W, Seidel D (1985): Effects of medrogestone & conjugated oestrogens on serum lipid & lipoprotein concentrations. *Maturitas* 7:343–350.

875. Thallasinos NC, Gutteridge DH, Joplin GF, Fraser TR (1982). Calcium balance in osteoporotic patients on long-term oral calcium therapy with and without sex hormones. *Clin Sci* 62:221–226.

876. Thom M, Chakravarti S, Oram DH, Studd JWW (1976): Effect of hormone replacement therapy on glucose tolerance in postmenopausal women. *Br J Obstet Gynecol* 84:776–783.

877. Thompson B, Hart SA, Durno D (1973): Menopausal age and symptomatology in a general practice. *J Biosoc Sci* 5:71–82.

878. Thomson J, Maddock J, Aylward M, Oswald I (1977): Relationship between nocturnal plasma oestrogen concentration and free plasma tryptophan in perimenopausal women. *J Endocr* 72:395–396.

879. Thomson J, Oswald I (1977): Effect of oestrogen on the sleep, mood and anxiety of menopausal women. *Br Med J* 2:6098:317–319.

880. Thuesen L, Henriksen LB, Diet C, Engby B (1986): One-year experience with a low-fat, low-cholesterol diet in patients with coronary heart disease. *Am J Clin Nutr* 44:212–219.

881. Tiefer L, Melman A (1987): Adherence to recommendations and improvement over time in men with erectile dsyfunction. *Arch Sex Behav* 16:4:301–310.

882. Tikkanen MJ, Kuusi T, Nikkila EA, Sipinen S (1987): Post-heparin plasma hepatic lipase activity as predictor of high-density lipoprotein response to progestogen therapy: studies with cyproterone acetate. *Maturitas* 9:1:81–86.

883. Tikkanen MJ, Kuusi T, Vartianien E, Nikkila EA (1979): Treatment of post-menopausal hypercholesterolaemia with estradiol. *Act Obstet Scand* Suppl 88:83–88.

884. Tobachman JK, Tucker MA, Kase R, et al (1982): Intra abdominal carcinomatosis after prophylactic oophorectomy in ovarian cancer prone families. *Lancet* 8:795–797.

885. Tonelli M, Cucinotta D, Gnudi A, et al (1970): Intestinal absorption of radioactive calcium in old patients with osteoporosis treated with medroxyprogesterone acetate. *Giornale di Gerontologia* 18:420–425.

886. Transbol I, Christensen MS, Jensen GF, Christiansen C, McNair P (1982): Thiazide for the postponement of postmenopausal bone loss. *Metabolism* 31:4:383–386.

887. Treloar AE (1981): Menstrual cyclicity and the premenopause. *Maturitas* 3:249–264.

888. Treloar AE, Boynton RE, Behn DG, Brown BW (1967): Variations of the human menstrual cycle through reproductive life. *I J Fertil* 12:77–126.

889. Treloar AE (1974): Menarche, menopause and intervening fecundability. *Human Biology* 16:89–107.

890. Trowell H, Burkett D, Heaton K (1985): Definitions of dietary fibre and fibre-depleted foods, chapter 2 in Trowell H, Burkett D, Heaton K (eds): *Dietary Fibre, Fibre-Depleted Foods and Disease.* New York, Academic Press, 23–29.

891. Tsang R, Glueck CJ (1979): Atherosclerosis, a pediatric perspective. *Current Problems in Pediatrics* 9:3:3–11.

892. Tulandi T, Lal S (1985): Menopausal hot flush. *Obstet & Gynecol Survey* 40:9:553–563.

893. Tulandi T, Murphy BEP, Lal S (1985): Plasma cortisol concentrations in women with menopausal flushes. *Maturitas* 7:367–372.

894. Turner J, Roy D, Irwins G, Blaney R, Odling-Smee W, Mackenzie G (1984): Does a booklet on breast self-examination improve subsequent detection rates? *Lancet* 337–339.

895. Tverdal A (1987): Systolic and diastolic blood pressures as predictors of coronary heart disease in middle aged Norwegian men. *Br Med J* 294:671–673.

896. Utian WH (1975): Effect of hysterectomy, oophorectomy and estrogen therapy on libido. *Int J Obstet Gyn* 13:977–100.

897. Utian WHS (1972): The true clinical features of postmenopause and oophorectomy and their response to oestrogen therapy. *S Afr Med J* 46:732–737.

898. Utian WH (1972): The mental tonic effect of oestrogens administered to oophorectomized females. *S Afr Med J* 46:1079–1082.

899. Utian WH (1974): Oestrogen, headache and oral contraceptives. *S Afr Med J* 48:2105–2108.

900. Utian WH (1975): Definitive symptoms of postmenopause— incorporating use of vaginal parabasal cell index. *Front Horm Res* 3:74–93.

901. Utian WH (1978): Effect of postmenopausal estrogen therapy on diastolic blood pressure and bodyweight. *Maturitas* 1:3–8.

902. Vallance S (1977): Relationships between ascorbic acid and serum proteins of the immune system. *Br Med J* 2:437–438.

903. Valle R (1978): Hysteroscopy: diagnostic and therapeutic application. *J Repro Med* 20:115–118.

904. Valle RF (1981): Hysteroscopic evaluation of patients with abnormal uterine bleeding. *Surgery, Gynecology and Obstet* 153:521–526.

905. Valle RF, Sciarra JJ (1979): Current status of hysteroscopy in gynecologic practice. *Fertil Steril* 32:619–632.

906. Van Beresteyn ECH, Schaafsma G, deWaard H (1986): Oral calcium and blood pressure: a controlled intervention trial. *Am J Clin Nutr* 44:883–888.

907. VanCampehout J, Choquette P, Vauclair P (1980): Endometrial pattern in patients with primary hypoestrogenic amenorrhea receiving estrogen replacement therapy. *Obstet Gynecol* 56:349–355.

908. VanKeep PA, Serr DM, Greenblatt RB, Kopera H (1978): Effects, side-effects and dosage schemes of various sex hormones in the peri and

postmenopause. Workshop Report in Female and Male Climacteric. *Current Opinion 1978.* Baltimore, University Park Press.

909. Van Keep PA, Wildemeersch D, Lehert P (1983): Hysterectomy in six European countries. *Maturitas* 5:69–75.

910. Varma SD (1987): Ascorbic acid and the eye with special reference to the lens. Third Conference on Vitamin C. *Ann NY Acad Sci* 498:280–306.

911. Veith JL, Anderson J, Slade SA, Thompson P, Laugel GR, Getzlaf S (1984): Plasma β-endorphin, pain threshholds and anxiety levels across the human menstrual cycle. *Physiol Behav* 32:31–34.

912. Verbeek ALM, Hendriks JHCL, Holland R, et al (1984): Screening and breast cancer. *Lancet* 9/22:690.

913. Vermeulen A, Deslypere JP (1985): Testicular endocrine function in the aging male. *Maturitas* 7:273–279.

914. Vermeulen A, Rubens R, Verdonck L (1972): Testosterone secretion and metabolism in male senescence. *JCEM* 34:730–735.

915. Villeco AS, deAloysio D, deLiverali E, Ferrari G, Mauloni M (1985): High blood pressure and ischaemic ECG patterns in climacteric women. *Maturitas* 7:89–97.

916. Vinson JA, Bose P (1987): Bioavailability of synthetic abscorbic acid and a citrus extract. Third Conference on Vitamin C. *Ann NY Acad Sci* 498:525–526.

916a. Viswanathan M, Van Dijk JP, Graham TE, Bonen A, George JC (1987): Exercise and cold-induced changes in plasma β-endorphin and β-lipotropin in men and women. *J Appl Physiol* 62:622–627.

917. Vollman RF (1977): The menstrual cycle, vol 7 in *Major Problems in Obstetrics and Gynecology.* Philadelphia, Saunders.

918. Volpe A, Facchinetti F, Grasso A, Petraglia F, Campanini D, Genazzani AR (1986): Benefits and risks of different hormonal replacement therapies in post-menopausal women. *Maturitas* 8:327–334.

919. VonEiff AW (1975): Blood pressure and estrogens. *Front Horm Res* 3:177–184.

920. Von Schoultz B (1986): Climacteric complaints as influenced by progestogens. *Maturitas* 8:107–112.

920a. Vorherr H (1986): Fibrocystic breast disease: pathophysiology, pathomorphology, clinical picture, and management. *Am J Obstet Gynecol* 154:161-179.

921. Wahl P, Walden C, Knopp R, Hoover J, Wallace R, Heiss G, Rifkind B (1983): Effect of estrogen/progestin potency on lipid/lipoprotein cholesterol. *NEJM* 308:862–867.

922. Wahner HW (1985): Endocrine symposium: assessment of metabolic bone disease: review of new nuclear medicine procedures. *Mayo Clin Proc* 60:827–835.

923. Wahner HW, Dunn Wl, Riggs BL (1984): Assessment of bone mineral: part 2. *J Nucl Med* 25:1241–1253.

924. Waldron I (1982): An analysis of causes of sex differences in mortality and morbidity, in Gove WR, Carpenter GR (eds): *The Fundamental Connection between Nature and Nurture.* Lexington, Mass, Lexington Books.

925. Walker A (1985): Mineral metabolism, in Trowell H, Burkett D, Heaton K (eds): *Dietary Fibre, Fibre-Depleted Foods and Disease.* New York, Academic Press, 361-375.

926. Wallace RB, Hoover J, Barrett-Conner E, et al (1979): Altered plasma lipid and lipo-protein levels associated with oral contraceptives and oestrogen use. *Lancet* ii:112–114.

927. Walter S, Jensen HK (1977): The effect of treatment with oestradiol and oestriol on fasting serum cholesterol and triglyceride levels in postmenopausal women. *Br J Obstet Gynaecol* 84:11:869–872.

928. Walton J, Dominquez M, Bartter FC (1975): Effects of calcium infusions in patients with postmenopausal osteoporosis. *Metabolism* 24:7:849–854.

929. Wardlaw SL, Wehrenberg WB, Ferin M, Antunes JL, Frantz AG (1982): Effect of sex steroids on $\beta$-endorphin in hypophyseal portal blood. *J Clin Endocrinol Metab* 55:877–881.

930. Ware MD, Thomas EK, Notelovitz M (1985): Serum hormone levels in men exposed to vaginal oestrogen cream: a preliminary report. *Maturitas* 7:373–376.

931. Wasnich RD, Ross PD, Heilbrun LK, Vogel JM, Yano K, Benfante RJ (1986): Differential effects of thiazide and estrogen upon bone mineral content and fracture prevalence. *J Obstet & Gynecol* 67:4:457–462.

932. Wassertheil-Smoller S, Romney SL, Wylie-Rosett J, et al (1981): Dietary vitamin C & uterine cervical dysplasia. *Am J Epidemiology* 114:714.

933. Watson RC (1973): Bone growth and physical activity. *International Conference on Bone Mineral Measurements* 380–385.

934. Webb P (1986): 24-hour energy expenditure and the menstrual cycle. *Am J Clin Nutr* 44:614–619.

935. Wehrenberg WB, Wardlaw SL, Frantz AG, Ferin M (1982): β-endorphin in hypophyseal portal blood: variations throughout the menstrual cycle. *Endocrinology* 111:879–881.

936. Weinsier RL, Boker JR, Feldman EB, Read MS, Brooks CM (1986): Nutrition knowledge of senior medical students: a collaborative study of southeastern medical schools. *Am J Clin Nutr* 43:959–968.

937. Weinstein H, Slenker L, Porges RF (1977): Diagnostic vacuum aspiration curettage. *NY State J Med* 77:373–376.

938. Weir RJ, Briggs MA (1974): Blood pressure in women taking oral contraceptives. *Br Med J* 1:533–535.

939. Weisberg M (1984): Physiology of female sexual function. *Clin Ob/Gyn* 27:697–705.

940. Weiss NS (1975): Risks and benefits of estrogen use. *NEJM* 293:1200–1202.

940b. Weissman C, Goldstein S, Askanazi J, Rosenbaum SH, Milic-Emili J, KinneyJM (1986): Semistarvationandexercise. *Am Physiol Soc* 2035–2039.

941. Wentz WB (1974): Progestin therapy in endometrial hyperplasia. *Gynecol Oncol* 2:362–367.

941a. Wentz WB (1985): Progestin therapy in lesions of the endometrium. *Seminars in Oncology* 12:23-27 Supp. 1

942. West CP, Lumsden MA, Lawson S, Williamson J, Baird DT (1987): Shrinkage of uterine fibroids during therapy with goserelin (Zoladex) a luteinizing hormone-releasing hormone agonist administered as a monthly subcutaneous depot. *Fertil Steril* 48:1:45–51.

943. Whipple B, Komisaruk BR (1985): Elevation of pain threshhold by vaginal stimulation in women. *Pain* 21:357–367.

944. White SC, Wartel LJ, Wade ME (1971): Comparison of abdominal and vaginal hysterectomies: a review of 600 operations. *Obstet Gynecol* 37:530–537.

945. Whitehead MI, McQueen J, Minardi J, Campbell S (1978): Clinical considerations in the management of the menopause: the endometrium. *Postgrad Med J* 54:2:69–73.

946. Whitehead MI, Minardi J, Kitchin Y, Sharples MJ (1978): Systemic absorption of estrogen from Premarin vaginal cream, in Cooke ID

(ed): *The Role of Estrogen/Progestogen in the Management of the Menopause*. Baltimore, University Park Press, 63–72.

947. Whitehead MI, Townsend PT, Pryse-Davies J, Ryder TA, King RJB (1981): Effects of estrogens and progestins on the biochemistry and morphology of the postmenopausal endometrium. *NEJM* 305:1599–1605.

948. Whitehead MI, Townsend PT, Gill DK, Collins WP, Campbell S (1980): Absorption & metabolism of oral progesterone. *Br Med J* 289:825–827.

949. Whitehead MI, Townsend PT, Pryse-Davies J, Ryder T, Lane G, Siddle NC, King RJB (1982): Effects of various dosages of progestogens on the postmenopausal endometrium. *J Repro Med* 27:8:539–548.

950. Whitehead MI, Townsend PT, Pryse-Davies J, Ryder T, Lane G, Siddle N, King RJB (1982): Actions of progestins on the morphology and biochemistry of the endometrium of postmenopausal women receiving low-dose estrogen therapy. *Am J Obstet Gynecol* 142:791–795.

951. Whitehead MI, Fraser D (1987): The effects of estrogen and progestogens on the endometrium. *Obstet Gynecol Clin N Am* 14(1):299–320.

952. Whiting SJ, Draper HH (1980): The role of sulfate in the calciuria of high protein diets in adult rats. *J Nutr* 110:212–222.

953. Williams AR, Weiss NS, Ure CL, Ballard J, Daling JR (1982): Effect of weight, smoking, and estrogen use on the risk of hip and forearm fractures in postmenopausal women. *Obstet Gynecol* 60:695–699.

954. Williams PT, Krauss RM, Kindel-Joyce S, Dreon DM, Vranizan KM, Wood PD (1986): Relationship of dietary fat, protein, cholesterol and fiber intake to atherogenic lipoproteins in men. *Am J Clin Nutr* 44:788–797.

955. Wilson PWF, Garrison RJ, Castelli WP (1985): Postmenopausal estrogen use, cigarette smoking and cardiovascular morbidity in women over 50. *NEJM* 313:17:1038–1043.

956. Wingo PA, Layde PM, Lee NC, Rubin G, Ory HW (1987): The risk of breast cancer in postmenopausal women who have used estrogen replacement therapy. *JAMA* 257:209.

957. Wiseman RA, MacRae KD (1981): Oral contraceptives and the decline in mortality from circulatory disease. *Fertil Steril* 35:277–283.

958. Wiske PS, Epstein NH, Bell NH, Queener SF, Edmondson J, Johnston CC (1979): Increases in immunoreactive parathyroid hormone with age. *NEJM* 300:1419–1421.

959. Wood K, Coppen A (1978): The effect of estrogens on plasma tryptophan and adrenergic function in patients treated with lithium,

in Cooke ID (ed): *The Role of Estrogen/Progestogen in the Management of the Menopause*. Baltimore, University Park Press, 29–38.

960. Woodruff JD, Prystowsky H, Telinde RW (1966): Postmenopausal bleeding. *South Med J* 51:302–305.

961. Wren B, Garrett D (1985): The effect of low-dose piperazine oestrone sulphate & low-dose levonorgestrel on blood lipid levels in postmenopausal women. *Maturitas* 7:141–146.

962. Wright RC (1969): Hysterectomy: past, present and future. *Obstet Gynecol* 33:560–563.

963. Wuest JH, Dry TJ, Edwards JE (1953): The degree of atherosclerosis in bilaterally oophorectomized women. *Circulation* 7:801–809.

964. Wylie-Rosett JA, Romney SL, Slagle NS, et al (1984): Influence of vitamin A on cervical dysplasia and carcinoma in situ. *Nutr Cancer* 6:49–57.

965. Wynn V (1982): Effect of duration of low dose oral contraceptive administration on carbohydrate metabolism. *Am J Obstet Gynecol* 142:739–746.

966. Wynder EL, Escher GC, Mantel N (1966): An epidemiological investigation of cancer of the endometrium. *Cancer* 19:489–520.

967. Yen SSC, Tsai CC (1971): The effect of ovariectomy on gonadotropin release. *J Clin Invest* 50:1149–1153.

968. Ylostalo P, Kauppila A, Kivinen S, Tuimala R, Vihko R (1983): Endocrine and metabolic effects of low dose estrogen-progestin treatment in climacteric women. *Obstet Gynecol* 62:682–686.

969. Zamah NM, Dodson MG, Stephens LC, Buttram VC, Besch PK, Kaufman RH (1984): Transplantation of normal and ectopic human endometrial tissue into athymic nude mice. *Obstet Gynecol* 149:6:591–597.

970. Zannoni VG, Brodfuehrer JI, Smart RC, Susick RL (1987): Ascorbic acid, alcohol, and environmental chemicals. Third Conference on Vitamin C. *Ann NY Acad Sci* 498:364–388.

971. Zemcov A, Barclay LL, Sansone J, Metz CE (1985): Receiver operating characteristic analysis of regional cerebral blood flow in Alzheimer's Disease. *J Nucl Med* 26:1002–1010.

972. Zauner CW (1985): Physical fitness in aging men. *Maturitas* 7:267–271.

973. Zemel MB, Schuette SA, Hegsted M, Linkswiler HM (1981): Role of the sulfur-containing amino acids in protein-induced hypercalciuria in men. *J Nutr* 3:545–552.

974. Zussman L, Zussman S, Sunley R, Bjornson E (1981): Sexual response after hysterectomy-oophorectomy: recent studies and reconsideration of psychogenesis. *Am J Obstet Gynecol* 140:725–729.

# Index

*Page numbers in italics refer to figures and tables.*